Blood Saga

One source of ethnographic data frequently absent in anthro-pological analysis is the response of the people studied to the ethnographer's description and the interpretation of the meaning of their lives. For the most part anthropologists (as well as communities studied) have been shielded from any local appraisal and aftershocks resulting from publication because we have traditionally worked in "exotic" cultures and among preliterate people. . . . Such invisibility, and hence invulnerability, has not been the fate of those who have studied modern cultures and self-reflexive people.

Nancy Scheper-Hughes, *Saints, Scholars, and Schizophrenics: Mental Illness in Northern Ireland*

Blood Saga

Hemophilia, AIDS, and the Survival of a Community

Susan Resnik

UNIVERSITY OF CALIFORNIA PRESS

Berkeley / Los Angeles / London

University of California Press
Berkeley and Los Angeles, California

University of California Press, Ltd.
London, England

© 1999 by
The Regents of the University of California

Library of Congress Cataloging-in-Publication Data

Resnik, Susan, 1940-
    Blood saga : hemophilia, AIDS, and the survival of a community
/ Susan Resnik.
        p.   cm.
    Includes bibliographic references and index.
    ISBN 0-520-21195-2 (alk. paper)
    1. Hemophilia—United States—History.   I. Title.
RC642.R47 1999
362.1'961572'00973—dc21   98-14150

Printed in the United States of America
9   8   7   6   5   4   3   2   1

The paper used in this publication meets the minimum requirements of
American National Standards for Information Sciences—Permanence
of Paper for Printed Library Materials, ANSI Z39.48-1984.

This book is dedicated to the U.S. hemophilia community. As a participatory social history, it serves as a conduit for the voices of, shapers of, and witnesses to scientific and technological breakthroughs and defining events. Among the most important of these voices are those of succeeding cohorts of men, who share their perceptions of growing up with hemophilia during the 1940s, 1950s, 1960s, and 1970s and thus chronicle the emergence, empowerment, and transformation of this community.

The book is also a memorial tribute to all those who have perished, in particular to seven of the informants: "Brett H.," "Cliff H.," "Eugene H.," "Harold H.," "Kent H.," "Lloyd H.," and "Mindy H." "Brett H." felt passionately about the importance of chronicling this community's history. He served as a member of my doctoral dissertation committee and participated in the review process, contributing his skills as a historian and his knowledge as a community member until he died on May 6, 1993—my birthday. His guidance and caring will never be forgotten.

I also wish to dedicate this book in loving remembrance of other individuals involved in my research who have passed away: Samuel Wolfe, M.D., a leading figure in U.S. public health, the senior tenured member of my doctoral committee and a caring mentor; and my dear aunt, my role model, Dorothy Turberg Biltchik, who shared the task of audit editing with me.

A special dedication honors my late grandfather, Phillip Turberg, a gentle, wise Talmudic scholar, who nurtured my love of learning and encouraged me to ask questions. I promised him that someday I would write a book.

Contents

Preface   ix

Acknowledgments   xi

1.
Introduction   1

2.
The Dismal Era:
Because the Blood Comes from the Woman   8

3.
The Years of Hope, 1948–65   20

4.
A Research Milestone Heralds the Golden Era,
1960–65   37

5.
The Hemophilia Community Enters Politics:
The Late 1960s and Early 1970s   56

6.
Politics and the Blood Business in the Golden Era   73

7.
The Meanings of the Golden Era   90

8.
The AIDS Era Begins:
The Years of Confusion and Denial, 1980–82   109

9.
The AIDS Era, 1982–85: Tension Mounts, Conflicts Erupt   125

10.
The AIDS Era, 1985–88:
The Hemophilia Community Rises to the Challenge   137

11.
"A Vote for the Status Quo," 1988–92   150

12.
Approaching the Biotech Century:
Out with the Old, In with the New, 1992–98   169

13.
Conclusion: Lessons to Be Learned   192

Appendixes

A. Glossary of Terms and Acronyms   199
B. Research Methods   221
C. Informant Interview Discussion,
   1990–92   230
D. Informants   233
E. Linguistic Markers along
   Historical Pathways   238
F. Federal Hemophilia Program Regions   240
G. Changes In Death Rates and Causes of Death
   in Persons with Hemophilia A, 1979–89   241
H. Hemophilia Treatment Center
   Data Collection and Presentation:
   A Historical Overview   243

   Notes   255

   Bibliography   275

   Index   283

Preface

It was in 1989, a time when technology had gone awry and medical heroes were increasingly perceived as villains, that I decided to become the conduit for voices telling a story that had to be told, to be heard and preserved. These voices belonged to members of a community that had been my "home" for ten years, a community that appeared about to become a ghost town, about to lose 70 to 90 percent of its members. This is not a geographic community but one defined by shared bonds of disease, gender, and outlook, and by its history of suffering, endurance, and sometimes triumph. The story is that of the hemophilia community in the United States.

I had entered this community by becoming the education director of an education project designed for patients and their families at the National Hemophilia Foundation in 1979. That was the "Golden Era," when doctors were called "treaters" and were viewed as heroes and leaders, and patients called each other "blood brothers." Thanks to a "miracle treatment," those patients were the first generation of adult men with hemophilia to live long enough to share in the American Dream—an education, employment, marriage, and perhaps raising a family.

In the summer of 1982, just at the time when I decided to return to Columbia University to resume my graduate education in public health and anthropology, everything changed. The best of times rapidly became the worst of times. The AIDS virus had infiltrated their miracle treatment, the pooled plasma products used to treat bleeding episodes. As a result, by 1989, a majority of community members knew that they were HIV-positive, and they—and their families—were facing the specter of sickness and death. Realizing that no one had previously attempted to chronicle the social history of this community, I chose this history as the basis for my doctoral dissertation. The result, "The Social History of Hemophilia in the United States (1948–1988): The Emergence and Empowerment of a Community," forms the basis for chapters 2–10 of this book.

Since 1988, instead of collapsing and disappearing, the hemophilia community has adapted and metamorphosed. Its members, who had been called "canaries in the mine shaft," testing the blood of our nation and perishing as a result, have changed leadership, come out of their medical closet, and emerged as "the town criers," issuing a warning, taking a place at the table, reframing their disease, and shaping the nation's blood safety policies to prevent further tragedy. I relate these developments in chapters 11–13, based on updated research to cover the years 1988–98.

This is a story that touches all those connected by bonds of blood and has many lessons to teach us.

Acknowledgments

This book was written in two separate places at two times. My doctoral dissertation, entitled "The Social History of Hemophilia in the United States (1948–1988): The Emergence and Empowerment of a Community," forms the basis of chapters 2 through 10. I did the research for and writing of this portion from 1989 to 1994 while living in New York City, completing my doctorate in public health at the Columbia University School of Public Health. Under the auspices of the University of California Press, I revised the first section and drafted the update section (chapters 11 through 13) during the seven months from March through September 1997, while living in Del Mar, California. Thanks to the support and dedication of those who have been involved, I have been able to include additional updates through June 1988.

During both periods of time, I have had the benefit of a wonderful support system. Family, friends, mentors, and colleagues have provided emotional, intellectual, financial, and technical support. Thanking each one of them here would add another lengthy chapter to this book. I shall try instead to summarize their contributions to my work as briefly as possible.

I deeply appreciate being selected as a recipient of a doctoral dissertation research grant awarded by the U.S. Agency for Health Care Policy Research (Grant 1R03HS06596–01). This award provided funding used to travel, tape-record, transcribe, and audit-edit (that is, edit the transcript while listening to the tape) the informant interviews and life stories gathered over a two-year period. Ralph Sloat, director of grants administration, and project officers Mim Kelly and Eleanor Walker also provided guidance and demonstrated their interest in my topic both during and after the completion of the funding period.

All of the members of my doctoral dissertation committee maintained their interest and availability throughout this lengthy and complex undertaking. I wish to thank Sheila Gorman, Larry Brown, Lambros Comitas, and Annette Ramírez de Arellano. All have served as mentors, providing guidance, setting standards, and opening doors to the acquisition of knowledge and the development of skills. Each of their unique perspectives has contributed to enriching the process and to improving the final product.

Ronald Grele, director of the Columbia University Oral History Office, contributed advice and wisdom. He, Mary Marshall Clark, and their staff also provided assistance that enabled me to produce archival quality materials. I am gratified that the Columbia University Oral History Collection will serve as a future home for all of the audiotapes and transcripts from my dissertation research and for the audiotapes of additional interviews conducted in 1997.

I appreciate the cooperation of all of the agencies and institutions that furnished access to their files. I am especially grateful to the informants and their families, who granted interviews and furnished materials from personal files and who are listed in Appendix D. They have shaped this participatory social history by contributing their voices and thoughts.

Many individuals contributed their skills during the various stages of development of the dissertation. Jeffrey Resnik, Scott Pearson, Max Ramírez de Arellano, and Esther Newton furnished initial assistance and guidance in the selection of appropriate computer hardware and software. Scott Pearson also provided ongoing assistance in the production of the dissertation. Transcription and editing were accomplished by Adele Oltman, Nationwide Transcribers, Inc., and Dorothy Turberg Biltchik. Mike's Print Shop was an invaluable resource for reproducing all transcripts and the manuscript.

Readers and editors who contributed their skills and time during the final stages of the dissertation are "Adam H.," Bettijane Eisenpreiss,

Laurie Norris, Martine La Tour, Lucie Kassabian, Lucy Rector, Melanie Dreher, Rose Dobrof, Anne Foner, Eileen Koski, Betsy Randall-David, and Betsy Kase. Mindy Wexler-Marks typed the final version. I am profoundly grateful to them all for their commitment and contribution, which enabled me to produce the completed dissertation, submitted in September 1994.

In April 1994 Alan M. Brandt, a medical historian from Harvard Medical School who heard me present a paper based on my research at a meeting of the American Association of the History of Medicine, expressed interest in my work and alerted the Institute of Medicine Committee studying HIV and the U.S. blood supply about the dissertation. The committee subsequently used it as a resource. I also appreciate his encouragement that I seek publication and his guidance in directing me to the University of California Press.

After I moved to California in late September 1994, I received additional encouragement to submit the manuscript, as well as an offer to help during the revision phase, from Michael Davidson, professor of American literature and writing at the University of California, San Diego. During the period of submission, acceptance, revision, and updating, I have had the further benefit of a warm welcome, enthusiastic support, and timely guidance. Meeting Jim Clark, director of the University of California Press, and Katherine Bell, assistant to the director, face to face energized me as I began the revision process. Katherine's ongoing communication, constructive criticism, and feedback enabled me to move toward completion in a timely manner. Dan Dixon's expertise in communication and legal matters has enabled me to move forward in an appropriate fashion.

Just as in the original phase of research and production in New York, there has been a host of supporters in California helping me along. In addition to Jim Clark and Katherine Bell's reading of my draft revisions, Michael Davidson has devoted considerable time, critiquing both the content and the style, giving my work line-by-line attention. He also shared his perspective as a person living with hemophilia, an added bonus in this endeavor. Another member of the UC San Diego faculty, Steven Epstein, assistant professor in the Department of Sociology, has offered his thoughtful criticism and shared his research, helping me to make links and clarify issues.

Sheldon Margen, M.D., Fred Rosen, M.D., and Virginia Oleson, University of California Press readers who critiqued my manuscript, also provided direction and specific suggestions. I appreciate their positive comments and have endeavored to respond to them by altering or adding material as the case may be.

My book has also been enriched by the addition of new material furnished by Stephen Pemberton, a historian from the University of North Carolina, Chapel Hill, regarding the research of Kenneth Brinkhous. I appreciate his sharing his perspectives, both on paper and in our phone conversations. By furnishing photos of the "bleeder dogs," he has enhanced my ability to tell this part of the story.

Thanks to phone, fax, and e-mail, my bicoastal connections have remained strong. Fred Rosner, M.D., shared telephone conversations and faxed updated materials that allowed me to provide more accurate information about ancient Talmudic writings concerning hemophilia. Lambros Cornitas and Larry Brown have continued to provide support and feedback during this new research phase. Mindy Wexler-Marks has been available and helpful in smoothing the transition between computer systems.

In Del Mar, I want to thank my friend Debbie Coburn for doing needed secretarial and clerical work. Also, Shirley and Rufus Abelsohn and Paul Brookes and the rest of the staff at CLONE Duplicating and Printing have been extremely helpful regarding duplication needs. The chief orchestrator of the transformation of dissertation into book via the computer is Rob Healey, truly a Renaissance man. Rob has spent innumerable hours translating the documents and teaching me how to use my new technology and has contributed his creativity in the production of both written and illustrative material. I am also in debt to Peter Glaser, friend and engineering expert, who has guided me in the purchase and use of hardware and software and enabled me to surmount challenges and obstacles as they occurred. I thank Abbie Cory, doctoral candidate in English at the University of California, San Diego, for her assistance in last-minute research and fact checking.

From April through September 1997 I conducted interviews and required rapid replication of archival quality audiotapes and production of archival quality transcripts. The entire staff at Moonlight Video, Encinitas, did a superb job, with quick turnaround of tapes. Linda Luke, professional transcriber, friend, and fellow Del Mar Historical Society member, produced excellent transcripts overnight. Her speed and accuracy enabled me to keep up the momentum and to progress on schedule.

I also wish to thank the members of the hemophilia community and, in particular, members of the National Hemophilia Foundation staff who have contributed additional materials to the book. Nelson Escoto of the Hemophilia and AIDS/HIV Network for the Dissemination of Information (HANDI) provided ongoing help in responding to my requests promptly and accurately. Jodi Corngold has selected photos and made them available. Steven Humes and Anthony Ramos also furnished important materials and suggestions. Ann-Marie Nazzaro took the time to read the dissertation and to furnish me with some phone numbers of contacts. Other photos and printed materials for the revision and update were furnished by Shelby Dietrich, Donna Boone, Mary Gooley, Bruce Evatt, Mike Soucie, and Sally Crudder.

Thanks also to Del Mar friend, artist, and professor of botany, Brian Capon, who drew the composite chart illustrating Queen Victoria's lineage.

The San Diego hemophilia community has also been welcoming and supportive of this project. The local NHF chapter has offered help and invited me to speak at their board meeting. In particular, I would like to thank Cathy Glass, R.N., George D'Avignon, M.D., Adam Milgram, and Leon and Judy Faitek. I am looking forward to adding their stories to the Hemophilia Community Oral History Collection.

I have been fortunate in the team that has guided me to the "light at the end of the tunnel": project editors Mimi Kusch and Jean McAneny at University of California Press and manuscript editor Ellen F. Smith. Mimi offered sound guidance and supportive and flexible encouragement during the editing process. Ellen's rapid comprehension and editorial skills have transformed my manuscript into an accessible book for both academic and general readers. Jean has directed the project through its final stages.

The greatest gift that a loving family can offer is ongoing encouragement and support. My husband, Hal Resnik, has been a partner in this process. I thank him and all of my children and grandchildren, who have been my cheering section during the entire period of producing both the dissertation and the book: Wendy Lee Goodfriend and Kim

Crowder; Marsha, Scott, Shawn, and Kyle Summers; Claire, Jeffrey, Laura, Julie, Denise, Rob, Allyson, and Matthew Resnik.

I also wish to thank my cousins' support systems, extended family, and friends and colleagues who have sustained and supported me with love and encouragement for the duration.

CHAPTER 1

Introduction

What is often lost sight of . . . is the process of disease definition itself, and second, the consequences of those definitions once agreed upon in the eyes of the individuals in the making and discussing of social policy, and in the structuring of medical care. We have, in general, failed to focus on that nexus between the biological event, its perception by the patient and practitioner, and the collective effort to make cognitive and policy sense out of these perceptions.

Charles E. Rosenberg, "Disease in History:
Frames and Framers," *Milbank Quarterly*

After thousands of years, hemophilia, an incurable, inherited disease, has been transformed into a readily manageable chronic illness. Currently, the possibility of a cure seems imminent, due to the development of gene insertion therapy. However, this history of success also includes tragedy, vulnerability to the plague of our times due to technology gone awry. The pooled plasma products that contributed to the successful management of the disease also carried the AIDS virus to the hemophilia population and to their sexual partners. In the 1980s, the quest for a cure for hemophilia became intertwined with the battle to halt the spread of AIDS. It seemed at first that this tragedy would demolish the hemophilia community, but like a phoenix rising from the ashes, it has adapted, selected new leadership, and reemerged,

1

transformed with even greater strength and influence. The community has metamorphosed from being seen as the "canaries in the mine shaft" who perished in order to warn others of the danger in our blood supply to outspoken activists signaling danger before it becomes disaster. This book tracks the story of these developments chronologically and concludes by identifying the lessons that they offer to various groups within society and to society as a whole.

How did the small hemophilia population (1 out of 7,500 live male births, a total population in the United States of approximately 15,000 to 20,000) attain the ability to experience "the American dream," with a normal life style and the expectation of a normal life span within a brief period?[1] What were the scientific breakthroughs and innovations in how care was delivered that initiated changes in the way the disease was perceived, experienced, and treated? How and by whom has this disease been defined and "framed" in the past?[2] What cultural factors may have contributed to the creation of a climate that permitted the community to be exposed to the AIDS virus? What strengths enabled this community to adapt, progress, and survive? What lessons can we learn, and for whom is this story significant?

I have searched for answers to these questions and in the process have identified the emergence of other salient issues, using the anthropologist's methods and tools and the oral historian's strategies and technology. My focus, or "unit of analysis," is the hemophilia community. The hemophilia population, consisting for thousands of years of isolated families, evolved initially into a community of fate. Anthropologists describe this configuration as a "communitas," a community of sufferers, of empathy.[3] During the second stage of its development, the community was transformed into an organized, politically vocal constituency with a significant involvement in United States health care systems and agencies. The third stage was characterized by initial divisiveness, followed by expansion, empowerment, and democratization. And finally, the community now faces a new possibility of scientific breakthrough to a cure. My discussion of this transformation in the nature, composition, size, and organization of the hemophilia community occurs within the framework of a chronological narrative across five major periods: the Dismal Era, before 1948 (Chapter 2), the Years of Hope, 1948–65 (Chapter 3), the Golden Era, 1965–82 (Chapters 4–7), the AIDS Era, 1982–88 (Chapters 8–10), and Approaching the Biotech Century, 1988–98 (Chapters 11–12).

Since the hemophilia community is situated within U.S. society and culture, it has both been shaped by and contributed to that larger sphere throughout this fifty-year time span, and these contextual influences are discussed in each portion of the historical narrative. At times the hemophilia community has served as a leader, establishing a health delivery model and, as noted, acting as "the canaries in the mine shaft" by testing the nation's blood. And at times the hemophilia community has emulated other communities of interest, as in the arena of political advocacy.

This study also focuses on the existence of a specific hemophilia culture. As discussed in Chapter 2, the hemophilia community takes pride in ownership of a special early history, a language rich in linguistic markers delineating specific periods in time, and an outlook molded by sharing bonds of blood, gender, and suffering. This shared worldview coexists with varying perspectives and senses of meaning expressed by the community's subcultural groups and hemophilia age cohorts. References to both shared and varied perceptions are highlighted throughout the book. The subcultural segments of the hemophilia community include persons with hemophilia, their families, a full range of multidisciplinary health care providers, agency and program directors, and plasma industry executives and representatives. Physicians are classified as researchers, treatment center medical directors, and treaters. These varied groups generate marked diversity in interpretation of scientific breakthroughs, delineation of time frames, and experience of treating the disease and living with the illness. New voices and ideas have also emerged as the community has expanded and changed over time.

Throughout the book, political and scientific developments combine with economic, cultural, and social forces to shape this story. The relevance of these contextual elements is reflected in the expressed values, attitudes, and beliefs that enter into the making of decisions and the establishing of policies.

The Research Approach

When I began my research, I found there was no written history of the U.S. hemophilia community. Rather than relying on the medical literature or interviewing only physician leaders who would serve as surrogates, I chose to develop a participatory social history that would reflect the views of all segments of the community. I approached this task both as an "applied anthropologist," using an ethnographic approach and an "emic" orientation (that is, attempting to "see through the eyes" of the informants), and as an oral historian, using a tape recorder. In this way, I captured the views and voices of the shapers and the witnesses in the U.S. hemophilia community. Both informant groups were presented with a core list of issues that covered the evolution of the community and were encouraged to introduce other issues of importance to them. As frequently mentioned topics emerged, they were added to the original list of items. (For a more detailed description of how I carried out my two phases of research, in 1989–94 and in 1997, and a linear account of what I studied, see Appendix B. For a list of the issues discussed with informants, see Appendix C.)

A total of forty-eight informant interviews were conducted for the first phase of my research in 1990–91. The sample consisted of thirty-six leaders, shapers, and witnesses (among them hemophilia treatment center providers, agency leaders, program directors, and plasma manufacturing executives) as well as twelve persons with hemophilia in their twenties, thirties, forties, and fifties, representing the range of age cohorts that grew up with hemophilia prior to the 1980s. At the time of their interviews, two of the older men were acknowledged as community leaders. (As described in Appendix B, I used code names for these informants with hemophilia, an arbitrary first name and the initial "H." for "hemophilia.") Initially, I employed a purposive sampling strategy. During a period of exploration before selecting my informants, I both read about and discussed early scientific discoveries and defining events with two physicians, Frederick Rickles, M.D., and Charles Abildgaard, M.D., and one person with hemophilia, "Brett H.," who was familiar with the history of hemophilia research. They assisted me by identifying pioneer researchers, specifying defining events, and delineating time frames. When I contacted suggested informants, they, in turn, recommended others for me to contact. I also employed a snowball strategy.[4] I selected as a "key informant" a person with hemophilia, "Adam H.," who was then in his mid-forties and widely acknowledged as a community leader. He both offered comments on my researcher selections and guided me to other informants. "Adam H.," "Brett H.," and Drs. Rickles and Abildgaard collaborated with me in the selection of the remainder of informants. Some of the informants have played an active role in the hemophilia community throughout the entire fifty-year time span; others were present for only limited periods of time. Many of the informants who described developments at the local level in the early years became leaders and advocates on the national level and helped make policy decisions in the later years.

Beginning in 1948, when the Hemophilia Foundation was incorporated, the national and local levels of activity were intertwined. Both medical and lay leaders traversed local, national, and international levels. The small size of the affected population, the strong sense of "blood brotherhood" and community, and the personal, nonbureaucratic style of relating by government agency and program directors fostered a climate of informality and interconnectedness. This study, too, considers all levels in order to capture a holistic sense of the community over time.

What Is Hemophilia?

Hemophilia is currently defined as "a genetic blood clotting disorder" that affects about 15,000–20,000 Americans, with an estimated incidence of 1 in 7,500 live male births. Hemophiliac bleeding does not occur faster than in people with normal levels of clotting factors, with which the body is able to stop bleeding, but it is prolonged. The clinical disease is a sex-linked recessive disorder, usually occurring in males, because the defective gene that causes it is on the X chromosome. (Indeed, hemophilia was one of the first diseases known to follow classic Mendelian laws of heredity.) Males have one X chromosome and one Y chromosome that occur as a pair; females have two paired X chromosomes. In the male with hemophilia, the X chromosome contains an abnormality, which may be either a deletion or a defective segment, in one of the genes; the Y chromosome cannot counteract it, as would a second normal X chromosome in a female. This defective gene restricts the production of one of two essential clotting factors, known as Factor VIII and Factor IX. Lack of Factor VIII (also known as antihemophilic factor or AHF) results in what is called hemophilia A or "classical hemophilia"; lack of Factor IX (or plasmathromboplastin component) causes hemophilia B, also known as "Christmas disease," after a British family that had this form of the disease. The disorder is usually carried by mothers to their sons, since the son's X chromosome comes from the mother. For a woman who is a carrier of one defective X chromosome, there is a 50 percent chance that a son will have hemophilia and a 50 percent chance that a daughter will be a carrier. Approximately one-third of cases are born to women with no known history of hemophilia in their families. However, some of these women are true hemophilia carriers, who may have received an abnormal gene transmitted through many generations of females in their families but not seen in male members, or they may have had affected relatives whom they did not know or who died as infants. Other cases may be caused by spontaneous mutation. All daughters of men with hemophilia will be carriers, because the father's sole X chromosome carries the defective gene. Though extremely rare, we now know that there can be females with the disease. In what is known as "excessive Lyonization," a symptomatic carrier inactivates the good X chromosome and presents like a severe hemophilia patient. Another genetic defect that can cause hemophilia is Turner's syndrome, in which a female has only one X chromosome (XO) rather than two (XX) and that X chromosome carries a trait for the disease. And if a woman who is a carrier marries a man with hemophilia, the daughter can inherit the damaged X chromosome from both.[5] (Until modern treatment became available, of course, few men with hemophilia lived into healthy enough adulthood to consider marriage and family.) Hemophilia affects all socioeconomic levels, races, and ethnic groups. The glossary contained in Appendix A offers further details and definitions of important terms; it also explains abbreviations and acronyms.

Hemophilia is divided into three levels of severity: severe, moderate, and mild. The level of clinical severity, meaning how much bleeding occurs, usually depends upon the amount of active clotting factor present in the blood. In severe hemophilia, where clotting factor is less than 1 percent of the normal range, bleeding occurs spontaneously into the joints and muscles. Injury, surgery, and dental procedures thus present significant problems. In moderate hemophilia, clotting activity is between 1 and 5 percent of the normal range. Spontaneous bleeding does not usually occur, but minor injuries can cause prolonged bleeding. In mild hemophilia, clotting activity ranges from 5 to 50 percent of normal.

People with mild hemophilia do not bleed into their joints, but serious bleeding can occur as a result of trauma or surgical or dental procedures. The majority of persons with hemophilia are in the severe category—and most of my hemophilia informants were also in this category.

These definitions and descriptions present a clinical picture of hemophilia as a disease. It is much more than that. For those who have it and those who treat it, it is an illness—a social, psychological, and economic experience. For those who legislate about it or fund and administer programs for it, it is a health care system. Its meaning has changed over time, shaped by these hemophilia community members. I invite you to share their social history, a half century of living with hemophilia.

CHAPTER 2

The Dismal Era

Because the Blood Comes from the Woman

*For it was taught: If she circumcised her first child and he died
[as a result of bleeding from the operation] and a second one
died [similarly], she must not circumcise her third child.*

Locating the earliest descriptions of human hemophilia requires exploring writings from the far distant past. The epigraph to this chapter is the earliest known mention, attributed to R. Judah, the Prince, redactor of the Mishnah, and is in the tractate Yebamot 64b in the *Babylonian Talmud,* a compilation of Jewish law dated to the second century.[1] A famous Islamic surgeon of the tenth century, Albucasis, also referred to a condition interpreted by scholars as hemophilia in his encyclopedic work on medicine and surgery, *Al Tasrif.* In twelfth-century Spain, Maimonides, a physician and Talmudist, drawing from the ancient writings and his own observations, included a discussion of this bleeding problem in relation to circumcision in *The Mishneh Torah,* his fourteen-book codification of Biblical and Talmudic law. Maimonides augmented R. Judah's words by saying that this rule should hold true whether the third child was from a woman's first or second husband, confirming the notion of maternal transmission. The most important code of early Jewish law, the *Shulhan Arukh* (The Prepared

Table, 1565), compiled by R. Joseph Caro, also recommends that the sisters of a woman whose son died as a result of circumcision should not have their sons circumcised, with two additional rabbinical scholars reconfirming the assumption by stating "because the blood comes from the woman."[2]

Scholars attribute these rabbinical dictates to a remarkable perception of the genetic transmission of a familial bleeding disorder, probably hemophilia.[3] (All of these writings were, of course, proscriptive and descriptive; no treatments were offered for this condition during these darkest of ages.) Since circumcision is considered the most important ritual in the Jewish religion, which places a high value on the birth of a male, a rabbinical directive to set aside this ceremony is most unusual. That this condition was discussed in these ancient holy writings and was considered to be significant to the point of making an exception to performing this ceremony has contributed to the hemophilia community's sense of having a "special" history and culture.

The Nineteenth Century: Physicians Contribute to the Medical Literature

Physicians in the United States and Europe began to write about families of "bleeders" in the early 1800s. In 1803 John Conrad Otto, a Philadelphia physician, provided the first accurate description of hemophilia in the modern medical literature, reporting on families from Maryland and New England with "unaffected mothers" and sons who were "bleeders." Otto's report and one written in 1813 by John Hay, another American physician, suggested that the condition must be inherited from just one of the parents—that is, a carrier female paired with a normal male or a normal female paired with a bleeder male. (These represent two of the five possible combinations in sex-linked inheritance.) By 1820 a German physician, Nasse of Bonn, had formulated observations on inheritance into what is known as "Nasse's Law," that hemophilia is transmitted entirely by unaffected females to their sons. In 1828 another German physician, Frederick Hopff, credited his teacher, Schoenlein, with using the term "haemophilia" and also with proposing transfusion therapy.

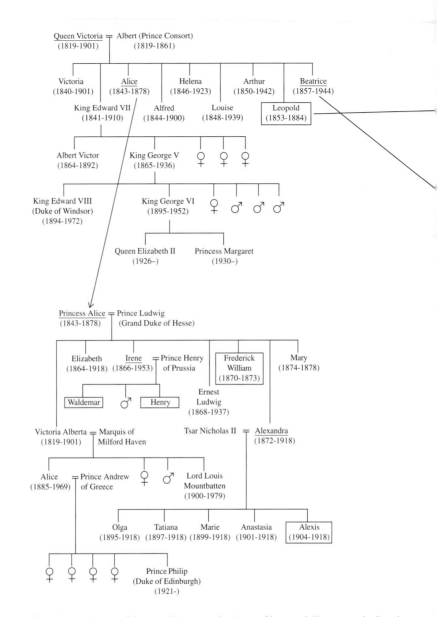

Figure 1 The descendants of Queen Victoria. Carriers of hemophilia are underlined, persons with hemophilia are boxed. Dashed lines indicate an uncertain diagnosis. Genealogies adapted from: Miller, Connie, PhD., *Inheritance of Hemophila* (New York: National Hemophilia Foundation, 1998) and Potts, D.M. and W.T.W. Potts, *Queen Victoria's Gene* (Phoenix Mill: Sutton, 1995).

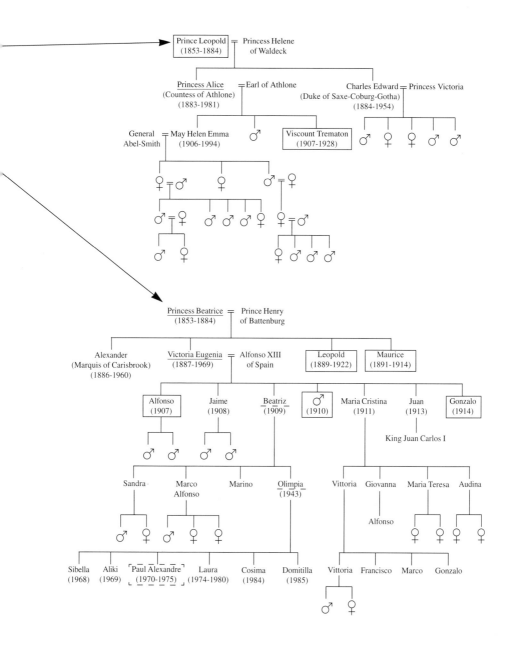

Transfusion was actually attempted in 1840, although a time lag in communication probably accounted for a comment in the literature in the late 1840s that, although transfusion had been suggested, it had not yet been attempted. By the end of the century, in 1893, the first recorded observation of prolonging clotting time in a capillary tube was published in England.[4]

These initial attempts to analyze blood coagulation and subsequently to provide therapeutic intervention for the disease known as "haemophilia" provided the foundation for the research and treatment attempts that were to increase substantially in Europe and in the United States in the twentieth century. The description and definition of hemophilia, however, would remain essentially the same for the next fifty years.

"The Royal Disease"

Until the end of the nineteenth century, awareness and recognition of hemophilia were confined primarily to the medical profession, who either saw it in their patients or read about it in the literature. As often happens, hemophilia became more widely known once it affected a well-known person. Although communication was slow in the 1800s, hemophilia gained prominence when the most famous monarch in Europe carried the gene, which her progeny passed on throughout the ruling dynasties of the entire continent. Queen Victoria, the world's most renowned carrier of hemophilia, gave birth to two carrier daughters, Alice and Beatrice, and a hemophilic son, Leopold, the Duke of Albany. Her description of having a son with hemophilia is probably the first personal, nonmedical documentation of the disease. In a letter written to her prime minister, Benjamin Disraeli, she said that Leopold, who was then twenty years old, "had been four or five times at death's door and was never hardly a few months without being laid up."[5]

Alice's daughter Alexandra became the consort of Czar Nicholas II of Russia and gave birth to Alexis, who "is probably the world's most famous hemophiliac."[6] In Alexis's case, the disease may have directly shaped history: according to Pierre Gilliard, his tutor, hemophilia "was one of the main causes of the Tsar's fall."[7] The family's anguish over the situation and their reaching out to Rasputin for help was common knowledge. From that time forward, hemophilia has remained in the public mind as "the Royal Disease." This label, with its connotation of aristocracy, has also become a linguistic marker within the hemophilia community's culture.

The Twentieth Century Begins: Pedigrees, Research, and Treatment

In 1911 Drs. W. Bulloch and P. Fildes published their "monumental review of pedigrees of families with bleeding disorders."[8] They also defined and stabilized hemophilia on the "triad of symptoms, sex incidence, and inheritance."[9] Their citations extended back to 1519, and they provided an annotated bibliography of over forty-four pedigrees. As G. I. C. Ingram states, "For students of haemophilia, it is at once their Shakespeare for its drama and human warmth and their Bible for its towering authority—or at least, shall we say their Old Testament, for in 1911 Bulloch and Fildes could only deal with haemophilia clinically and genealogically, the Law and the Prophets so to speak; the Grace of laboratory diagnosis and blood product therapy could then be only dimly foreseen."[10] In the same year, however, coagulation research demonstrated that the formation of thrombin in hemophilia blood was abnormally slow and that adding traces of plasma to it shortened clotting time.[11]

Descriptions of various hemophilia treatments were published in the United States and England in the 1920s and 1930s. In 1926 the hemophilia section of the *U.S. Surgeon General's Catalogue*, a guideline for health providers, contained a long list of treatments including "injection of sodium citrate, calcium lactate, Witte's peptone, anaphylaxis, splenectomy, and the galvanic needle." In Britain in the 1930s, R. G. MacFarlane, a prominent hematologist, treated hemophiliacs with a topical solution of snake venom. In the 1950s he wrote a paper that included a self-critical appraisal: "The main value of [a historical story] is that one sees that the growth of knowledge is hampered by prejudice and the failure to recognize one's own ignorance, as well as the misuse of words and the mixing up of facts and theories. Having seen that, one resolves to do better in the future."[12]

The next major step forward was the introduction by D. R. Feissly of Lausanne, France, of plasma for transfusions. In an article published in the *Journal of Clinical Investigation* in 1937, A. J. Patek and F. H. L. Taylor demonstrated that the intravenous administration of redissolved plasma precipitates shortened blood clotting time.[13] Oscar Ratnoff, M.D., recalls working with Patek in 1939, just after Ratnoff's graduation from Columbia University Medical School. Both were at Columbia's Research Division of Chronic Diseases (now Goldwater Hospital) where Patek was then studying liver disease, following a training period at the Thorndike Laboratories at Harvard under Dr. George Minot. Ratnoff recalls, "What [Patek] did was to be the first person to demonstrate that you could take a fraction [a chemically separated constituent] of normal plasma and correct the defect, both in the test tube and in the patient himself. A similar fraction of hemophilic blood didn't work in the test tube—I don't think he tried that on patients. That was the critical experiment in the development of knowledge about hemophilia."[14]

In the 1930s Kenneth Brinkhous, M.D., also entered the world of coagulation research. He recalled his introduction to the field:

I was approached during my late sophomore year in medical school [at the University of Iowa] by a newly arrived chairman of pathology, Dr. Harry P. Smith, who had just come from the laboratory of Nobel laureate George H. Whipple in Rochester. He was looking for someone to help him clean up the laboratory and get it established, and I was looking for a job, and this is the way I got started. He was interested at the time in blood clotting and in fibrinogen, and I would say that the start of my work in blood clotting was in the summer of 1930, which I guess is now over sixty-one years ago. Many people have told me, "You certainly got in a rut early, and you're still in it!"

Blood clotting at that time was not well understood. The people who were in it were thought to be cantankerous and disagreeable. Nobody could seem to agree on much of anything. Some of my friends said: "Why don't you get wise (so to speak) and go into something important like cancer?" But I persisted along that line.

The scientific climate in the 1930s was quite different from that of today. Remembering a meeting of the Federation of American Societies for Experimental Biology in Toronto in 1939, Brinkhous described how the research team was regarded in those days:

I showed very clearly that there was a deficiency in the plasma factor. It wasn't until the [1980s] that I realized how important the publication itself was. I called that a few years later the "antihemophilic factor" for the first time, and Webster's dictionary attributes that to my paper. Today it is known as Factor VIII.

Most papers had single authors or maybe two. Here we had a group of five people where we could contribute various parts to a single project. . . . People would raise their eyebrows and say: "Well, they probably couldn't get there on their own so they had to join a group." This was the first team research in blood clotting, and many, many things came out of that; the characterization of Vitamin K and obstructive jaundice, and mechanisms of heparin function. . . . We published in the *Journal of Biological Chemistry*.[15]

Between 1900 and 1940 funding for projects in clotting research, as for all basic research, came primarily from private sources, mainly foundations and universities. Not until after World War II did the U.S. government provide much funding for medical research efforts. Until then, federally funded research focused on projects with commercial or military applications, and the Department of Agriculture was the government's leading scientific research agency. (Not yet urbanized, the United States valued its farmers and their products.) In 1938, the budget for the U.S. Public Health Service was $2.8 million, in comparison with $26.3 million for the Department of Agriculture.[16]

Both Drs. Brinkhous and Ratnoff recalled the poor quality of life for persons with hemophilia during those times. As Brinkhous stated:

They [persons with hemophilia] were admitted to the hospital because they were very sick. I think hemophiliacs were a sort of fatalistic group at that time. They knew, in fact, that it was better to do nothing than to try to do something that might not turn out. For instance, death from teeth extraction was very common at the time. It was . . . dismal.[17]

Peter Levine, M.D., remembered hearing about "the bad old days of hemophilia" from his mentor, Anthony Britten, M.D., who had started a small hemophilia center at the New England Medical Center Hospital:

There was a group of patients whom Dr. Britten treated who were victims of the sort of the end of the spectrum of lifelong, severely debilitating chronic illness, who handled it by acting out. I think it could be safely said that these were extraordinarily sociopathic individuals. They'd come and have brawls on the medical floors. They would regularly loot the narcotics cabinet. They would throw glassware around and were frequently arrested and taken out of the hospital to jail. This was, of course, in the "bad old days" when the treatment was so terrible.[18]

One of the rare survivors to old age, Ben Lederman, who was born in 1913, became the official keeper of the history of the hemophilia community. He was the "griot," or community story teller:

Indulge an old fogy while I reminisce about the "bad old days" in hemophilia therapy as it applies to surgery. When I was eight days old I was circumcised. The experience was terrifying for my parents. They feared I would bleed to death as had two of my grandfather's male siblings. Being congenitally contrary and blissfully ignorant of both history and hemophilia, I survived. No further surgery was done for sixty years.[19]

Using both sarcasm and humor, Lederman described the "witches' brews" concocted by the researchers of the 1930s:

Let's start with the simpler recipes devised for the palates of the poor bloody victims of hemophilia. *Calcium phosphate* and *milk sugar* could do no harm; and if it was fortified with *Vitamins A, B, C, D,* it might even help. Mixed *alkaloids* were then proposed. Later *brewer's yeast* (very popular for acne in those years) was given. And of course, *cod liver oil* (children cried for it, billboards proclaimed) so it ought to be good for pediatric bleeders. . . . *Fasting* for 48 hours was naturally the final prescription for getting a good clot. P.S. Did you know that a few years after Dr. Howell's article was published, a subcutaneous injection of cottonmouth moccasin venom was given? Some of us are still hissing.[20]

Throughout the first half of this century the quality of life for hemophiliacs, known as "victims" or "bleeders," remained essentially unchanged. They struggled with pain and crippling resulting from spontaneous internal hemorrhaging into soft tissues and joints. They were unable to obtain an education because of excessive absences from school. Their parents lived lives of isolation and desperation, with no expectation of a future for their sons, for they knew that most boys with hemophilia died between the ages of twelve and nineteen. Indeed, there was very little difference between the excessive mortality of the nineteenth century and that of the 1930s.[21] However, coagulation research before 1940 paved the way for developments that would dramatically change the prospects for children born with hemophilia in the next thirty years.

The Early and Mid-1940s:
The Light at the End of the Tunnel

Advances in the technology of blood storage and transfusion were concurrent with developments in coagulation research. The first permanent blood bank in the United States was established in 1937 at Cook County Hospital in Chicago, Illinois, by Dr. Bernard Fantus, who set the model for sterile procedures, record keeping, and observation of patient reactions.[22]

Medical progress has always accompanied the horror of war.[23] During World War II the American Red Cross sponsored the development of a new system for treating shock with plasma. At its pilot center for American blood needs at Presbyterian Hospital, New York, Dr. Charles Drew set the standard for collecting, storing, transporting, and administering plasma under battlefield conditions.[24] The technology was further developed by a Harvard biochemist named Edwin Cohn, who focused on separating specific proteins from dried plasma. This fractionation process produced albumin, which proved enormously effective in preventing shock.[25] When the prominent Philadelphia surgeon Isidore S. Ravdin, M.D., was called to Pearl Harbor to treat the wounded in December 1941, he brought a satchel of fifty bottles of Cohn's albumin with him. Ravdin's reports of dramatic success spurred the government to a national mobilization for albumin, with Cohn in charge.

Cohn realized that he would need industry's help and insisted that seven major pharmaceutical companies send chemists to Boston, where he and his staff trained them in the fractionation technique. Cohn provided these companies with his formula on the condition that he maintain quality control of the process; every time a company produced a batch of albumin, it sent a sample to Cohn's lab to be tested for purity. By September 1943, the lab and its affiliated companies had sent more than 60,000 units to the military. By November that number had doubled. The combination of plasma and albumin created "a sensation" on the battlefield among medical officers, though the press usually described them both simply as "plasma."[26] Spurred on by the proven usefulness of these blood components, coagulation researchers, who now became known as "clotters," pursued a variety of research pathways after the war.

As the production of albumin moved ahead, Cohn and his colleagues at Harvard had begun to explore ways in which the discarded blood fractions could be put to use. In 1946 they demonstrated that one of those fractions, called Cohn Fraction I, indicated antihemophilic activity.[27] In 1947, Dr. Kenneth Brinkhous and his group published the finding that platelets separated from the blood of hemophiliacs reacted normally and that the hemophilia defect was in the plasma. Using different methods Dr. Armand Quick came to the same conclusion during that year.[28]

Although there is little recorded information concerning the quality of life for youngsters with hemophilia during World War II, two informants offer a glimpse into childhood with hemophilia before the 1950s. Frank Schnabel was born in 1929 in Spokane, Washington. Thirty years later he would become the founder of both the Canadian Hemophilia Society and the World Federation of Hemophilia. During an interview in 1959, he recalled that his mother, Mazie, decided that the best way for him to live was "to accept as much of life as he could take, . . . to have him shoot the rapids and live, rather than paddle in the backwaters and merely die." He noted that she "rounded off all the sharp corners in the house, but cotton wool was alien to her spirit." When Frank was old enough to ride a tricycle, he was given one, and he added that "I might not have climbed as high in the tree as my friends, but I'd climb. I'd jump off a fence but not a roof." In a diary he kept beginning in 1941, he wrote: "Played hockey. . . . Had a pinecone fight. . . . Had a big battle at snowforts. . . . Did not go to school because tooth was loose and gum was bleeding. . . . Played baseball. . . . Got another nosebleed. . . . Had a sore leg from sliding into base. . . . Went to the hospital had a transfusion. . . . Wasn't as bad as I'd thought. . . . Allied troops trying to escape by Dunkirk. . . . Memorial Day. . . . Had another bloody nose. . . . Shot off some firecrackers. . . . Neighbors complained." In his interview, Frank described "days in bed, repeated transfusions, and nights of pain," but recalled learning to endure the pain without sedatives because his mother had been warned by the doctor that "once Frank started taking them, he would need them increasingly."[29]

"Adam H.," a "key informant" in this study, was also a child with hemophilia in the 1940s. His earliest memories of an awareness of his condition were "when I fell on the kitchen floor . . . at about four or five. . . . I fell and hit my cheek and it blew up and I ended up hospitalized," where "the treatment was [a transfusion of] whole blood." Understatement is evident in his description of "a knee bleed": "You wouldn't bleed to death from a bad knee—but the pain would be rather unpleasant. When it got really bad, you'd call one of the doctors. He'd come out at midnight and give me a shot of morphine. On a few occasions when even that didn't work, my rabbi would come over and almost literally spend the night with me. I guess in many respects it wasn't a very pleasant childhood." "Adam" remarked that "If you close your eyes, it's very hard to relive the pain that you've had—or, as some people say, the people who continually relive the pain go crazy."[30]

Clearly, both of these men experienced what many refer to as "the bad old days" of hemophilia during their childhood years. The way they express themselves shows a combination of courage, optimism, and denial that became the coping mechanism for many such children. Hospitalizations and treatment with whole-blood transfusions interrupted activities and required many days out of school. Scientific and technological progress had not yet improved the quality of their lives. In addition, parents had to absorb the financial burden of whatever course of treatment was available. American health insurance consisted of a varied assortment of plans shaped primarily by "piggybacking on existing organizations such as voluntary hospitals, the medical profession, and the life insurance industry." In contrast to the development of health insurance in European countries, which began with the working class and concentrated first on income maintenance and then expanded coverage, American health insurance grew by "responding to the needs of the middle class requiring funds during the Depression."[31] Quality and accessibility of insurance coverage varied tremendously, and geographic location and socioeconomic status were key determinants of both coverage and access to care. Not for many years would the political, economic, and cultural climate foster developments that would eventually change the childhood experience of living with hemophilia.

CHAPTER 3

The Years of Hope, 1948–65

Nineteen forty-eight marked the beginning of a "golden decade" for coagulation research.[1] Symbolized by the creation of the National Institutes of Health (NIH), the postwar economic and political climate nurtured young medical researchers returning home from the war, fostering the continuation of work begun in the 1930s. Nineteen forty-eight was also a defining year for hemophilia. On June 15, Robert Lee Henry, an attorney who had a son with hemophilia, filed a certificate of incorporation in the New York Department of State, creating the Hemophilia Foundation.[2] By the 1950s, this organization, renamed the National Hemophilia Foundation (NHF), would emerge as the sole national voluntary health agency associated with this disease and would become a powerful voice in Washington, advocating for funding to support coagulation research.

A "Golden Decade"
for Coagulation Research, 1948–58

Both of these organizations contributed significantly to the scientific career of Dr. Kenneth M. Brinkhous.[3] In particular, he cites 1948 as a personal milestone in his professional development, the year that he acquired an NIH grant.[4] (Brinkhous's association with the NHF is discussed at the end of the chapter.) Having studied plasma since 1939, he was able to do some coagulation research in the early 1940s while directing the Southwestern Pacific field medical laboratory under General Douglas MacArthur. Following the war, he resumed his hemophilia clotting research at the University of North Carolina Medical School in Chapel Hill, but with the NIH funding he was able to transform his laboratory studies by purchasing and maintaining hemophilic dogs. According to Stephen G. Pemberton, Brinkhous's laboratory-based studies made the "canine hemophiliac" an integral feature of postwar research on bleeding disorders. By framing the dogs as "patients," Brinkhous created a unique clinical situation. His research has been described as creating a link between laboratory research discoveries and treatment for people with hemophilia and accelerating the pace of transfer from research to treatment. It also has been touted as a "proven" example of how animal research can benefit humanity.[5] Brinkhous's grant, entitled "Coagulation in Hemophilia," is the longest-running NIH grant, continuing through the present.

Brinkhous's plasma studies drew on his own wartime research and also on the work of Dr. Edwin Cohn at Harvard Medical School, which represented the major coagulation research effort of the war years and which, as we have seen, had focused on plasma fractionation. For their experiments Brinkhous's research group was able to purchase Cohn Fraction I in the marketplace. Brinkhous recalled that at that time there was no method for measuring antihemophilic factor (AHF, now known as Factor VIII), so their research involved a lot of trial and error. "If you were making something and you had no test on the bench that would tell you how much was there, you could go down all sorts of pathways, and I think that's what happened." He adds that his group developed the more precise measurement methods that came to be widely used.[6]

In addition to their work on plasma fractions, Brinkhous has credited his group's success in making scientific discoveries to having an animal model for hemophilia, the hemophilic dogs. As he related the story, the dogs had belonged to a woman in Ithaca, New York, who raised Irish setter show dogs. She had noticed that a certain number of male puppies in her litters would develop swollen joints and die by the age of three months. When a test administered by veterinarians from Cornell revealed a lengthy clotting time for blood from these dogs, one of the owner's relatives, who was a medical resident at Duke University, suggested that the dogs might have hemophilia. Although the owner did not have any "living bleeders" at that time, she did have two females, Nora and Lynn. Brinkhous commented, "Lynn was pregnant and she was the excitable one, and Nora was the placid one. We bought a pig in a poke." When Lynn gave birth to twelve puppies, Brinkhous's group was able to use the male bleeders among them to test the effects of administering plasma and the various plasma components they were studying. Brinkhous said emphatically, "I still believe firmly that the way you do this is you test in animals and then you test in people." He noted that they had "a perfect setup, going from laboratory bench to Nora and Lynn and their offspring and then to the clinic." He derives an added measure of satisfaction from being able to raise adult animals with no joint disease. He clearly savors his memories of those beginning years, emphasizing that they were "golden."[7]

This "golden decade" is also described by Frederick Rickles, M.D., another researcher informant, as "the time when protein chemistry came into being," when "people began to understand more about plasma proteins of all sorts and the clotting proteins were model proteins to work with." He added that "Lots of capable biochemists tried to isolate factors out of plasma. Since then a whole series of clotting proteins have been isolated, purified, and characterized."[8]

By 1952 rapid scientific progress in protein chemistry led to a change in the definition of hemophilia. Four significant, independent publications reported evidence of another plasma clotting activity separate from that involving Factor VIII, the component of plasma that is inactive or missing in classical hemophilia. From that point on, hemophilia was described as "a blood clotting disorder affecting males with two possible major protein deficiencies, either Factor VIII [hemophilia A] or Factor IX [hemophilia B]." In 1952, Oscar Ratnoff, M.D., and his colleague Gerald Rosenbloom, M.D., discovered still another clotting activity, which they named Hageman Factor after their patient who manifested this coagulation deficiency. It ultimately became known as Factor XII.[9] In 1953 Brinkhous and his colleagues showed that Factor VIII and Factor IX deficiency were the two major separate types of hemophilia.

Another sign of progress in 1952 was acceleration of precision in measurement, with the development by Brinkhous's research group of an

accurate test for measuring Factor VIII. Although the British coagulation researchers R. G. MacFarlane and Rosemary Biggs had previously developed a measurement technique, the Chapel Hill Group's
thromboplastin generation test, a one-stage method, was generally
adopted because of its relative simplicity.[10]

As noted above, shortly after the end of World War II, the federal
government opened up its pocketbook to fund scientific advances. Until the 1940s, basic research had been sponsored primarily by private
foundations, universities, and pharmaceutical companies, who hired scientists to do research in their own laboratories. During the war, the
battlefield benefits of blood components and new medications helped
shape an appreciation of the research that led to these new treatments
and changed the attitude about the federal government's responsibility
toward medical research. In the postwar years, this new way of thinking
was reflected both within and outside the government. Within the government itself, restructuring of agencies and establishing of new priorities led to a new emphasis on medical research. The United States Public Health Service (PHS), which had been administering health grants
to the states and sponsoring intramural research in the National Institute of Health (NIH), was authorized by Congress in 1944 to make
grants for outside investigation in medicine (other than for cancer).
When the Office of Scientific Research and Development became the
National Science Foundation after the war, its Committee on Medical
Research was moved into the NIH. As a result of the transfer, the NIH
budget grew from $180,000 in 1945 to $4 million in 1947. In 1948 the
National Institute of Health became the National Institutes of Health,
incorporating the "categorical disease" approach and subsuming the
National Heart Institute and five other categorical institutes. The NIH
budget grew to $46.3 million by 1950.[11]

These structural changes and budget allocations reflect a dramatic
change in attitude. Throughout our nation's history, American culture
has often reflected skepticism of big government, in keeping with fundamental values of individual liberty. These values have contributed to
generating legislative decisions and establishing policies, affecting both
public and private sectors, that generally maintain a stance of governmental noninvolvement. The postwar years reflected a shift in the climate of thought that supported the federal government's emphasis on

and generosity to medical research. It was a time of optimism and economic expansion, a time when, in Paul Starr's words, "modern medicine became a metaphor for progress without conflict."[12]

In addition, the United States had emerged from World War II as an international leader, as a result of both its economic and its military strength. With the European economies devastated, the United States became the "leader of the free world" and assumed the responsibility of fostering both economic and medical advancement.[13] The cold war competition with the Soviet Union in the 1950s created an exciting opportunity for medical researchers to emerge as victors on a new battleground. Richard Carter's biography of Jonas Salk, who produced the vaccine to combat polio, the leading cause of crippling in children throughout the first half of the twentieth century, captures the excitement and victorious spirit of the time. When it was announced that research trials had demonstrated the vaccine's effectiveness, the entire nation paused to mark the moment: "More than a scientific achievement, the vaccine was a folk victory. People observed moments of silence, rang bells, honked horns, blew factory whistles, fired salutes, kept their traffic lights red in brief periods of tribute, took the rest of the day off, closed their schools or convoked fervid assemblies therein, drank toasts, hugged children, attended church, smiled at strangers, forgave enemies."[14] Researchers savored their new-found prominence and looked forward to other triumphs. With available funding, they hoped to discover other "magic bullets."

Two other developments also combined to change the way Americans thought about government involvement in medical care. Since the use of antibiotics had diminished the impact of most infectious diseases, other kinds of conditions were gaining greater attention. Mary Lasker, a New York social activist and philanthropist whose husband had made his fortune in advertising, became a general, leading her troops of doctors into the fray to conquer these new enemies. Lasker believed that doctors and research scientists were used to "thinking small" and encouraged medical researchers to request large amounts of money. In addition, she and her husband organized a lay lobby, known both as "the noble conspiracy" and as "Mary and her little lambs," which helped establish an entirely new advocacy pattern as they spearheaded fundraising for the American Cancer Society. Efforts by other "categorical illness" advocacy groups—including the National Hemophilia Foundation—soon followed. Moreover, by funding categorical illness research, members of Congress who were opposed to the idea of national health insurance could maintain the status quo by voting instead for research appropriations.[15]

Changes in Medical Care: Hospital Expansion and Specialization

During these prosperous years, government policies also fostered progress in other domains of health care. Funding led to hospital construction and the financing of medical education for returning veterans. This support and expansion of existing institutional and professional structures further enhanced medical authority. In *The Social Transformation of American Medicine,* Paul Starr describes these as "the liberal years," in which "liberal opinion held that America had transcended the need for drastic political reform by incorporating change into free institutions. Medical science epitomized the postwar vision of progress without conflict. There was an alliance between liberalism and medicine which bolstered professional authority and medical autonomy. All could agree about the value of medical progress (that is, if they could afford the cost, as the advocates of national health insurance would add)."[16]

Indeed, Rosemary Stevens remarks that, instead of World War II providing for a structural realignment of health services, it had the reverse effect, in that programs introduced during the war and in the immediate postwar years approached health services piecemeal.[17] What did change dramatically was the location of these services. Before the war, most doctors had gone into practice after an internship of one year and then practiced independently. In 1930 only one physician in sixteen worked in a hospital full-time, and four out of ten doctor-patient encounters took place in the patient's home.[18] In 1946 Congress enacted legislation fostering the centralization of medical education, research, and delivery of patient care within the walls of hospitals. The Hill-Burton Act, which Stevens calls "the most important piece of health legislation in the postwar decade," provided funding for massive community hospital construction on a nationwide basis.[19] By the 1950s, most doctors spent at least three years in a hospital residency after completing their internship, and one doctor in six worked full-time in a hospital.[20]

During the postwar years the Veterans Administration (VA) Hospital System also expanded. Its new leadership fostered affiliations with medical schools, using the hospitals for clinical research and training. As part of this strategy the VA promoted the locating of its facilities in urban areas. The affiliated medical school committees were granted the right to vote on appointments for the hospitals' medical staffs, paving the way for the increasing power of the medical school faculty in the hospital setting.[21]

As academic medicine flourished, an increasing emphasis was placed on specialization. Until the 1930s most doctors were general practitioners, but in that decade groups of physicians "began to carve up medicine into specialty divisions." The American Medical Association's (AMA) Council on Medical Education and Hospitals, along with the AMA specialty sections and the four examining boards then in existence, issued standards for examining boards and settled jurisdictional disputes among specialties. The first edition of the *Dictionary of Medical Specialists* was published in 1940, granting elite status, at least on paper. But the reality at that time was that AMA general practitioners were still powerful enough to set limits on opportunities for special practice, and the relationship between general practitioners and specialists was still "loosely defined."[22] During World War II, however, "properly certified specialists" had received a higher rank, which as Stevens notes, "gave doctors a healthy respect for the value of board certificates."[23] After the war, the VA ruled that no doctor would be treated as a specialist without board certification in that specialty. The proportion of physicians who reported themselves as full-time specialists rose from 24 percent in 1940 to 37 percent by 1949.[24] Although this shift began to affect patterns of health care delivery, it did not reach all strata of our population.

Hemophilia Patients: A Tough Group of People

While researchers were savoring their "golden decade," most physicians and hemophilia patients were still frustrated. In the late

1940s and in the early 1950s many physicians remained unaware of scientific advances in coagulation research and in the potential of using plasma and its components. For the most part, boys with hemophilia who sought medical care were treated by pediatricians or general practitioners who gave them transfusions of whole blood to control bleeding and kept them in the hospital for lengthy periods. Not until the 1960s, when the National Hemophilia Foundation's developing network of physicians disseminated coagulation research results and the use of new orthopedic procedures, was there much allure in becoming a specialist—a hematologist or an orthopedist involved in treating hemophiliacs.

The first group of new specialists to treat hemophiliacs in the postwar years told stories that were similar to the early clotters' tales of the "bad old days." Dr. Marvin Gilbert, an orthopedist, described the hemophilia family in those days as "a tough group of people," probably because they had suffered so much pain. He emphasized that most physicians did not know anything about hemophilia. Indeed, one patient referred to an ear, nose, and throat specialist was asked by that doctor when he had developed the condition! According to Gilbert, at that time there was little trust of doctors and little that doctors could do to ameliorate the situation for the patients. Patients "felt that they knew more than the doctors; when treatment improved, patients became easier to deal with. It's easier to deal with somebody when you can do something for them."[25]

Only those patients fortunate enough in socioeconomic status and/or proximity to a pioneering treatment center received plasma, which was then administered as a liquid transfusion extracted from a single unit of whole blood. Whole blood remained the standard, and home treatment was a rarity. There were, however, exceptions. One of the first hemophilia treatment centers was based at the Rochester General Hospital, in Rochester, New York. In 1948, Mary Gooley, a laboratory technician, had come to work in the hospital's blood bank and in the intravenous therapy department. She described her first experience with hemophilia patients:

I didn't know what hemophilia was. It could have been a Greek race horse as far as I was concerned. . . . Patients were coming in with huge, swollen, boggy knees or major hemorrhages; most of them sitting at home in wheelchairs until the pain and the bleeding got to the point where they had to come in to have something done. It was really crisis management, and we didn't have very much to manage them with.

I remember that the first patient that I saw was a young man who had been in another hospital emergency room where he had gone through twenty-two venipunctures. He was very chubby, six or seven years old.

They were called "sufferers" or "bleeders," rarely "hemophilic patients." They had a very strange disease which few people understood. It was almost a mystical kind of thing. We were all very insecure, and to give them whole blood would take a very long time. They were very reactive to the whole blood. There were all kinds of reactions. They could very easily be overloaded with pulmonary edema. [The most common reaction was hives, but transfusions could also result in excess fluid, especially in children, with their smaller systems.] And we weren't doing them very much good.[26]

While providers of care for hemophilia patients expressed feelings of impotence and frustration, persons with hemophilia described how attempts to have a normal life were often thwarted by the disease. Men in the oldest informant cohort were children during the 1940s and 1950s. They share memories of isolation and pain that they might rather forget. They all refer to "horror stories" and call other men with hemophilia "blood brothers." Recalling being forced to eat large quantities of peanut butter, in every imaginable form, brought chuckles. It had been touted as "a miracle cure" in the 1950s; and of course it wasn't. All remember the number of days that they were absent from school; in one case it was more than 80 out of 180.

The golden decade and the flourishing of medical specialization did not cast any glow on these informants. "Cliff H." (Charles Carman), a person with severe hemophilia, was born in a little town in New Mexico. He wasn't diagnosed until he was four years old because "it took that time to get the appropriate diagnosis"; when it was finally made, "they still didn't want to call it hemophilia." He recalled his doctor:

There was a family doctor who was my physician during all of my growing up years—he was just a family physician, not a specialist. Certainly he did not know a lot of things that he probably should have known at that time, and frankly, probably made some errors. But by the same token, he did a lot of things right. Right in the sense that he always advised me that the person who should know the most about the disease is myself. He used to give me articles he had at the time, and his counsel was "I don't know everything that we should be doing, but we'll do the best we can." He used an awful lot of heating pads in those days that should never have been used. And that complicated a lot of factors. But for the most part all we had was whole blood, narcotics, and bed rest.[27]

"Irwin H." (Richard Johnson), a severe hemophiliac who is African American, grew up in an inner-city housing project in Pennsylvania. He recalls being treated with whole blood "that would drip maybe four or five hours in the back laboratories in the hospital." He had four cousins with hemophilia who died because "they believed in faith and religion and weren't treated." He recalled missing school and once staying in the hospital for a year and a half. Describing himself as "rebellious," he spoke of gangs, shootings, and stabbings, noting that he "came from a very poor neighborhood where there were very few fathers."[28]

The hospital wanted his mother to find blood donors to "supplement how much blood we were taking in, my brother and myself," but "people from the inner-city projects don't think in those terms; these people were struggling day to day to just eat." To cover their expenses they had Department of Public Assistance (DPA) support, in effect welfare, which covered both medical and dental expenses within certain limits. The hospital helped them deal with those limits by sending "Irwin H." home for a day and then bringing him back, so that coverage would begin again. The welfare allowance wasn't sufficient to provide him and his brother with enough food; they ate "beef, rice, and, of course, peanut butter, but there wasn't enough." He spoke of the frustration of feeling tethered to the hospital, yet also felt that the hospital introduced him to a world beyond the ghetto:

It gave me experiences different than what I would have got directly or just being in the projects. It gave me a different perspective on life, because I met a lot of kids who had come from very affluent families, and they would talk about things that I didn't even know anything about—like a person who waits on them in their house or a father who has so much money that he can actually hire people to donate blood to his children only. . . .
[In the hospital] they would just give me something, and I would take it and it would make my body stop hurting. It stopped the hemorrhaging, and it stopped the pain in my joints, so that I would just take it—where their families actually orchestrated what their kids were going to get and even had special people donate it for them.[29]

In marked contrast to these informants the experience of "Adam H.," a person with severe hemophilia from suburban New Jersey, highlights how different the quality of health care and the quality of life were then for more affluent members of our society. (Unfortunately, though to a lesser extent, they still are.) He traces the inheritance of his condition to his mother's family, "a traditional upper-middle-class German-Jewish family." His mother grew up in Connecticut and went to college. His father's family, of poor Russian-Polish background, had prospered in the hotel business, becoming "one of the wealthiest families in the area." While money did not ease the pain, it cushioned many of the effects of the disease and allowed "Adam H." to remain free of worries over access to blood and medical care.

We were particularly not poor in many of the kinds of things that made life easier for me as a person with hemophilia. And the reason for the importance of the hotel business is that I was able to get a lot of the personal services that I needed.
    . . . In my junior year of high school it came time to take the National Merit Scholarship Qualifying test. . . . The problem was that at the time of the test I wasn't walking, . . . there was no way that I could get to the school even though I lived no more than two or three blocks away. . . . It was nice having a station wagon from the hotel, a bellhop from the hotel who could carry me from upstairs where my bedroom was, down to the car, drive me over to the school, and carry me to the principal's office, wait there for two hours while I took the test, and then carry me back home again.[30]

He recalled being treated with "shots made from some component of plasma which had been thawed and that they had extracted a concentration of the plasma, taking each unit of plasma and extracting two or three doses of concentrate and injecting it on a weekly basis." Bellhops picked him up at school and drove him to his weekly appointments. His physician was a specialist, and there was no problem with obtaining a supply of blood:

At the hotel we had a whole bunch of blood donors. They were used to donating blood, because once a week we sent a truck to the Bowery to pick up people to serve as porters or dishwashers for the week. We had our own chicken coops. Later we turned these chicken coops into housing facilities for what we now call the homeless. They used to stay there for a week or two until we paid them and they could get drunk and go back to New York City and we'd send the next truck in. . . . There was a ready supply of blood donors.[31]

Viewing childhood in postwar America through the eyes of "Irwin H." and "Adam H." brings socioeconomic and racial differences into sharp focus. The disparity in quality of life in general and in health care in particular echoes in their voices. They seem to speak from different places and times; yet they are the same age and lived less than two hours apart. Beneath the surface of an egalitarian society with the best medical care in the world lay a lack of safety nets, racial discrimination, and barriers to access to "a gold standard" of health care for all. In the 1950s when—or so we wanted to believe—father knew best and all moms smiled and baked apple pies, these problems were not openly discussed. For the most part, the veneer of good care for all remained intact.

The Blood Services and Insurance Industries

At the same time that societal values led to promoting research programs, the mainstream of American culture also fostered entrepreneurial achievement. Since both blood banking and health insurance were considered "industries," government assumed a hands-off policy. Good business was considered to be good for the country.

Blood services in the United States include resources for collecting, storing, and transfusing blood. Generally speaking, blood banks, both nonprofit and commercial, handle whole blood and plasma. Plasma manufacturers collect and market plasma and its component products. In *The Gift Relationship: From Human Blood to Social Policy*, Richard Titmuss's seminal study comparing the value systems of societies through the case studies of their blood donation and transfusion systems, the United States is described as "an immense country with a great variety of social institutions, practices, and customs, a fundamental reality of size and pluralism which must constantly be borne in mind in any attempt to generalize and draw comparisons with countries the size and homogeneity of England and Wales. . . . Unlike England and Wales, there is no national or even state blood program and no single responsible authority on the state or local level."[32]

The first attempt to collect data on the supply and transfusion of blood in the United States was made in 1956–57. Although he states that information was "of varying quality and had many gaps and discrepancies," Titmuss reports that in the United States in 1956 there were more than 5,100,000 units of blood collected and some 4,500,000 transfused. The gap between the amount collected and the amount transfused was termed "wastage." Titmuss suggests that the greatest proportion of this could be termed "administrative waste," resulting from defects and inadequacies in planning, administration, and organization: failures to match demand and supply; the over-ordering of blood; the hoarding and regular wastage of blood by hospitals and blood banks; incorrect estimates of blood from different groups; delays in transportation; and many other factors in the system itself not connected with the quality of blood or its actual use by physicians in hospitals. In his analysis, Titmuss notes a growing trend toward larger blood banks, "particularly the commercial banks, and other banks who pay the suppliers of blood."[33]

In the now famous Kansas City case of 1962, two commercial blood banks in that city complained to the Federal Trade Commission about the Kansas City Hospital Association, maintaining that the association had refused to use them and had given all its business to the Community Blood Bank. The commercial blood banks argued that the result was a monopoly. The judge ruled in favor of the commercial blood banks, even though they were located in what was described as "a slum area, displaying a sign saying 'cash for blood' which drew blood donors described as 'skid row derelicts.'" This decision made it illegal to take part in a collective decision not to purchase blood commercially, "despite the weight of evidence that it carried a greater hepatitis risk." Clearly, this judgment in effect marked one state's acceptance of less than adequate standards for blood safety from that time on. It also reinforced the concept that blood was increasingly considered to be "a product," subject to the rules of the marketplace, rather than a public good, subject to monitoring and regulation.[34]

The rise of the U.S. plasma industry further reinforced this concept, as plasma and its components also came to be seen as products. The value of albumin had been demonstrated during World War II, and international demand for albumin after the war spurred the growth of the plasma manufacturing industry in the United States. The subsequent development of the plasma byproduct gamma globulin, which proved useful in the prevention and treatment of a number of diseases, in turn encouraged the development of other byproducts. From these initial years, "the blood business" expanded within an international context and became a major component of the hemophilia culture.

Another American industry of importance to family health care in the postwar years was the health insurance industry, which included an assortment of companies primarily shaped by established institutional structures and their geographical location. This model was very different from health insurance in European countries, which began as part of general national programs of social insurance that focused on income maintenance for the industrial working class. Although the American Association for Labor Legislation (AALL) had hoped to emulate the European model and institute compulsory health insurance as early as 1915, such proposals were regularly defeated.[35] It was primarily in response to the needs of the middle class, who required funds during the Depression to pay hospital bills, that private health insurance developed in the Blue Cross system, under the control of hospitals and doctors.

Once Blue Cross demonstrated its feasibility, commercial carriers became interested, and the system expanded through a series of competitions between "the Blues" and commercial plans in a pattern that "piggy-backed itself on preexisting organizations . . . the voluntary hospitals, the medical profession, and the life insurance industry."[36] Disorganization and skyrocketing costs in the health insurance arena had a tremendous impact on all families, particularly on those dealing with chronic illness. Lack of access to insurance coverage and inadequate coverage increasingly became major concerns for hemophiliacs and their families. However, before 1948 there were no organized efforts to promote access to blood or insurance coverage for the hemophilia population. Families dealing with the disease usually lived in isolation, only coming in contact with others who shared their situation within their own families or in hospital emergency rooms.

The Beginning of Hope: The End of Isolation

Although new treatments were slow to disseminate, in another sense the plight of hemophiliacs did begin to change in 1948. Two years before, in 1946, Robert Lee Henry, a wealthy lawyer from the North Shore of Long Island who had a son with hemophilia, read an article in the *New York Daily News* describing an accident that happened to a young boy from the nearby community of Glen Cove. Like his son, the boy had hemophilia, but the family was not as fortunate as the Henry family. This article provided the stimulus for Henry to create the Hemophilia Foundation, officially incorporated in New York in 1948.[37]

Shortly before his death in 1987, Henry described his vision in an interview with "Paul Phillips," the then executive director of the National Hemophilia Foundation (and an informant who preferred the use of a code name): "As a result of my son Lee having to live with hemophilia, I decided that something had to be done in the way of a more permanent approach to dealing with the needs of those affected by hemophilia. What I hoped for was that the organization would promote different areas that would lead, quite naturally, to the cure."[38] The certificate of incorporation was written in the spirit of the foundation's creator, stating its mission as "To make grants and donations for research and clinical study of hemophilia, abnormal blood conditions, and similar ailments; to publish information and knowledge related to the prevention and treatment of these diseases; to provide medical scholarships; to provide funds for persons suffering from hemophilia and kindred ailments."[39] Henry's wife, Betty Jane, has described her own sense of priorities: "At that time we wanted to help whoever needed to stop the pain first. The first thing was that the pain was so terrible. Everybody thought of hemophilia as blood gushing all over the place, but nobody knew about the pain."[40] Establishment of the foundation created an identifiable base, a nexus and a pivot for developing networks and support groups of hemophilia families and for the dissemination of information to physicians and families. In addition, it was granted tax exemption under the Internal Revenue Code as a charitable organization.

This beginning was in marked contrast to other chronic illness associations founded in that time period, which tended to be provider-driven. For example, the American Diabetes Association, created in 1940, was started by twenty-five physicians, who cited the need "for an exchange of ideas among physicians and research scientists."[41] In contrast, the Henrys and their friends took charge of the foundation. From the beginning, parents had power, largely because physicians had little to offer in the way of treatment or technical expertise; clinicians were virtually powerless. Mary Gooley recalled that Robert Lee Henry was willing to put all his financial resources to work in research to find a cure. The Henrys and their friends epitomized the spirit of voluntarism and *noblesse oblige* among upper-class Americans. Mrs. Henry took immediate steps to raise money to finance the operation of the foundation and to help families in need. She involved friends of the same social set and planned fund-raising events. She noted that "A big bundle came in from a patient of Dr. [Henry] Jordan's (an orthopedist from Lenox Hill Hospital); I think it was $100,000 . . . and the money accomplished so much. It took care of the children." Remembering treatment in those days, she added: "The blood was taken care of at Mt. Sinai and the joints at Lenox Hill."[42]

After telling their son's story to a reporter from *McCall's Magazine* in 1951, the Henrys were deluged by letters from "throughout the country and all over the world." For the first time families who had felt isolated and powerless heard about others like themselves and began to communicate with each other. Local chapters of the foundation were formed in Rochester, New York, Chicago, and Los Angeles. While most other national organizations that came into being at that time had strong central organizations and required that local contributions flow into national headquarters, the Hemophilia Foundation functioned as a loose federation of allied groups and required no prescribed amount of monetary support from its chapters.[43] The organization was set up in this fashion both to minimize expenditures for a central office staff or operations and to encourage local units to fill local needs. Chapter meetings provided a forum where parents traded "horror stories" over coffee, held tense discussions of how to recruit blood donors, and found a safe place to release pent-up anxiety. The chapters were, in the words of one participant, "mutual commiseration societies."[44]

Moving Ahead

While most families were taking their children to the hospital for transfusions, a few pioneers were doing things differently. After learning about the use of fresh-frozen plasma in Chapel Hill and Mount Sinai through the hemophilia network, Mary Gooley was among the first to use the new product. Of this time in the late 1950's, she recalls,

Because most of our patients had no insurance and no way of getting to the hospital, some of them who lived outside the city were in pretty bad shape. We took the plasma home with us to our home freezers and planted it among the peas and the strawberries, not worrying about hepatitis or any of the things we should have been thinking about and traveled on our own time to transfuse those patients out of their homes.[45]

In addition to progress at official hemophilia treatment locations, I learned via the informal hemophilia network of an amazing "unofficial" story about a woman referred to as "a pioneer parent." After locating her, I discovered that she was indeed a pioneer. In the 1950s Mrs. J. Green's sons were patients at the Carter Blood Center in Fort Worth, Texas, where the progressive physician Dr. Richard Halden encouraged parents to learn to infuse (that is, to administer plasma intravenously) their hemophilic sons at home and keep them out of the hospital. (At that time the medical establishment would not condone parents or adult patients treating themselves. Physicians or nurses treated persons with hemophilia, usually in a hospital in-patient setting.) After the family moved to Chicago in 1961, Mrs. Green would take the long railroad trip back and forth to Texas to get the necessary supplies and would secretly infuse her sons in their back bedroom. This activity went on for several years, until eventually Mrs. Green began to share her secret with other mothers.[46]

Institutional innovation in the structure of delivery of hemophilia still awaited the 1960s. In the interim, the National Hemophilia Foundation (renamed in 1956) fostered the dissemination of information about hemophilia and reported the strides being made in plasma research. When Kenneth Brinkhous's wife read a magazine article about the Henry family and the new foundation, she showed it to her husband, who proceeded to visit the headquarters during a trip to New York City.[47] This meeting began a fruitful relationship between the NHF and the group in Chapel Hill. Brinkhous became the first chairman of the NHF Medical and Scientific Advisory Council (MASAC), and the foundation became a vehicle to disseminate information and education about hemophilia research to physicians throughout the United States and abroad.

CHAPTER 4

A Research Milestone Heralds the Golden Era, 1960–65

Coagulation research flourished in the 1960s, supported both by government funding from the NIH and by the growing plasma industry. NIH student research grants combined with the lure of future professional recognition and economic rewards to encourage young medical students to become specialists in hematology, which had become an exciting field. Frederick Rickles, M.D., now medical director of a hemophilia treatment center, recalled that in those days medical school tuition was $150 per quarter and that's exactly what his grant provided, but he also noted that it was only when the National Institutes of Health came into being as a substantial agency that funding became available for research into diseases like hemophilia.[1]

The Growth of Research

NIH grants enabled the handful of pioneer "clotters" with their own labs to nurture a growing cadre of future coagulation researchers. In addition to Kenneth Brinkhous at the University of North Carolina at Chapel Hill and Oscar Ratnoff at Case Western Reserve University in Cleveland, Fred Rabiner and Irving Schulman, who were both originally at New York Hospital and later at different institutions in Chicago, offered early training to several young hematologists who play a major role in the field today. This training helped establish a career path that combined research and clinical practice within academic medical centers.

Frederick Rickles had had the opportunity to work summers in Rabiner's lab at Michael Reese Hospital in Chicago in the 1950s while he was still a teenager. In the 1960s, when he attended medical school at the University of Illinois, he worked part-time in the lab there directed by Schulman's junior colleague, Charles Abildgaard. He remembered that his project involved analyzing Factor VIII inhibitors in patients to see if they crossreacted in Factor VIII in animal species, using blood from chickens, cows, and other species. He also recalled that during those years all of the patients they treated who were over the age of twenty-five were in wheelchairs.[2]

Charles Abildgaard, also the medical director of a hemophilia treatment center, had welcomed the opportunity to work with Schulman, because he was one of the three researchers who, working independently, had separated Factor VIII from Factor IX at about the same time. He noted that "Schulman did it in New York and pretty much with his own hands in the lab." Abildgaard began his hematology fellowship with Schulman in 1960 at Children's Memorial Hospital in Chicago, where, in 1961, they experimented with one of the first concentrates for Factor VIII, known as AHF-rich fibrinogen. The study involved only one or two patients because the researchers were still uncertain exactly how to use it and in what dose. At about the same time they learned that Hyland Laboratories, in Los Angeles, California, had developed a Factor VIII concentrate, called Hemofil, which they hoped might be helpful for a patient of theirs with thrombocytopenia, a condition characterized by a low platelet count. Initially the people at Hyland, who were not familiar with either Schulman or Abildgaard, were reluctant to provide the concentrate. However, Schulman and Abildgaard discovered that Hyland was about to start clinical trials of Hemofil and informed the company that they were working with a large population of children with hemophilia.[3] They convinced Hyland they could contribute by providing patients and as a result became participants in the first clinical trial of Factor VIII in this country.

Another hemophilia treatment center medical director, Margaret Hilgartner, M.D., had become interested in hemophilia as a third-year medical student at Duke University. She was one of the first people trained in the newly emerging subspecialty of pediatric hematology and one of the first two hundred to become board certified. Her initial interest had been sparked by the case of a patient with hemophilia who had been admitted to the dental service for an extraction and had not revealed his condition to the oral surgeon. The patient subsequently suffered a great deal of bleeding and developed an inhibitor, or antibody to clotting factor, when he was treated for the bleeding. Hilgartner followed his case with her mentor, "one of the well known clotters," until the patient died. She recalled "vowing then and there that I would never have another patient go through the same horrendous bleeding and dying from this disease, if there were something that I could possibly do about it." After completing her internship, Hilgartner went to New York Hospital, where she received further training in coagulation research from Schulman and Rabiner. She followed them to Chicago to continue her laboratory training. After five years she returned to New York Hospital to organize the Pediatric Hemophilia Clinic there.[4]

While the climate of the early 1960s provided an opportunity for these young physicians to hone their research skills in the laboratories of the leading coagulation researchers of the day, it also set limits on the scope of academic medicine. At that time the scientific culture frowned upon certain trappings of success as not appropriate for academia. According to Kenneth Brinkhous, "if a faculty person discovered something and patented it, many colleagues looked upon him as greedy." As a result, products developed in the labs of medical schools were most often turned over to industry. Brinkhous's Chapel Hill group developed a relationship with Hyland Laboratories, in what Brinkhous calls "the Los Angeles–Chapel Hill Axis."[5] Founded by Dr. Clarence Hyland, who had been the Director of Laboratories at Children's Hospital in Los Angeles, the firm's initial business was provision of the albumin component of plasma in wartime.[6] Following the war, as researchers began to explore the other plasma components, Hyland Laboratories recognized an opportunity to increase profits by marketing plasma components that had been previously discarded. The marketplace became driven by the potential of marketing these by-products on a national and international basis.

In addition to conforming with academic norms, Brinkhous felt that involvement with industry could change the lives of people with hemophilia: "I knew that back in rural Iowa, where I came from, it didn't make a darned bit of difference what I did. If it was not somehow available through standard channels to a physician, it wasn't going to help those people. They were going to have to travel long distances to a specialized center. That was basically my thinking."[7] Thus Brinkhous viewed the commercialization of blood components as a means to a desirable end, a way of distributing blood products through "standard channels to physicians" to be used as a treatment controlled by physicians. By entrusting the plasma industry with the opportunity to fulfill this vision, he also expressed confidence in the private sector's ability to do an effective job.

Hyland was not the sole manufacturer of blood products. Other entrepreneurs, aware of potential national and international markets for plasma products, entered the "blood business." Cutter Laboratories, Inc., of Oakland, California, collaborated with Stanford University in attempts to fractionate Factor VIII from plasma, a relationship that would lead to a scientific milestone in 1965.

The Discovery of Cryoprecipitate

Charles Abildgaard, a medical resident at Stanford in the mid-1960s, remembered coagulation researcher Judith Graham Pool, Ph.D., and the project that led to the discovery of cryoprecipitate:

> They obtained frozen plasma in very large containers that they got from Japan. They would thaw that and send her [Pool] samples of the liquid parts to assay. She wasn't really finding very much Factor VIII activity, and then someone mentioned to her that when they thawed this large amount of plasma, there was always some mucky stuff at the bottom of it, and she said, "Well, send me some of that, too."
> She found that at least half of the Factor VIII activity was in the residue. What was happening was that, because of the large volume, as the mass thawed, it stayed cold. So this was cryoprecipitate.[8]

Pool immediately published her results and has subsequently been credited with this scientific breakthrough, the use of cryoprecipitate to treat bleeding episodes. Both Brinkhous and Ratnoff noted that scientists had recognized for several years that a cold precipitate of plasma contained a high concentration of clotting material (AHF, or Factor VIII).[9]

However, Pool's discovery "of this simple approach" that could be used for the treatment of hemophilia was a milestone.

Apparently others had also been close to achieving this result. Rickles recalled:

> I often tell one of those famous stories about missed opportunities in that Charlie Abildgaard and I discovered cryoprecipitate and I didn't know that we had!
>
> I made a mistake in an experiment, and instead of putting frozen plasma back in the freezer at the end of the day's experiment, I instead stuck it in the refrigerator. When I came in the next morning, there was all this junk in the bottom of the tube which I spun out, and I used the plasma for my experiment. My experiment didn't work because there was no Factor VIII in it. And I went back and fished the junk out of the trash and assayed the junk and got these outrageously high values for Factor VIII in the junk, and neither Charlie nor I believed it, and so it was one of those things. And sure enough, about a year later Judith Graham Pool discovered cryoprecipitate.[10]

In 1990 Ratnoff learned from a European colleague that a medical student in France, working on a project to earn his medical degree, had made a similar discovery before Pool did. The project "consisted of separating out a cold precipitable protein, which turned out to have the property of correcting hemophilia." Ratnoff noted that the student "not only did this [corrected hemophilia] in the test tube; he did it in patients," but his discovery was never published in the medical literature, because he was killed in an automobile accident.[11]

News of Pool's discovery was disseminated through National Hemophilia Foundation channels. Cited as a significant breakthrough by scientific journals, industry publications, and the media, word spread quickly that "the outlook for treatment improved almost overnight." Cryoprecipitate was adopted widely for routine treatment of hemophilia, marking an end to risky high-volume blood transfusions.[12] It could be easily produced in hospitals and blood banks from single units of blood, refrozen, and stored for up to a year. It was described as safe, inexpensive, and effective. Interestingly, a major contribution to the diffusion of this procedure was the development of technology for the production of plastic bags. According to Abildgaard:

> Without plastic bags, the single-donor production of cryoprecipitate at the blood bank level would have been impossible, but since they had the plastic

bags, they could separate the blood and keep it. They could separate the plasma, freeze it, and then thaw it in the refrigerator so that the cryoprecipitate developed. Then they would have these frozen bags of cryo. . . . This provided a very inexpensive sort of homemade treatment at the blood bank level.[13]

Local chapters of the NHF worked out arrangements to obtain cryoprecipitate (popularly known as "cryo") from blood banks. They solicited donors, who would come either directly to the blood banks or to mobile blood processing facilities. Chapters had already been mobilized around blood drives, but the incentive of access to cryo fostered increased activity. Some chapters worked with hospitals to have the processing of cryo accounted for as a by-product of processing of other blood products from whole blood, enabling the hospitals to provide the cryo to hemophiliacs "as essentially a free good."[14] In addition to single-donor cryo, large amounts of Factor VIII could be obtained by cryoprecipitation of multiple bags of fresh-frozen plasma and then pooled. For the first time, a patient's level of Factor VIII could be sufficiently elevated to cover major surgical interventions, dental extractions, and trauma treatment at a very low cost.[15]

These benefits described by physicians and the literature tell part of the story. Listening to the words of hemophilia informants recalling their experiences and recollections adds other dimensions. For "Adam H.," who was a college student in the mid 1960s, the discovery of cryo led to his involvement with the Metropolitan New York Chapter of NHF, because, as he put it, "I made a decision that my future was too important to leave in the hands of others . . . and it was a means of knowing what was going on and being able to be somewhat in control." He worked with the New York Blood Center to bring in donors in exchange for cryo. Although he spent his share of time "in playing political games and in student politics at school," working on "donor plans was a big part of being a person with hemophilia." But the sense of control was still limited. Recalling that "there was not much home care at that time," he remarked, "Who cares whether it's concentrate or cryo if you are going to the hospital emergency room" to receive it?[16]

"Adam" was one of the first young patients to represent his own needs at a time when parents still led the hemophilia community. Initially he worked at the local level, joining the parents who formed the local chapter. Early on he expressed his dissatisfaction with the limitations of hospital-based treatment, foreshadowing the quest for a mode of treatment independent of the hospital setting. Adam's ability to articulate concerns and his self-confidence in asserting himself with older adults may be seen as, in part, a reflection of his privileged socioeconomic status.

Before the use of cryo, most boys with hemophilia born in the 1950s, the next cohort younger than "Adam H.," had generally been treated with fresh-frozen plasma rather than whole blood. However, few were treated at home, and frequent trips to emergency rooms and long hospital stays were still the norm. As "Daniel H." (Glenn Pierce), an informant with severe hemophilia who grew up in a blue-collar neighborhood in northern Ohio, remembered:

I think that there have been three periods in my hemophilia life. The first period was from birth until I was about twelve years old when cryoprecipitate became available. Prior to that time I had been hospitalized approximately sixty-five times. I had missed tremendous amounts of school and in many ways I had been deprived of a normal childhood.

The second period was ushered in when cryoprecipitate came. I was able to go from being confined to a wheelchair with braces and casts that would remain on for months and months to being able to rehabilitate myself. With the help of treating bleeding episodes with cryo [I was able] to become a normal walking person who was able to function productively, miss less school, and reach a point where I could go to college and do well.[17]

"Daniel H." recalled that his main childhood socializing experiences had been in the hospital, where he met other boys with hemophilia, and at a hemophilia camp called "Camp Cheerful." He found he enjoyed "being around other people with hemophilia. . . . We felt a camaraderie." As he "became more mobile" as a result of treatment with cryo, his social activities began to include others who did not have hemophilia. But his experiences with cryo were not straightforward:

There were some problems with cryo, although I alluded to it as a miracle cure. There were a lot of unknowns at the time, and a physician who I happened to get during this time, a pediatric hematologist, [when I was] between eighth and tenth grades, decided that cryo was not a particularly good thing to use. He was concerned about inhibitor development, which of course, was absolutely untrue. . . . I didn't have the kind of access to cryo that I needed, so I wound up getting into trouble with bleeding.

He thought I should tough it out with ice, bandages, and elevation, unless it was really a severe bleed. Then [I'd] get into an argument with him about what was a severe bleed. . . . By the time I got to eleventh grade, he had actually committed suicide. Then I had another physician who was more liberal about cryo. So there was a big change in philosophy, and I became more aggressive about treating bleeding episodes with cryo.

I went on to a rehabilitation program myself in eleventh and twelfth grades, and somehow I managed to find the discipline to really exercise on a regular basis and took advantage of receiving even more cryo, knowing I wouldn't bleed. So I was able to build up my arms and legs and actually got rid of my last crutch in the twelfth grade. . . . I didn't really have a social life until the twelfth grade, and things started to pick up a little bit.[18]

Another informant with severe hemophilia born in the 1950s grew up in Pennsylvania. Describing his experience with the condition, "Lloyd H." said:

My first recollection of hemophilia is lying in a hospital when I was about two and a half [years old], receiving transfusions of whole blood, then lying there and receiving transfusions of plasma, then lying there and getting transfusions of cryoprecipitate. . . . I would have to go to the hospital either as an inpatient or as an outpatient and have someone else administer the blood.

. . . In those days . . . we had to get the approval of a physician to get a transfusion, and it had to be at "normal hours." So if you had a bleed at midnight, you had to wait until about six-thirty or seven o'clock to get the approval of a doctor, because they would not trust the patient to just come in and say he's bleeding and needs a transfusion. The doctor would never see me. He would just talk to my parents over the phone. So there was in those days a tremendous control by physicians over every aspect of a hemophiliac's treatment.[19]

"Lloyd" remembered that his parents helped form the Central Pennsylvania Chapter of the NHF and served as officers. For him this meant that his parents had to constantly call people up asking them to give blood, and then he had to write thank-you notes to those who responded. He recalled this happening both during the time when he received plasma and later when he received locally made cryo.[20]

These remembrances clarify why the discovery of cryo heralded "the beginning of the Golden Era" for researchers; but its impact on boys with hemophilia and their families represented more of a stepping-stone than a solution. In addition to socioeconomic differences, geographical location and individual treatment philosophies determined how the condition was managed. For most, it still meant trips to the hospital and dependence on medical judgment regarding each bleeding episode. Home therapy remained a rarity; insurance coverage was a widespread problem; and unevenness in quality of care continued to be the norm.

These inequities were not unique to the hemophilia population in the 1960s, as both Paul Starr and Charles Rosenberg describe the health care climate then. Starr notes that although the early 1960s are generally thought of as "a time of promise," when John F. Kennedy's "New Frontier" was followed by Lyndon Johnson's "Great Society," American medical care was, in fact, becoming a symbol of "the continuing inequities and irrationalities of American life." The power of the "medical school empires" had increased in metropolitan areas, but all too often literally adjacent to those "gleaming palaces of medical science" were neighborhoods that had been "medically abandoned." Rural areas also suffered from shortages of doctors and nurses. Quality of care was left in the hands of the increasingly powerful medical establishment, and hospitals became "the institutional center of our health care system."[21]

But according to Rosenberg

The American hospital became a problem. It has remained one. Depending on the critic's temperament, politics, or pocketbook, the hospital appeared a source of uncontrolled inflationary pressure, an instrument of class and sexual oppression, or an impersonal monolith, managing in several ways to dehumanize rich and poor alike.

To many detractors it seemed the stronghold of a profession jealous of its prerogatives and little concerned with needs that could not be measured, probed, or irradiated. Meanwhile, hospital costs mounted inexorably.[22]

On the ongoing problem of health insurance coverage, Starr presented disturbing data:

If a family's income were among the highest rather than the lowest third of the population, it was twice as likely to have some insurance (80 versus 40 percent). When the main earner was fully employed, the probability of having some insurance was 78 percent. When the main earner had only a temporary job, the probability was only 36 percent, if retired 43 percent, if a housewife, just 32 percent. When the main earner was employed in manufacturing, the chance of having insurance was 91 percent, when employed in construction 65 percent, and in agriculture, forestry, or fishing, only 41 percent. If the family lived in a metropolitan area, its chances of having insurance was 75 percent, if they lived in a farm area, 44 percent. Two thirds of those who lived in the Northeast, Midwest, or the West had some insurance. But only about half of those who lived in the South did.[23]

Health insurance loomed large then, as it still does today, as a central problem for people with hemophilia and their families. "Gregory H.," another person with severe hemophilia born in the 1950s, resided in a suburban area near New York City. He stated that:

In the United States there was always a battle between two things [quality of care and financial concerns]. In other words, the physicians were always nice and wanted to help you, and then the insurance people or the finance people at the hospital were always pounding on you. Of course, they didn't pound on me as a child; they pounded on my parents. . . . In the U.S. there was a crazy kind of patchwork quilt. A lot of the care that you got depended on the kind of noise that your parents could make. It was, and it still is, unfair.[24]

The families coping with the financial, emotional, and medical aspects of hemophilia were clearly not represented as players on the national level in the 1960s. Assertive parents striving to maximize the quality of life for their children while surviving financially were doing so on a case-by-case basis on the local hospital level. The local NHF chapters, increasingly supported by the NHF's professional central office staff, focused their efforts on developing linkages with the Red Cross, hospitals, and blood banks to help the families. By joining the National Health Council and the newly organized World Federation of Hemophilia (WFH), the NHF took initial steps in raising the agency's profile. However, it had not yet begun to find its political advocacy voice.

The NHF continued to disseminate information to its lay and professional constituency about developments in research and treatment, primarily through its quarterly bulletin. First held in 1953, the NHF annual meeting became an event that not only augmented the spread of information but also provided a setting for informal networking among parents and medical leaders and became the key point of reference for remembering new developments, emerging problems, and changes in leadership. These meetings also provided the forum for local chapter leaders and medical researchers to discuss important issues of the day. By the mid 1960s representatives from forty-one chapters in thirty-two states attended these meetings.[25] A quote from the president's report for 1964 captures the flavor and facts of hemophilia and the NHF at that time:

Looking back to 1962, the first annual meeting which I attended, I cannot help but compare that meeting with this. . . . Today in place of one room in the Statler Hotel in New York, we are occupying most of the Mayflower Hotel in Washington, D.C. Paralleling the growing interest of medical and research scientists in hemophilia is the public interest. . . . Important problems remain to be solved; foremost is the securing of funds necessary to carry out the objectives of the Foundation, namely to provide better care for the sufferers of hemophilia and support research to cure the disease.[26]

The report also noted that in 1965 research would be bolstered by "the NIH spending over 4 million dollars on blood coagulation research, with a good percent of this being spent in areas related to hemophilia and research efforts sponsored by the American Red Cross, Cutter, Hyland, and Merck."[27]

Using Cryoprecipitate to Produce a Coagulation Concentrate

Although the discovery of cryoprecipitate was heralded as a medical milestone, it was nonetheless time-consuming to administer and required special refrigeration. People with hemophilia still looked forward to a day when stable and easily stored coagulation concentrates could be manufactured.[28] That day seemed to come when, under the auspices of Hyland Laboratories, a biochemist named Murray Thelin combined Pool's discovery of cryoprecipitate with the methods for concentrating plasma developed by Brinkhous and his group at Chapel Hill. Thelin, himself a hemophiliac, had come to the University of North Carolina at Chapel Hill to study for a doctorate with Kenneth Brinkhous and biochemist Robert Wagner, who had worked together on developing a concentrate of AHF or Factor VIII. In their early efforts, Brinkhous and Wagner discovered that attempts to remove the plasma fluid also destroyed the delicate clotting protein. In 1957, Wagner suggested a new technique that allowed them to preserve the AHF during the plasma fractionation and that was shown to cause no harmful side-effects in tests. Using this method, the group began to produce a substance that could be concentrated. By 1962 they were able to use the concentrate "to get antihemophilic factor up in a patient to twice the normal levels, 200 percent"; before that time they had been able to achieve levels of only 40 or 50 percent of normal. They celebrated the event—and decided that industry should take the next steps. Noting that "all of the original work: the toxicity, the compatibility, the dosing, and the clinical testing on patients had been done at Chapel Hill," Brinkhous remarked, "that was handed to them [Hyland] on a platter."[29]

After completing his studies, Thelin was hired by Hyland, and he brought the Chapel Hill method with him. When Pool discovered cryoprecipitate, the next steps were clear to Thelin, who began to work with cryo, using the Wagner method to concentrate the product. Shortly after he began to test this substance, he had a brain hemorrhage and decided to risk using the new concentrate on himself. After the first transfusion, his Factor VIII levels "soared," and in ten days "he walked out of the hospital smiling." When Thelin experienced another life-threatening bleed, a peptic ulcer, he used the substance once again with success. Then he and the medical director of Hyland, Dr. Edward Shanbrom, decided to test whether the concentrate could be used to prevent prolonged bleeding. Shanbrom administered daily and then weekly injections to Thelin. "The results seemed miraculous: weeks passed without a bleed."[30] But since hemophiliacs can go through cycles of diminished bleeding, there was still no proof that it was the concentrate that was making the difference.

Shortly afterward an unexpected incident presented them with an opportunity to establish proof. Thelin was injured in an automobile accident, and he and Shanbrom agreed to withhold the concentrate to see what would happen. The bleeding resumed. This provided the evidence that Hyland used to release the product for testing. As Dr. Brinkhous observed, in those days, researchers did not have to go through the clinical trial phases required today; they "could forge on ahead." Confirming evidence came from hospitals in Chicago, Boston, and New York. For the first time surgeons were able to perform major surgery on hemophiliacs and find "the operation was nearly as simple as if the man had been normal."[31]

The impact of concentrates was particularly significant for orthopedics. When he was first introduced to the use of concentrates in 1965–66, Marvin Gilbert, who later became medical co-director of the Mount Sinai Hemophilia Treatment Center, was a resident in orthopedics at Mt. Sinai. He recalled the limits of orthopedics in the years before this breakthrough: "The orthopedist couldn't do very much. The patients bled into their joints, and the only way you could really stop it was to give them fresh-frozen plasma—and if you overloaded their circulation, they went into heart failure. . . . Dr. Henry Jordan [chief of Orthopedic Surgery at Lenox Hill Hospital] made a true art out of bracing joints to keep them from bleeding. However, he had patients that were walking around with stiff arms and legs."[32]

Gilbert had begun to take care of hemophilia patients who were under the care of Louis Wasserman, then chief of the "very strong" Department of Hematology at Mt. Sinai and an "internationally known" physician, according to Gilbert. (Wasserman was also on the NHF board and a member of the Medical and Scientific Advisory Council and had sponsored the placement of Martin Rosenthal, a hematologist in his department, as the first medical director of the NHF.) In order to learn more about the state of the art of orthopedics and hemophilia, Gilbert read widely and observed other orthopedists working with the hemophilia population. He started by reading Jordan's treatise, *Hemophilic Arthropathy* and then began to go to Lenox Hill Hospital on a weekly basis to work with Jordan. He also visited orthopedists on the West Coast of the United States and abroad. When an opportunity to study in England presented itself, he went for three months. There he discovered that total hip replacement, an exciting procedure developed in England in the mid-1960s, could change the lives of men with hemophilia whose hips had been severely damaged.[33] Another surgical breakthrough, knee replacement, followed shortly.

The new surgical techniques, coupled with the availability of concentrates, made it possible to transform the lives of young men who had been crippled by arthritis caused by bleeding that began at an early age. Grateful patients and their families pursued what had been only a dream a decade before, life without a wheelchair. The demand for orthopedic intervention multiplied. Access to technology and concentrates brought feelings of satisfaction and success. Recruitment to the specialty became easier. The Golden Age for orthopedists working with hemophilia had begun.

When Henry Jordan retired from Lenox Hill, Mt. Sinai became the place to go on the East Coast for both "joints and blood," and Marvin Gilbert became the specialist to see. What he learned during a trip to the West Coast in the mid-1960s would represent another major avenue to be pursued in the future. Gilbert went to observe physical rehabilitation methods that were being used with hemophilia patients as part of a funded demonstration project based at the Los Angeles Orthopaedic Hospital, under the direction of Shelby Dietrich, M.D.

The Multidisciplinary Team Approach:
The Template for Comprehensive Hemophilia Care

In Los Angeles Gilbert and his colleagues discovered not only the use of physical therapy, but also an innovative way of organizing and delivering hemophilia health care. What they were witnessing was the beginning of another significant part of the hemophilia success story, the comprehensive care model using a multidisciplinary team approach, which was originated by a pediatrician named Shelby Dietrich. Dietrich started treating hemophiliacs in the summer of 1957, when she became the director of a small outpatient clinic in Los Angeles. She discovered that the clinic had signed an agreement with the Southern California Hemophilia Foundation, founded in 1955, "to try to secure for the member hemophilia patients medical services and particularly plasma administration in a coordinated centralized setting." The agreement with the clinic was to provide care for the pediatric patients, "since there were so few adults that little thought was given to their care."[34]

Dietrich said that at that time what she knew about hemophilia "was from the film *Rasputin*—the original—and a little bit from medical school . . . people bled; that was the sum total of my knowledge." But her skills lay in "doing exquisite IVs on infants," and since "that was the only skill really needed, plus the general pediatric ability to render care," she became one of the two pediatricians hired. At the time there were approximately fifty patients with hemophilia being cared for by the clinic, and the treatment was reconstituted "freeze-dried whole plasma," which was supplied by the Red Cross but had been processed by the nearby Hyland Laboratories. For Dietrich, that original experience was "not a happy time." It was "marked by death, bleeding, terrible catastrophic problems, overwhelming blood loss, and occasionally screaming children." Sometimes the doctors used whole blood. She remembered that their maxim was "when in doubt of the diagnosis, give whole fresh blood."[35]

Dietrich also recalled that the financial problems were enormous. A year or two after she arrived, the Red Cross withdrew from its part of the arrangement and would no longer supply the dried plasma manufactured by Hyland. Since "there were no programs like MediCal and private insurance was rudimentary," the Foundation often had to pay the bills. It was her "first inkling of the financial problems that have been characteristic of the hemophilia terror ever since."[36]

An orthopedist on the staff of Los Angeles Orthopaedic Hospital who worked with the clinic suggested that they move their location, which they did in 1962. Dietrich recalled that "Orthopaedic Hospital had a wonderful Department of Physical Therapy which emphasized rehabilitation therapy," an approach she thought had great potential benefits. She had admitted her first patient for physical therapy in the late 1950s, at the suggestion of a physical therapist, and had also written a proposal concerning the applicability of vocational rehabilitation to hemophilia, which she submitted to the Division of Vocational Rehabilitation in Washington. Dietrich noted that the medical director of Orthopaedic Hospital happened to be a friend of the director of the division.[37]

The climate of the 1960s had fostered further expansion of federal funding, beyond research to other kinds of programs based in hospitals and communities. By providing "seed money" for such hospital-based projects, the federal government was bypassing the state and assuming a role formerly taken by philanthropic foundations. To Dietrich's "enormous shock and surprise," she received a telegram in the fall of 1963 stating that the Orthopaedic Hospital Hemophilia Treatment Center had been awarded "what was then a giant sum of money for the first grant for rehabilitation in hemophilia." She attributed the award to the influence of the director of Orthopaedic Hospital and his connection to the director of the Division of Vocational Rehabilitation. Feeling that her own efforts had little to do with it, having her name on the grant "was a shock that I will never forget."[38]

Having previously worked in special education in the Pasadena school system, Dietrich was aware of "the team concept." She also felt that "by nature and temperament doctors alone didn't accomplish what they wanted to do," and she perceived that hemophiliacs were "terribly crippled in social, economic, and personal" ways. In proposing a team approach to demonstrate the possibilities of known rehabilitation techniques applied to individuals with hemophilia, her project had the unique aspect of the simultaneous coordination and use of these techniques in one setting.[39]

One hypothesis of the proposal was that the team approach to rehabilitation would be more effective than the individual consultant approach because the medical and psychosocial aspects of the disease are so delicately interwoven that "successful management of the patient is not possible unless all the specialists involved meet and share planning ideas in person." Another hypothesis stated that "early and basic medical care would prevent crippling as well as morbidity and mortality."[40] Dietrich described the initial team as:

composed of two pediatricians, one internist, the orthopedist from the other hospital (we persuaded him to come); a physical therapist whom I stole away from the California Hospital (this was my first lesson in recruiting and pirating personnel away), . . . a social worker, . . . a vocational counselor, and a psychologist who was a personal friend of mine from Pasadena. The social worker was the father of a patient of mine. The dentist was a friend of somebody else's. . . . I look on those first six years as our "Camelot Days."[41]

Dietrich recalled that the demonstration project's "Camelot Days" contrasted vividly with the clinical experience of just a few years earlier. As project director, she made weekly team meetings mandatory; those who didn't attend could not remain on the staff. She said, "That was a huge step for me: the first time that I realized that directors really have power!"[42]

The *Los Angeles Times* ran a feature story in August 1965 showing Shelby Dietrich and a patient exercising. The boy's mother described her son's prospects for "a nearly normal life span" as a result of the treatment and exercise at Orthopaedic Hospital.[43] During that same year, however, difficult experiences contrasted with the successes. One of Dietrich's "cruelest and saddest memories" was when they had access to "a few hundred units of Hyland's first Factor VIII," which was used in an appendectomy for a boy with acute appendicitis. There was no postoperative bleeding, but the concentrate ran out, and two weeks later the boy began to bleed and died.[44]

By 1966 Hyland was ready to announce the commercial availability of concentrate. The *Los Angeles Times* featured an article with the headline: "Normal Lives Possible: New Shots Protect Hemophilia Victims."

A Los Angeles firm is about to market a blood extract that may do as much for people suffering from hemophilia as insulin does for diabetics—make it possible for them to live normal lives except for shots.

Dr. Shelby Dietrich, Director of the Hemophilia Rehabilitation Project at Orthopedic Hospital, said that the Hyland Laboratories . . . will soon make an anti-hemophilic blood concentrate available for the first time. . . . For those already crippled by hemophilia, the Hyland extract of blood plasma will make surgical corrections possible for the first time.[45]

The *Washington Post* picked up the article and ran a story on the first page headed: "Blood Shots Will Help Hemophiliacs." But Dietrich felt that "the real event that occurred was when concentrate was licensed" in the spring of 1968. In an article featured in the *Wall Street Journal,* she went on to say: "By that time the National Hemophilia Foundation had heard of us. . . . They organized a meeting in Los Angeles, and everyone on earth seems to have attended. We were not really being displayed, we were being grilled. . . . They couldn't help but understand that we were doing something, since we had a lot of patients, a lot of records, and, obviously, a well organized staff."[46]

Dietrich's group issued a report entitled *Hemophilia: A Total Approach to Treatment and Rehabilitation* in August 1968. Accomplishments listed included: "a marked decline in the number and duration of hospital admissions and stays. The number declined by 36 percent in 1967, and the hospital days were reduced by 40 percent." The introduction to the report states:

Historically, the critical concern of the physician treating hemophilia has been the preservation of life. With the advent of anti-hemophilic plasma, this consideration, while still important, particularly when bleeding occurs internally, is equaled or overshadowed by the problems inherent in survival; bleeding into the joints with resulting orthopedic and neuromuscular residuals, and/or emotional problems secondary to the life-long disease process of clinically unstable character. Therefore habilitation as well as rehabilitation now becomes important and is paramount in the complete management of the patients with the disease.

The report went on to emphasize that only because there had been advances in medical technology, "principally the large supplies of AHF plasma," was it feasible to utilize known rehabilitation techniques which had been developed in other severely disabling conditions. In addition, the costs of rehabilitative care would be less expensive in the long term than would welfare support for disabled young men with hemophilia.

The authors also expressed a belief in the importance of keeping patients out of the hospital because "hospitalization is not a normal way of living, especially for children and adolescents."[47]

While this treatment was transforming the lives of the boys with hemophilia and their families living in the Los Angeles vicinity, the publicity had created interest among families who could afford to travel to California for consultations. "Lloyd H.," who lived in Pennsylvania, spoke of his experience at Orthopaedic Hospital as part of gaining his "freedom." From the time he was six years old, his parents had taken him to Lenox Hill Hospital in New York City, because "they were concerned about getting me an orthopedist who knew things about hemophilia." As a result of the customary treatment offered, he had leg braces from the age of seven to eighteen. He recalled that there were hemophiliacs "from all over the country and all over the world" who came to see Dr. Jordan. When his parents learned of "a new method out in Los Angeles at Orthopaedic Hospital which used factor and exercise to strengthen the limbs so that my legs could do without braces," they wanted him to go there. "Lloyd" recalled that Dr. Jordan told his parents if they took him to California, he would never treat him again.[48]

"Lloyd" did go to Los Angeles for an evaluation while he was in high school and finally "ended up going out there for college and law school." He describes the treatment as "a total comprehensive system that was different than anything we knew about." He had never been treated by an orthopedist and a hematologist and seen a social worker " . . . and all in the same facility." He described the physical therapy as "having an attitude not to coddle the hemophiliacs but to make sure they had adequate factor to prevent bleeds and to exercise them very hard so that limbs became strong and would not be susceptible to bleeding." He added:

Going to L.A. was probably the biggest change in my life, because not only did my medical care improve, but they had a very strong attitude of teaching independence and self reliance which was very different from the attitudes that I had seen from my doctors before. . . . I was eighteen and it was a natural time for independence. . . . I can say those were the best years I've ever had, plus the fun of going to college and meeting people.[49]

"Lloyd's" parents' ability to financially support the travel, living expenses, and medical care was, of course, not the norm. Most teenagers with severe hemophilia were not so fortunate. Recognition of the need to provide access for hemophiliacs throughout the country to concentrates and comprehensive care came through the new medical leadership at the National Hemophilia Foundation. By 1968, Martin Rosenthal had been succeeded by new medical co-directors, Dr. Marvin Gilbert and "Dr. Marcus Victor" (an informant who requested the use of a code name). "Victor," a platelet physiologist who had become director of the Mt. Sinai Hemophilia Clinic after training at Strong Memorial Hospital in Rochester, New York, and at the National Institutes of Health, described himself as "captivated by the challenges of hemophilia, both in terms of health care delivery and of economics." His impressions of the model, gained during the NHF meeting held in L.A., dovetailed with Gilbert's admiration: "The visit to Orthopaedic Hospital made it clear to me that this multidisciplinary, lifelong approach to hemophilia was the way to go." Noting that "Shelby Dietrich had not really recognized the potential of her own way of doing business"[50] "Victor" saw the potential for national and worldwide proliferation of the comprehensive care model. In order to reach these goals, NHF and its constituency would have to use political avenues to acquire the necessary funding from both state governments and the federal government. The synergy between scientific and structural health care delivery innovations of the 1960s paved the way for the political activism that would characterize the 1970s.

CHAPTER 5

The Hemophilia Community Enters Politics

The Late 1960s and Early 1970s

Evolving Leadership in the Hemophilia Community

Parents continued to lead the hemophilia community on both the local and national levels from the late 1940s through the late 1960s, but the founding group of wealthy New Yorkers, led by Robert Lee Henry and Betty Jane Henry, began to lose their clout as the Foundation became more professionally organized and chapters proliferated throughout the country. The overriding concern of parents representing local chapters was obtaining an adequate supply of blood for their sons, while Henry insisted on retaining the primacy of research as a national focus. In 1956, the year when the Hemophilia Foundation officially changed its name to the National Hemophilia Foundation (NHF), as Henry continued to resist pressure from chapter leaders "to convert the Foundation into a professionally staffed operation raising substantial funds for program and services," he was ousted from the presidency. The annual meeting where the decision was made became known as "the Palace Revolution."[1]

To meet the demand for more services, the number of paid staff increased, and they became an accepted part of the growing community. The professional staff expanded the Foundation's focus to include the emotional, social, educational, and vocational aspects of living with hemophilia, organizing conferences and disseminating information on these issues. Pioneering work done in the 1960s by David Agle, M.D., a psychiatrist working with Oscar Ratnoff in Cleveland, described both the psychological features of the bleeding disorder and patient and family adaptation to this chronic disease, For example, Agle described a "counter-phobic" behavior in some hemophilic boys, whereby they would indulge in dangerous behaviors in an attempt to ward off their fear of injury. These studies led to counseling approaches that included family systems therapy. Agle joined the slowly growing cadre of medical specialists who were becoming part of the hemophilia community. Under the aegis of the NHF, they formed the nucleus of what was known as "the Hemophilia Flying Circus," sharing their growing expertise with physicians and parents throughout the country through a "road show" that traveled to NHF chapters to discuss new findings and give advice.[2]

From its earliest days the NHF did not attempt to become involved with organizations that dealt with other chronic illnesses, reflecting the sense of "specialness" that families dealing with hemophilia describe. The Foundation did, however, maintain a relationship with the American Red Cross, which has persisted over time. When the officials of both organizations met to discuss their current and future relationship in 1967, NHF chapters expressed the hope that the Red Cross would be able to supply cryoprecipitate. The Red Cross agreed to fill this need and also to initiate programs to collect plasma through the process known as plasmapheresis, in which, unlike a standard whole blood donation, the plasma is separated from the drawn blood as it is collected and the remaining blood components are immediately reinfused into the donor. Although certain matters regarding credit exchange for blood remained unresolved, NHF members who attended the meeting found it "impressive" that the Red Cross had kept up-to-date with the changes in therapy in the field of hemophilia.[3]

By 1968, new tensions in the organization began to appear. The NHF's structure at that time consisted of a board of trustees, officers, and nine regional chapter directors. Each chapter president was considered a trustee, and additional trustees were nominated and elected at the annual meeting. (This structure was to prove problematic; see the comments of G. William Bissell in Chapter 7.) Following the recommendation of the nominating committee, the trustees then elected the officers: a president, four vice presidents, a board chairman, three vice chairmen, a secretary, and a treasurer. These officers, in concert with the nine regional representatives and the chairman of the Medical and Scientific Advisory Council (MASAC), made up the Executive Committee.[4]

Money in particular became an issue. At that time, NHF spent about 15 percent of its budget on meetings and travel, which was twice as much as most voluntary health agencies.[5] Meanwhile, in a change of policy from the early days, local chapters were now expected to contribute 25 percent of their income to the national organization. Added to the rising cost to families for blood products following the development of concentrates, this was placing a strain on chapters, and they turned to NHF for relief. When the response was that chapters should solicit door-to-door for contributions rather than looking to the national leadership to find ways to lower the cost of blood products and raise money, the chapter leadership became increasingly frustrated, and charged the executive director with incompetence. The professional staff was also proving to be inadequate, and the ranks of local parent leaders had not produced anyone with either the ability or interest to take on the task.

There was also a change in the medical leadership of NHF in 1968 with the appointment of Dr. Marvin Gilbert and "Dr. Marcus Victor," as medical co-directors, succeeding Dr. Martin Rosenthal. Gilbert and "Victor" were also co-directors of the Mt. Sinai Hemophilia Clinic. "Victor" offered an especially broad perspective on hemophilia treatment; after attending a meeting of the World Federation of Hemophilia, he reflected that "some of the issues that I thought were national were international, as well. Within a very short time I was recognized as someone who could look with some perspective as to what the hemophilia issues were around the world."[6]

On July 29, 1969, Gilbert and "Victor" were among the featured players at "The Greystone Conference," the first annual conference of NHF chapter leadership. The chapters' charge to them was summarized in a lengthy poem, offered by Dr. Herbert Russalem, a participating behavioral scientist. Among the poem's messages was a call for increasing both the blood supply and research while "tak[ing] steps to keep costs reasonably low." In the context of rising costs and a shortage of concentrates there was a willingness to look toward the new young team of medical co-directors for leadership, but a hesitancy to place total confidence in them is revealed more than once in the poem. In it Russalem says the chapters must "find ways and means of coping with / The vagaries of medical prima donnas" and notes in the final lines, "Please do not mind us . . . when from time to time we take your pulse." The poem also raised questions on the relationship between the national organization and the local chapters (the "roots") and asked whether centers were needed in cities, cautioning that care should be taken "that community interest doesn't flag an itty-bitty."[7]

Clearly, the parents wanted Gilbert and "Victor" to solve existing problems, but they also wanted to assert their control of the Foundation. Ironically, the poem's concern about whether centers were needed in cities and how they might affect community interest was predictive of what was to come. As "Victor's" vision of comprehensive care centers, based on the model at Orthopaedic Hospital in Los Angeles, to be developed in major cities across the country (and abroad), was implemented, it did result in centers becoming far more powerful than chapters and in diminished interest in chapter activities.

At this conference, references to "the Hemophilia Community" were heard for the first time. In the United States the 1960s were a period of community organization, community activism, and the creation of community health centers. Perhaps the frequent use of the term during the meeting signaled another shift in direction of leadership, the readiness of the conference participants, who had identified themselves as members of a community of empathy, as parents of "sufferers" and "victims," to begin to view themselves as a politicized community. They began to organize to improve hemophilia health care for their entire national community, no longer confining their efforts to their particular local situation.[8]

Mary Gooley had become the executive director of the Rochester, New York, chapter and chaired the national Service Program Review. For her the Greystone meeting was a "landmark retreat," where medical and lay leadership of the Foundation and chapters "took stock of where we were and looked forward to the future of the Foundation."[9] An explicit indicator of the move toward organized political activity was the creation of a Legislation Committee, chaired by Dr. Margaret Hilgartner. She reported that her committee had a difficult time deciding what the Foundation should do regarding legislation. Many issues were raised but not resolved, including whether to join other groups such as "kidney, arthritis, and stroke" organizations; whether hemophiliacs should be declared "medically indigent and qualify under Medicaid"; and whether to advocate "an insurance-type program, with the government picking up the additional cost after a reasonable fee paid by the family for protection." (The committee stated that government expenditures were "fairly rigid but there might be some loosening up in the future.") The full conference summary report listed the priorities that emerged. Among the top ten were: a drive to improve the supply of blood, which ranked the highest; informing local doctors about improved treatment; and working toward a national health insurance program.[10]

Only four years later, the hemophilia community would reorder its priorities and unite in a concerted effort to seek federal funding from Congress for a national network of hemophilia treatment centers (HTCs). Primarily based in academic medical centers, the HTCs were to offer multidisciplinary comprehensive care and be directed, for the most part, by "hemophilia treaters." Both the climate established by the new Nixon administration and the leadership of the new NHF medical co-directors contributed to this shift in priorities.

The Nixon Administration's Influence on Health Care

During the same month as the Greystone meeting, July 1969, President Richard M. Nixon told a press conference: "We face a massive crisis. Unless action is taken within two or three years . . . we will have a massive breakdown in our medical system." The rhetoric of crisis adopted by the Nixon administration was familiar, as were many of its terms: "skyrocketing costs," over-specialization, and the need for redistribution of health manpower to underserved communities. Liberals wanting to extend reforms beyond Medicare were encouraged by the administration's expressed concerns. Advocates of the health team approach hoped that greater involvement of nurse practitioners, physicians' assistants, and other "physician extenders" would improve access and efficiency.[11]

In fact, the Johnson administration had enacted legislation that indirectly fostered the promotion of the health team approach, the Nurse Training Act of 1964. This law provided broad federal support for nursing care and aimed to increase both the number of nurses and the capability of nurses to provide quality care. It allowed schools of nursing to expand facilities, raise educational standards, and reorganize curricula to include new philosophies in nursing education, including the provision of expanding career ladders. The Health Manpower Act of 1968, Title II, broadened the scope of the program. In 1965, a demonstration project at the University of Colorado prepared professional nurses to give comprehensive well-child care in ambulatory care settings. These nurses were called "nurse practitioners," the first use of the term, and the project provided a training model for future programs in traditional collegiate settings.[12] Increasingly, the nurse practitioner training curricula came to focus on psychosocial aspects of care, health education, and counseling. By the 1970s nurses trained in these programs would find hemophilia treatment center directors eager to employ them as "clinical nurse coordinators"—when they could find the funding to pay them.

The Nixon administration explored other areas that might lead to cost containment. In a message on health care delivered to Congress on February 15, 1971, President Nixon stated:

The whole society has a stake in the health of the individual. Ultimately everyone shares in the cost of his illnesses or accidents. . . . Through tax payments, through insurance premiums, the careful subsidize the careless, the non-smokers subsidize those who smoke, the physically fit subsidize the rundown and the overweight, the knowledgeable subsidize the ignorant and the vulnerable. . . . Yet we have given remarkably little attention to the health education of our people. . . . There is no national instrument, no central force to stimulate and coordinate a comprehensive health education program.[13]

The president established a Committee on Health Education, charged with describing "the state of the art of health education in the United States by means of broad sweeping inquiries." The committee, composed of leaders representing health insurance companies, industry, unions, the media, advertising, and national health organizations, recommended the creation of a National Center for Health Education, which would "stimulate, coordinate, and evaluate health programs" and which would be financed by a combination of federal government and private sources. The group also recommended that "a focal point be established within the Department of Health Education and Welfare to work with all federal agencies to make the federal government's involvement in health education more effective and more efficient." In the letter of transmittal, the committee chairman stated: "we are convinced that . . . any change or improvements in the delivery and financing of health care will be virtually nullified unless there is, at the same time, an improvement in health education—which means not just supplying information about health to people but motivating them to accept the information and put it to work in their daily lives."[14]

A portion of the report addressed chronic illness, emphasizing that there should be "active participation of the people who will be the ultimate users of the health facilities" and that what is essential is education in "how to manage certain diseases that require special regimens including [learning] the frequency with which medications should be taken and [adhering to] rules about diet and exercise."[15] The increasing use of self-infused blood concentrates, which reduced the need for—and expense of—treatment by health professionals, highlighted the importance of having health education as an integral component of cost containment in the delivery of health care to persons with hemophilia. The choice of health education as a potential cost-cutting strategy exemplified the Nixon administration's philosophy of encouraging individual Americans to take responsibility for their own health. Cooperation between the private sector and government in general—and funding of the National Center for Health Education in particular—reflected the renewed emphasis on private sector responsibility. Awareness of this Administration's philosophy would influence the politically astute medical leaders of the hemophilia community as they planned for the future. Adaptation to the current climate, becoming aware of what would sell and what would work, became the hallmark of NHF's successful forays into politics.

NHLI Pilot Study of Hemophilia Treatment

Another concern of the Nixon administration, which directly involved the hemophilia community, was the marked expansion in use of human blood and blood products. The National Blood Resource Program (NBRP), a branch of the National Heart and Lung Institute (NHLI), contracted with the consulting firm Booz, Allen, and Hamilton to conduct three studies that would provide "comprehensive information and base-line data concerning the nation's blood resource." The resulting report, published in 1972, consisted of three volumes: the first concerns the supply and use of the nation's blood resource; the second focuses on the regulation of the blood resource; and the third was titled *A Pilot Study of Hemophilia Treatment in the United States*. The general preface to the report states: "Increasing demands for this resource [human blood and blood products] have led to the establishment of a vast complex of organizations that collect, process, and distribute blood and its products. However, comprehensive information about the nation's growing blood resource has not been available, and little had been known about what demand populations afflicted with several major types of blood disorders, such as hemophilia, might ultimately place on the blood resource."[16]

The *Pilot Study*, which was supposed to furnish Congress with information regarding this potential demand by hemophiliacs for blood products, focused on five principal areas of concern: the number of patients under treatment, the characteristics of physicians treating the patients, trends in organizing treatment, the use of blood and blood products in treatment, and "supplementary data" regarding patient experience (including "education, vocation, employment, financial experience, and experience in seeking and obtaining treatment"). In fact, this study was the first systematic attempt to determine the prevalence of hemophilia in the United States. Prior to the 1970s, a figure of 100,000 had been generally accepted as an estimate of the size of the nation's hemophilia population. The *Pilot Study* reported on responses to a nationwide mail survey of a sample of 5,486 physicians who were considered likely to treat the bleeding disorder itself (rather than its orthopedic or dental effects). Based on very high rates of response (from 64 to 90 percent in the different groups surveyed), the study estimated that 25,499 persons met the stated criteria of having either moderate or severe hemophilia A or B (Factor VIII or Factor IX deficiency), for a prevalence rate of 25.78 per 100,000 males. (There were 20,297 Factor VIII hemophiliacs and 5,202 Factor IX hemophiliacs.) The median age for this projected population was 11.5 years, in marked contrast with the median age of 26.8 for the entire U.S. male population at that time. Nearly 90 percent of the hemophiliacs were under the age of 25. The geographic distribution of the hemophiliacs tended to resemble the distribution of all U.S. males, except for a higher concentration in the Middle Atlantic regions, with 26 percent of the hemophilia population and 18 percent of the U.S. male population. The Pacific, New England, and West North Central regions also had a slightly higher proportion of hemophiliacs. Interestingly, the concentration of patients was discovered to relate directly to the concentration of hemophilia treaters.[17]

Among the supplementary data on the experience of patients and their families were the effects of hemophilia on work and school. Researchers surmised that many parents may have sought jobs that provided group insurance which would cover the cost of care, and many had to seek extra employment to meet the demands of the disease. More than one-third of the employed mothers cited their son's illness as the reason for working, and more than one-fifth of the fathers worked a second job to meet expenses. Some families who could not obtain good coverage reported spending as much as $65,000 a year and "quite obviously had to make extreme financial sacrifices in order to reduce or eliminate their debts for hemophilia treatment." For persons with hemophilia, both schooling and work were affected by the disease. Among adults, 44 percent were unemployed. Among severe hemophiliacs, 50 percent of those 16 years and older stated that their health prevented them from being employed; 23 percent of the severely affected children were unable to attend school.[18] These data would serve as a benchmark in future quests for funding by politically astute leaders of the hemophilia community.

An unexpected finding among the characteristics of physicians treating hemophilic patients was that hematologists were still in the minority among the estimated total number of 10,780 "treaters." The researchers had thought that hematologists, informally known as "clotters," would play the major role; instead the majority of the physicians were either internists or pediatricians. (In fact, only 6.8 percent of the physicians reported being "clotters"; at the opposite end of specialization, 8.6 percent reported being general practitioners.) This finding led the researchers to suggest that because hematology had only recently been listed as a subspecialty by the AMA, some specialists may have gone unreported. But perhaps more to the point was the fact that almost 60 percent of the total respondents had treated only one hemophiliac in 1970–71, while seven physicians reported treating 100 or more hemophilia patients. Specialized programs run by such physicians were primarily in major hospitals, and 42 percent of the hemophilia patients were cared for by "major treaters" in these programs.[19]

The study design reflected the researchers' assumptions that all decision making about treatments and blood product usage would rest with the treaters. Therefore, questions about preferences of blood products, reasons for determining their selection, and problems and concerns regarding blood products were administered only to the physician respondents. The study's selection of treaters as the primary respondents, with patients providing only "supplemental data," reflected the reality of who would make the decisions about purchasing blood and under what circumstances it would be administered. Over 60 percent of the physicians indicated that they preferred "physician administration" of the blood components—hematologists were a notable exception, preferring family- or self-infusion. Treaters reported that 90 percent of "episodic infusions" (that is, treatments for bleeding episodes) were administered in an institutional setting, usually a hospital, "by a physician or a trained clinician," as was required by statute in most states. In collecting data from the patients, the researchers noted that patients identified "nurses and other clinicians," rather than physicians, as the primary persons infusing them in the clinical setting.[20]

The Nixon administration's approach to assessing needs for the hemophilia community assumed that physicians would be the appropriate source of information. For populations affected by chronic illnesses such as diabetes and hemophilia, as technology developed and became more highly sophisticated, physicians who claimed ownership of the know-how and defined the market for the products selected became increasingly powerful.[21] At this same time, during the 1970s, the general public was beginning to question the judgment of physicians and to emerge as vocal consumers of health care. But in chronic illness families, where the patients were children and the prospect for life-long care depended upon the relationship with the treater, parents were rarely assertive. Although by this time, well into the Golden Era, treaters were actually able to improve the lives of their patients, the new

developments remained very much within the framework of the traditional model of medical authority.

At the time that the *Pilot Study* was conducted, 36 percent of the Factor VIII patients were receiving cryoprecipitate and 22 percent were using concentrates. (The remainder were treated with whole blood or
plasma—or received no treatment.) Only 6–7 percent of these Factor
VIII patients, all of them young adults, were either family- or self-
infused; 97 percent of the children under ten years of age were reported
as "physician infused."[22]

When physicians expressed their choice of treatment preferences,
they cited convenience, ease of administration, predictability of response, and price as the chief criteria. In response to another query, they
chose high cost as the biggest problem: "consideration for the cost of
blood products was determined to be the major problem which pre-
vented [physicians] from prescribing what they considered ideal treatment for their patients." At that time the possibility of blood-borne
hepatitis infection was not listed as a top-priority problem.[23] These responses from hemophilia treaters are very relevant as harbingers of the
future. Using cost as a key determinant in making decisions about patient treatment has played, and continues to play, a significant role in establishing policies, at both treatment center and NHF levels.

The *Pilot Report* noted that the threat of post-transfusion hepatitis
had made the national blood resource a major issue, and more than forty
bills that sought to regulate some aspect of the blood resource had been
introduced by the Ninety-Second Congress.[24] Yet, as just noted, the
possibility of contracting hepatitis was not among the most pressing
problems listed by the hemophilia treaters responding to this survey.
Resignation to the possibility of contracting hepatitis as "a necessary
evil," albeit rarely life-threatening, seems to have become part of the
mindset shared by both the provider and the consumer. The dramatic
changes in lifestyle and life span offered by the use of pooled plasma
concentrates made the risk of hepatitis seem a small price to pay in the
minds of most of the physicians and patients who had experienced the
"bad old days."

One physician who took exception to this stance from the beginning
was Oscar Ratnoff, who saw the risk of the spread of hepatitis through
pooling blood products as a serious problem and as an indicator of other

potential threats to the hemophilia population. He refused to put his patients on pooled plasma concentrates, keeping them on cryoprecipitate from the time that it became available, even though patients "had a passion to go on home therapy." Before his work with the hemophilia population, Ratnoff had done fibrinolysis (dissolving of clots) research and worked on a hepatitis project for four years at Johns Hopkins. Having also become "very familiar with the hepatitis literature," he was very much aware of the risk of pooling plasma and rejected use of the freeze-dried fractions needed for home therapy because "they came from lots as large as ten to twenty thousand plasmas." He mentioned that even in his own setting he was the exception; the pediatricians at his hospital treated children with lyophilized (freeze-dried) plasma products. He was well aware of the unpopularity of his stance, with both other physicians and patients, but he stuck by his beliefs. He describes himself as "a Cassandra," able to predict the future, but dismissed by all.[25]

Ratnoff made a point of the very broad training he had received, "which you can't get any more because of the pressures of life, partly economic and partly the desire to put people in pigeonholes." He also said that he had been fortunate with his teachers. Trained in neurophysiology, immunology, and respiratory physiology, Ratnoff is an experimental pathologist. In his lab, where he and his students are involved in coagulation research, he creates a climate "where [one] doesn't buy everything that [one] reads," and he speaks of his fellows as having "mind-sets with the willingness to do experiments." He feels that perhaps this atmosphere fostered the next major scientific development in the coagulation field, after the development of Factor VIII and cryoprecipitate. In 1970 Theodore Zimmerman, a research fellow in his lab who was trying to make an antibody to Factor VIII, discovered that Factor VIII had two components, the actual clotting protein itself and an associated protein. In "a landmark article" Zimmerman showed this associated protein was the substance deficient in persons with von Willebrand's disease, a closely related coagulation disorder that affects both males and females and that involves platelet formation.[26]

In discussing the projected needs and costs of future care for persons with hemophilia, the *Pilot Study* researchers specifically noted that they were not including von Willebrand's disease patients in the study sample—perhaps in response to the rapid dissemination of Zimmerman's research results. In addition, since the primary source of information projecting the future needs of hemophilia patients was physicians, persons whose hemophilia was mild enough that it was not being treated and members of groups who did not receive medical treatment for a variety of other reasons were also not considered in the totals to be used in planning for future hemophilia health needs. Even so, the projected needs and costs were considerable. Noting that "the 25,000 hemophiliacs and their families, along with third-party payers, blood banks, and hospitals, bore the expenditures at the present time," the *Pilot Study* estimated that from a minimum of $31 million to as much as $80 million in annual expenditures would be needed in the future for episodic care. If prophylactic (preventive) care were to be given, the estimate went up to from $58 million to $300 million. It further stated that the blood resources at that time had the capacity to provide an estimated 3 million whole blood units for episodic care; but if all severe hemophiliacs were to go on prophylactic care, 13 million units of whole blood would be needed, which would require over 76 percent of the plasma drawn in the United States to be fractionated to produce Factor VIII and Factor IX therapeutic agents. (It should be noted that although there were a few efforts made in administering clotting products prophylactically, most treaters at that time did not consider it.) The report noted that "at present, not all the plasma available is processed to provide blood coagulation factor concentrates, and major difficulties may exist in the delivery of these fractions to the patient."[27]

The Growth of Home Therapy
and Advocacy on the Local Level

During the years that the NHLI was conducting the *Pilot Study*, 1970–72, home therapy programs were slowly developing. The initial programs developed in Boston, Chicago, Fort Worth, New York City, Los Angeles, and Rochester, New York. Concurrently, the change of leadership at the NHF continued with the ouster of the president and the appointment of a new executive director, Kathryn Earnshaw, who had years of experience as executive director of the Cystic Fibrosis

Foundation. She and Drs. Gilbert and "Victor" worked effectively together as a team, encouraging local chapters to collaborate with hemophilia treatment centers in an activist role, initially to acquire state funding and then to join at the national level in an all-out advocacy effort for federal funding.[28]

Local efforts were guided by "how-to" packets, produced by NHF and designed to guide advocacy for state legislation and to provide coordination among chapters. The medical co-directors also "made numerous forays into chapters, answering questions, soothing feelings, providing help, carrying out training sessions, organizing medical advisory bodies, tasks extending far beyond the normal role of medical co-directors." "Victor" was described as having "an unusual combination of technical knowledge, political savvy, and energy," while Gilbert was considered "a perfect supplement to 'Victor,' . . . with qualities of geniality, broad experience, and persistence."[29]

The NHF chapters in New Jersey, Pennsylvania, and Ohio and the California Hemophilia Foundation chapters in that state were in the forefront of these efforts, and achieved notable successes. The New Jersey legislature passed a bill in 1971 authorizing the appropriation of $250,000 for a state hemophilia program. Pennsylvania followed in 1972, providing $2,000,000 for hemophilia care. In California, children with hemophilia had been covered by a state agency, Crippled Children Services (CSS), since the 1960s. In the 1970s, treatment centers and chapters undertook concerted advocacy efforts, arguing that dependence on the welfare system in order to meet the cost of expensive health care had become a common phenomenon among adolescents and young adults with hemophilia. Their efforts culminated in breaking the cycle of dependency by achieving the passage of the Genetically Handicapped Persons Program (SB 2265) in 1974.[30] Coverage would now be provided for employable adults who could become both consumers and taxpayers.

Similar "grassroots-level" advocacy for help with chronic conditions occurred for persons with diabetes, although here tensions led to a split into two separate organizations. The American Diabetes Association (ADA), originally created by physicians, had by 1970 become a voluntary organization incorporating "lay citizens." But an activist Pennsylvania parent, dissatisfied with the ADA's level of activism in seeking funding for research, started a new organization, the Juvenile Diabetes

Foundation, in 1970. The ADA has considered the newer organization "the competition" ever since.[31]

Nonetheless, both diabetes-focused organizations shared an appreciation of many of the same issues confronting the hemophilia community. One example in the early 1970s, a time when rights of the handicapped became a national issue, was whether or not to be considered under the rubric of "the handicapped," a philosophical dilemma for these populations in seeking coverage and funding.[32] Another similarity was an appreciation of the team model in health care, with the nurse playing a major role in educating patients for self-management of a chronic illness. Popular perception of the similarities between the two chronic conditions was reinforced by the press who would refer to "blood shots" used in hemophilia as analogous to insulin injections self-administered by diabetics. Although the voluntary agencies representing the two chronic conditions did not collaborate, they used some similar political strategies to achieve success in obtaining funding during this era, among them encouraging volunteers to become activists, maximizing the use of personal associations with legislators, and producing dramatic personal descriptions of the devastation wrought by lack of state-of-the-art therapy.

However, hemophilia treatment center directors were concerned about public perception of the similarity. Peter Levine, M.D., a treatment center director in Massachusetts, argued that there were vast differences between the two affected populations and in the costs involved. After an appeal to insurers for coverage for hemophilia patients involved in home therapy, he commented :

Almost without fail the initial response from all of them was negative. "We don't want to hear about this. If we do it for you, we'll have to pay for the home care of everyone with diabetes." And diabetes was thrown up by everyone. It was the huge roadblock. I mean, the differential cost between insulin and clotting Factor is probably 10,000 to 1. Nevertheless there are a lot of diabetics in the world, and people said, "We don't want to start paying for treatment at home. We only pay for what's done in the hospital."[33]

Ultimately, Levine managed to change their minds and to convince, in succession, the Blue Cross–Blue Shields of Massachusetts, New Hampshire, Vermont, Maine, and Connecticut "to make a special exception for hemophilia because of its unusual nature and cost." Levine's success in persuading insurers that "that this gamble was worth taking" was based on insights and observations he had made in developing his center's treatment plan. He had convinced his department chief to provide a half-time nurse and a half-time social worker skilled in reimbursement, by asserting that after two years he could pay for them, either by acquiring grants or by using the moneys generated by the center. He maintained that financially "it makes much more sense to educate the patients, provide them with therapeutic material at home and keep them out of the emergency rooms." By enlisting his nurse and social worker as data collectors, he was able to gather patient data on hospitalization, employment, and school attendance, which he used to document the cost-efficacy of using a comprehensive approach to hemophilia care, incorporating education for home therapy and self-infusion. He approached Blue Cross–Blue Shield with a comparison of current costs incurred by treating hemophilia patients in the hospital and the costs in his plan, using a system of health delivery that could measure both health outcomes and cost efficiency. His research was also published in the *New England Journal of Medicine* in 1973.[34]

The timing was perfect. By 1973, "Dr. Victor" had expanded NHF advocacy activities onto the national scene. With the support of the hemophilia community, he was pursuing his vision of creating a national network of hemophilia treatment centers offering comprehensive care. Levine's publication would prove to be a very effective piece of the NHF advocacy strategy. Seeking funding from Congress to support staffing the centers seemed less risky than looking for money to cover the use of blood products, and program evaluations were respected in the cost-cutting climate of the Nixon administration. Ironically, Levine "didn't know at the time that cost efficacy was going to turn out to become a major area. . . . It seemed from a scientific ground an intelligent thing to do."[35]

Once he realized the significance of cost efficacy, Levine convinced Blue Cross–Blue Shield to disseminate his findings via newsletters throughout the health insurance industry across the country—which provided "a springboard into the national limelight" for Levine and his program.[36] He joined "Victor," Gilbert, and Hilgartner as a leader of the hemophilia community and as a major player in the national politics of health care. Between 1973 and 1975, the hemophilia community's increasingly powerful medical leadership orchestrated a scenario that would result in the enactment of legislation leading to "one of the chronic-illness success stories of the decade."[37]

CHAPTER 6

Politics and the Blood Business in the Golden Era

When Marvin Gilbert and "Marcus Victor" became medical co-directors of the National Hemophilia Foundation, the organization faced bankruptcy. Fortunately they were saved in 1970 by the financial acumen and resources of the new chairman of the board, Lou Friedland, the father of a hemophiliac, who provided both personal funding and the financial know-how necessary to enable the Foundation to survive. Friedland, who was chairman of MCA-TV, declared, "The collapse of NHF was unthinkable, not only for the consequences of its chapters, but for the thousands of hemophiliacs who would lose the only national advocate for the money and treatment needed to bring better care within reach." In order to rectify matters, Friedland donated $94,000 worth of MCA stock and about $11,000 of other stock as collateral for a note, on the condition that the donated amount be used for research in the future. He also worked out a plan for additional participation assessments from the NHF chapters which would increase the national cash flow considerably.[1] This solution to the NHF's acute financial problems (if not its longer-term ones) allowed the organization to concentrate its energies on understanding the expanding "blood business" and on seeking state and federal funding for research and treatment.

Between 1971 and 1973 hemophiliacs, in large part because of their intimate connection to what was popularly called "the blood business," became more aware of the potential for entrepreneurial involvement. Plasma manufacturing companies "were hungry for sources of . . . antibody to hepatitis and other blood-borne diseases" for use in research, and many of those with hemophilia had been exposed to these diseases through the use of blood products, thus developing the desired antibodies. The process of plasmapheresis made it possible for persons with hemophilia to give plasma regularly. This plasma could then be sold for considerable money, either directly to blood banks or to "plasma brokers," who would handle the details of collection and the organization of payment.[2]

The desire for self-infusion and home therapy had also increased the demand for lyophilized, or freeze-dried, concentrates, which were produced only by commercial manufacturers. This aspect of the rapidly growing blood business also contributed to the changing roles and relationships between the manufacturers and the members of the community. As Nathan Smith, a member of the generation of older hemophiliacs, recalled, "In an earlier era when therapy was obtained by recruiting blood donors and receiving plasma from their donations, the relationship between hemophiliacs and their donors tended to be humanitarian. . . . Now those links of altruism were threatened. . . . Now they received products donated by faceless plasma sources of unknown quality, mediated by profit motivations and large corporations. . . . Now who knew or could tell about any of the processing that results in the concentrates now available?" He remembered the early 1970s as a time when hemophiliacs discussed the losses and the gains from the changing situation. There was a loss of "the gift relationship," which had been especially strong in small towns and rural areas. Concerns about "exploitation and profiteering" were balanced against an understanding that only industry had the equipment and personnel to produce concentrate on a sufficient scale for everyone with hemophilia to benefit.[3]

The Vision of Comprehensive Treatment Centers

The need for leadership both able and willing to tackle the economic and political problems in this increasingly complex situation helped pave the way for "Dr. Marcus Victor's" vision, stemming from his observations of the Los Angeles Orthopaedic Hospital Model Program, of creating a national network of hemophilia treatment centers, based primarily in academic medical centers and including the component of home therapy using concentrates. As part of this effort, "Victor" said that he sought both to make high-quality products available at the lowest prices and to be sure that no company would have a monopoly.[4] From the beginning, then, he "made sure to balance one manufacturer against another,"[5] and this practice set a precedent that was followed from then on, at both the treatment center level and the national NHF level. "Victor's" widely reputed negotiating skills did enable him to acquire products at the lowest prices within his treatment center and to receive an increasing supply of products from all of the manufacturers.[6] Although the NHF did not buy products directly, the Foundation's influence was increasingly powerful. "Victor's" leadership in both the political and the economic arenas created opportunities for the hemophilia community to succeed on both fronts and was generally well received.

As part of his efforts to advance comprehensive treatment and home therapy, "Victor" highlighted the accomplishments of the New England program under the leadership of Dr. Peter Levine and of the Rochester (New York) Hemophilia Treatment Center. In fact, "Victor" had trained at Rochester's Strong Memorial Hospital and was familiar with the treatment center's early forays into home therapy and its efforts to gain insurance coverage for persons with hemophilia in New York State. In 1971, Mary Gooley, by then director of the Rochester Hemophilia Treatment Center, had approached the manager of the Rochester Regional Blue Cross–Blue Shield offering to do a study, similar to Dr. Levine's, that would demonstrate that transfusion therapy and home care were cost-effective and could also save time and energy and prevent loss of jobs and days in school. She had asked for funds for 100 percent coverage for blood products plus the administration of the program, including training and supplies, to which the Blue Cross manager had agreed, in return for statistical documentation.[7]

During the early 1970s, a more grassroots political effort was also under way. NHF chapter leaders began to develop personal relationships with their local Congressional representatives, which helped pave the way to an effective presentation on the national level. Speaking about this period and how it was to culminate in the passage of federal legislation, "Cliff H." recalled:

The leadership of the patients and their families is a testimony to the principle that change can begin at the "grassroots level." People dedicated to a common cause can make a difference. . . . It would be difficult to count the hours that many patients and family members spent with doctors and state and national lawmakers urging them to take up our banner. The patient and his family have been members of a team that we now know has been successful in providing the current level of comprehensive care.[8]

A measure of this effectiveness can be seen in a comparison with the American Diabetes Association (ADA). During this same time period the ADA was also maximizing the use of physician leaders' relationships with legislators and galvanizing a groundswell of grassroots support in the form of "thousands of volunteers' signatures" for the Diabetes Detection and Education Act, originally introduced in 1972.[9] In 1970 the professional membership of the Diabetes Association was 9,000 and the lay membership 255,000. Although NHF records do not include membership numbers, in light of the small size of the total hemophilia population, the hemophilia community's ability to gain attention for its needs has been aptly characterized as "the effectiveness of a pygmy among the giants."[10]

The Changing Hemophilia Community

The NHF was so successful because it represented a self-defined, united community—but the configuration of that community was evolving. The original core group of parents who began the organization had multiplied, and the first cohort of boys with hemophilia had become young adults. Physicians and professional chapter and national staff had come aboard, and interconnections and informal networking had also increased as communication technology improved and NHF had developed printed materials. Despite the increasingly politicized nature of the organization, the spirit of "communitas," based both on genetic familial ties and on a shared cultural mind-set, still persisted. As "Adam H." stated:

I found at annual national meetings when I met people from different parts of the country or even from different countries, that there is a certain attitude towards life which is very common in people with hemophilia. It has to do with a number of things. . . . Number one: the ability to be flexible. . . . What I mean is, as a person with hemophilia you can't make plans for the future because you may have a sore knee and not be able to walk next weekend. . . . Wanting to maintain as much independence and self control as you possibly can. . . . Making your own decisions—every person with hemophilia has had the experience of going to the emergency room. Anybody who has been married and had kids has had the experience of being berated by some idiot resident or intern for ruining the gene pool of the country by having had kids. . . .

Another idea is understanding on one level that you could be dead tomorrow and somehow keeping that balance between living only for today and keeping in mind that there is a future, but don't count on it—but don't ignore it either. How you put that balance together leads to kinds of attitudes, at least in my experience, that cross cultural lines.[11]

Indeed, in addition to serving as a time to conduct important business, the annual NHF meetings had taken on the flavor of a large family reunion, as siblings and cousins from hemophilia families scattered across different parts of the country came together. Again, by contrast, although the ADA had recently been redefined as a voluntary organization, its medical model origins persisted. It described itself as made up of "physicians and interested laymen or volunteers," not as a single community.[12]

During the 1970s the hemophilia community became skillful at touching all bases in publicizing their plight and their needs. One strategy was to publicize their cost-effective health care delivery model, thus tapping into societal values and concerns about cost savings. NHF emphasized that the model was replicable, using data collection and program evaluation techniques to highlight the potential of saving dollars. It also used theatrical terminology and presentations that mirrored the communication style of the Nixon administration, with techniques drawn from the world of advertising. Working with connections in the advertising industry to produce a combination of strategies, the hemophilia community skillfully camouflaged the relatively minuscule size of the affected hemophilia population and created a dynamic presence.

Marvin Gilbert recalled gaining an awareness of Congress's fear of replicating the financial fiasco that occurred when kidney dialysis patients were made eligible for Medicare coverage in 1972. Because of a miscalculation of the numbers of patients with kidney disease who would survive with this new treatment, there was a vastly increased number of dialysis patients every year, which cost tremendous sums of money. Therefore, although many in the hemophilia community "really wanted money to cover the cost of Factor" (as freeze-dried pooled plasma concentrates of either Factor VIII or IX are known), it would not have been politically feasible in that climate to give the impression of a bottomless pit of financial need. Thus, as we have seen, the strategy of focusing on the need to provide comprehensive care by funding specific personnel in a specific number of treatment centers seemed far less likely to provoke legislators' anxiety.[13]

The treatment-center focus meshed with "Marcus Victor's" vision of comprehensive care. In his opinion, if the quest for federal funding had been confined to coverage of the blood products, "people would leave self-infusion as the only therapeutic modality and stay away from the comprehensive centers."[14] In fact, his concerns were well grounded. Some families who had acquired access to Factor were infusing their children at home and teaching others how to do it. "Adam H." recalled:

It was in 1971 that I started on home care. I went to "Nancy H.'s" house. She was out of the San Diego chapter, and she had two kids with hemophilia. . . . Eve and I went to her house, and she taught us how to do IVs. . . . It was parent teaching parent and person teaching person, with no medical training of any kind. Everything was done informally, catch as catch can.

We had all seen this being done when we were in the hospital emergency room. . . . Some people even learned to do IVs [all by] themselves, too. They found they were better than some of the "butchers" who called themselves doctors. It really wasn't very difficult to do.[15]

For the young adult hemophilia informants these initial attempts at self-infusion and home care were significant milestones in their lives. Not having to be in the hospital, "being able to sit up and not having to lie down, being able to do this myself and not have someone do it to me," brought a tremendous sense of liberation, a release from being "tethered to the hospital."[16] For these young men, their personal Golden Era began when they experienced these special moments of independence. The ability to "feel a sense of mastery," of "being in control," was very much intertwined with the use of Factor concentrates and self-care.[17]

A community-wide pragmatism ruled the day. Since the promotion of comprehensive care included the integration of education for family-

and self-infusion and the medical leadership stressed its support for promoting the independence of the person with hemophilia, the entire community rallied behind NHF to seek federal funding for the comprehensive care treatment center network. Lower prices for blood products and better insurance coverage would be pursued through other avenues. "Marcus Victor," who was perceived as having expertise in all of these matters, became "the man of the moment" in the 1970s.

The Enactment of Federal Hemophilia Legislation

As the hemophilia community geared up to lobby in support of federal legislation on hemophilia treatment, its visibility was enhanced by the publication in 1973 of *Journey* by Suzanne and Robert Massie. Well known as the authors of *Nicholas and Alexandra* (which they had also helped transform into a motion picture), the Massies' interest in hemophilia stemmed from their own experience as the parents of a son with the disease. *Journey*, which achieved instant popular acclaim, tells the story, seen alternately through the eyes of each parent, of raising a son with hemophilia in the United States. It paints a vivid picture of the impact of a multitude of obstacles, particularly the financial ones. The Massies augmented this personal saga with descriptive data supporting their criticism of both our government, for the lack of national health insurance, and the American Medical Association (AMA), for its lack of support for families with a chronic illness.

In its retelling of the parents' experiences from the earliest days of their son Bobby's life until he reached his teenage years, the book vividly captured the family's struggles and successes. Bobby's "journey"— from being educated at home because he was often too unwell to attend classes to becoming a self-sufficient full-time student—documents the progress in treatment, the importance of family support, and the dedication of hemophilia providers. Bobby began to transfuse himself at age thirteen, in 1970, as part of the home transfusion program established at New York Hospital by Margaret Hilgartner, and became a role model for young hemophiliacs. The icon of wheelchair-bound "poster boys" featured in hemophilia fund-raising campaigns of the 1960s was being replaced by pictures of Bobby and a photo of Lou Friedland's son during a Senate hearing, which was to become famous—new images symbolic of a promising future.

The hemophilia community rallied around its leadership to support S.1326, called the Hemophilia Act of 1973, which authorized the Secretary of the Department of Health, Education, and Welfare (HEW) to make grants and enter into contracts with public and nonprofit entities to establish comprehensive hemophilia diagnostic and treatment centers. The legislation was introduced by Senator Harrison Williams (D-N.J.), then acting chairman of the Subcommittee on Health of the Senate Committee on Labor and Public Welfare. Senator Jacob Javits (R-N.Y.) was the cosponsor. As informants report, in a scenario similar to that described by diabetes historians, the original groundwork was laid through the efforts of hemophilia advocates cultivating relationships with these key senators. Louis Friedland used his social capital, having "struck up a friendship with Senator Williams sometime earlier." The next step involved garnering the support of twenty-two senators "as a result of a vigorous legislative thrust by the chapters of the National Hemophilia Foundation across the country." The initial Senate hearing on the bill was scheduled for November 15, 1973. The arrival of a "great number of hemophilia patients, families, and supporters" the day before the hearing generated much energy and indicated a groundswell of support for the legislation. In contrast to many organizations described during this era, which emphasized professional networking, in this case it was well-informed hemophilia families that filled the Senate halls, creating the impression that hordes of people were advocating for this bill.[18]

The NHF had, however, hired John T. Grupenhoff of Grupenhoff and Endicott Associates (which represented the interests of its clients before Congress and federal agencies, especially on health issues) to create a legislative action plan. He met with the group as they arrived and guided them in their advocacy activities. Supplied with copies of draft legislation and the article by Peter Levine from the *New England Journal of Medicine*, these hemophilia community advocates met with "key Senate staffers." In particular, there were intense informal meetings, in hallways and then in a restaurant, with Senator Williams's legislative aide. Grupenhoff recalled considering "Dr. Victor" the driving medical force and Lou Friedland the driving layman behind the activity. And as a result of Friedland's input, the hemophilia community's dynamic presentation was shaped by the sophistication of the New York advertising and public relations industries. Grupenhoff recalled that the hearing room was packed with hemophiliacs and their parents and that both Senator Williams, who was presiding, and Senator Javits "were deeply moved" by the presentation. He described the hearing as "lasting only about an hour and a half, but it was one of the most extraordinary and successful hearings that I have witnessed." Grupenhoff described Friedland's testimony as particularly poignant:

Mr. Friedland first showed the committee a very large picture in color of his son at age 13 with swollen knees and elbows as a result of a recent occurrence of bruising. The large photo remained in front of the hearing Senators, but Mr. Friedland, taking a golf bag containing arm and leg braces that his son had used at age 13 to the front of the hearing room, asked Senator Javits to put out his arms. He then laid the braces one by one on the Senator's arms, indicating that even for the Senator, a strong and mature individual, the braces, which weighed over 30 pounds, were a heavy load. It was a dramatic moment, because shortly after the braces were removed from Senator Javits' arms, Mr. Friedland, a superb showman and publicist, indicated to the Senate that his son would now testify.

At this point, his son came forward, a remarkably healthy looking young man. He set up his infusion equipment and while he was infusing himself with concentrate, testified about the importance of getting this new therapy to all hemophiliacs. . . .

Senator Javits, leaving his chair, came down behind the witness and instructed a Senate photographer to take a picture. The Senator stated for the record: "I am going to keep this picture on my desk, and I won't take it down until the bill is passed."[19]

Marvin Gilbert also recalled the Senate hearing, noting that he has a copy of the photo of Friedland's son infusing. When it was his turn to testify, he said, "Orthopedics means 'ortho'—straight—and 'pedia'—child. The derivation of the specialty was to straighten the child. . . . In essence, I told the Senators that they had a chance to keep the child straight, to straighten him by providing Factor before he was ever bent."[20]

The beautifully orchestrated scenario impressed everyone who participated in it or viewed it. However, it was only a stepping-stone to the final passage of legislation that would benefit the hemophilia community. Discussions culminated in a decision to achieve passage by folding the measure into a larger package of legislation, a common practice in Congress. Grupenhoff credits Congressman Paul Rogers (D-Fla.) of the

Subcommittee on Health of the House Committee on Interstate and Foreign Commerce, with "shepherding it through."[21] During that same period, "in one of those fortunate accidents of history when events and people come together at an opportune moment," the American Diabetes Association was able to salvage components of its proposed bill and save it from "being buried in the categorical illness graveyard," through the efforts of "Representative Rogers, a personal friend of a new member of their Committee on Public Affairs."[22] Clearly Rogers was a key Congressional leader in the health arena during the 1970s—in Grupenhoff's words, "His leadership was everywhere evident, and he was trusted on both sides of the aisle."[23]

Eventually the hemophilia legislation was folded into H.R.14214, a bill containing formula grants to the states for health services, family planning programs, community mental health services, control of diseases borne by rats, home health services, and a center for the prevention and control of rape. Congress finally cleared the bill for the president's signature on December 19, 1974, and the House approved the final conference version on December 20, as the 1973–74 session ended. On December 23 the bill was vetoed by Gerald Ford, who had become president when Nixon resigned in August 1974. Because Congress had adjourned, there was no opportunity for the House and Senate to override the veto, and so the bill was laid over until 1975. Grupenhoff noted that there was "considerable unhappiness that the bill had been folded in with this larger piece of legislation, but because it was a comprehensive health act and the determination was made by the leadership of Congress, very little more could be done."[24]

In 1975 a new comprehensive hemophilia health care bill was introduced; it contained the same measures for hemophilia treatment as the former bill and also added the Nurse Training Program and extended the National Health Services Corps. The bill came to President Ford's desk in July 1975. He vetoed the bill on July 26, objecting to both the bill's cost and the extension of programs that his administration wanted to end.[25] The Hemophilia Program was not mentioned in the veto message.

The hemophilia community's committed and politically astute leadership continued to lobby vigorously and to use all available resources to maintain the momentum. Finally realizing that collaborating with others could be to their advantage, the NHF joined a coalition including the American Nurses Association, the National Association for Mental Health, Planned Parenthood, and other interested groups. Thus mobilized—and supplied with more cost-efficacy data accumulated by Peter Levine—their tenaciousness finally triumphed. In response to Ford's veto, the Senate agreed to reconsider the bill and overrode the presidential veto by a vote of 67 to 15, more than the two-thirds majority required. The lobbying intensified as the bill went to the House, which also voted to override the veto by 384 to 43, "a comfortable cushion."[26]

The passage of Public Law 94-63 on July 29, 1975, authorized appropriations for grants to hemophilia treatment centers (HTCs) offering comprehensive care. These moneys were to be used to pay personnel, such as social workers and nurses, who otherwise could not have been hired. In some cases the funds could supplement salaries so that part-time personnel could work on a full-time basis. Initially, funding was made available for twenty-six centers. With the passage of this legislation, the period known in the hemophilia community as "the Maternal and Child Health Years" had begun.

The Maternal and Child Health Years (1975–82)

For many of the directors of hemophilia treatment centers, the apex of the Golden Era is synonymous with the "Maternal and Child Health Years."[27] The Office of Maternal and Child Health (MCH), an agency of the U.S. Public Health Service, was given the responsibility for implementing the legislation for three reasons. First, hemophilia was viewed as a disease primarily affecting young boys and their families, thus falling under the aegis of MCH. Second, MCH had long experience with funding related to children. And third, it already had established working relationships with state Crippled Children's Services (CCS) programs, with which the new Hemophilia Treatment Center Program was to be affiliated. Indeed, the leaders of MCH were informed by a wealth of prior experience in both pediatrics and health services delivery, and this heightened awareness and background contributed from the outset to their provision of guidance and support to the hemophilia community.

Merle McPherson, M.D., who in 1990 was director of Habilitative Services of the Bureau of Maternal and Child Health, identified two particularly important health care developments that had already occurred and that would have a strong impact on the Hemophilia Treatment Center Program. First, significant biomedical innovations, such as the discovery of insulin and the development of renal dialysis, had "ushered in a revolution in care" and led to the extension of chronically ill children's lives. This, in turn, had led not only to greater concern for "the whole child"—the social, psychological, vocational, and medical needs—but also to the realization that the family as a whole was "the key to optimal care." Second, the development of regionally organized programs, such as the Regional Congenital Heart Disease Centers and later services in the area of perinatal physiology, highlighted the need to maintain "a balance between services within a tertiary-care center [caring for people managing chronic illnesses] and services at the community level, while maintaining effective communication between the two."[28] This experience enabled MCH leaders both to appreciate the steps already taken within the hemophilia community and to perceive gaps and needs that remained.

For its part, the NHF leadership understood immediately the importance of acquiring the cooperation of the MCH leadership in order to effectively implement the new program. The fact that, as "Marcus Victor" recalls, "comprehensive care methodology captivated Maternal and Child Health" helped establish the rapport between the NHF medical co-directors and the MCH leaders. "Victor" remembers "working with Vince Hutchins [M.D., Director of MCH] and Merle McPherson to convince them that this was a very sexy item that could be used as a prototype for chronic illness."[29] As a result, one of the early major activities was MCH visits to selected HTCs, such as Peter Levine's program in Massachusetts and the Rochester, New York, program.

In this way, the MCH reached out beyond the NHF leadership to develop relationships with other hemophilia treatment center directors—but there were some false steps. Mary Gooley offers an amusing recollection of the site visit made to the Rochester Center by Dr. Jack Hutchings of MCH:

He was asked to assess our rather unique program in Rochester because it was a chapter-run comprehensive care center located at the Rochester General Hospital. . . .

His first words to me when he sat down in my office were "I really don't know how to begin, Mrs. Gooley, because, number one, you're not a doctor and, number two, I have never dealt with a nonphysician director of a hemophilia care center. I know that the center has been here a long time and that you've been involved with it, but how did you become the director?" I reassured him that I had a lot of professional support and that my position had evolved over the years.[30]

Peter Levine's recollections are vivid and positive as he remembers visits from Donna O'Hare, M.D., the pediatrician who was first charged with the task of developing the hemophilia program. In those beginning days, Levine remarked, the MCH "spent a lot of time and asked a lot of wonderful questions. . . . It was clear that they were really interested in this." He added that "This was my first experience with people from any governmental agency who were really dedicated to doing something that was in the interest of health and had an eye to cost efficiency as well."[31]

This thinking had become particularly prudent in the mid-1970s. After 1974, a combination of recession and inflation marked the end of the postwar growth of entitlements and stalled the movement for national health insurance, despite the election of a heavily Democratic Congress.[32] Therefore, MCH regarded Peter Levine's center as one of the prototypes for delivery of comprehensive care. Representatives made frequent visits, expressing interest in the delineation of the professional roles and the face-to-face interaction on the team and in the "power, authority, and responsibility" of the nurses. They also involved Levine in writing protocols and guidelines, in keeping with the MCH style of fostering a feeling of inclusion among the HTC directors.

Working with MCH reinforced Levine's sense of the importance of his data collection and demonstration of cost efficacy. At the annual NHF meeting in 1975, at a get-together of treatment center directors, he proposed to coordinate responsibility for data collection at his center and encouraged all of the medical directors to participate. He argued that this would "be the only thing that will keep us alive"; otherwise they would "have a three-year grant or a five-year grant and it will dissolve." A subsequent NHF meeting of about fifty treatment center directors "hammered out a uniform data collection set." Levine agreed to mail it out once a year to all of the treatment centers with the understanding that people would take responsibility for returning it and he would not chase after them. He noted: "The one small stick in this stick-and-carrot act was that I would list on the first page all who had participated and would send a copy to the Feds." In addition to gaining the medical directors' cooperation, Levine involved the nurses, who "loved the collection of data." This gave them a whole new role that wasn't in the former job description: "Since data is power, it gave them a power that they didn't have before, another validation of their importance in the hemophilia world."[33]

Merle MacPherson held annual meetings of an ad hoc advisory committee, which included selected medical directors and the NHF leaders, another action that reinforced feelings of inclusiveness in shaping the development of the hemophilia program. Levine felt that these meetings were "real think tanks" and were extremely useful for bringing attention to emerging needs that could determine changes in the program.[34]

Within MCH's overall focus on building systems of care, the initial emphasis for the hemophilia program was on increasing the provision of comprehensive care, which was to include a home care component—that is, the promotion of family- and self-infusion. In addition, discussions of the ultimate goal of a national network revealed that there were areas of the country where no hemophilia expertise existed, which in turn led to emphasis on the need for regionalization. Encouraging progress in coagulation research, dealing with concerns about hepatitis, and ensuring the safety of the blood supply were not included in the mission of this government agency. In the community-wide enthusiasm and excitement of involvement in either delivering or receiving state-of-the-art care, these other matters would be put on the back burner, so to speak. A warning came from Oscar Ratnoff, but he remained "a voice in the wilderness."[35]

Focusing sequentially on priority concerns is part of the American cultural mind-set. In this case, the funding played a role in concentrating almost the entire hemophilia community's focus on either delivering or receiving comprehensive care and having access to affordable concentrates. The developing network of treatment centers provided opportunities for health care professionals to enter an exciting field and gave them the opportunity to do fulfilling work and to feel that what they were doing was important. Hematologists, who increasingly assumed the directorships of HTCs, felt both competent and important.

They had increasing access to and control over the plasma manufacturers' products that brought such a sense of freedom to patients, and this, in turn, enhanced the sense of power and appreciation they received from hemophilia families. They were also valued within their institutions for bringing in federal grants, making them "money getters," and for running cost-effective programs, making them "money savers" as well. In the academic medical center culture, these attributes, coupled with political know-how, increased their opportunities for recognition by promotion. Among these "treaters" achieving institutional recognition were the NHF medical co-directors, who became the acknowledged leaders in the hemophilia community.

The medical sociologist Elliot Friedson uses the term "the framework of practice" in analyzing the behavior of physicians.[36] The culture in academic medical centers contributed to shaping the specialists who were directing the hemophilia programs, just as the hemophilia programs contributed to the institutions in which they were based. This created a framework of practice in which research and specialization were revered and medical school faculty, who were chief physicians, were in control. When patients were involved, they were viewed not as "health consumers" but as recipients of care in a doctor-patient relationship. It was the norm for physicians who were HTC directors to speak of "my patients." For the medical directors and other health care providers, by-products of the Maternal and Child Health years included an increasing sense of both control and indispensability. Although the hemophilia treatment center grant renewals submitted to MCH emphasized the goal of enabling patients to live as independent and normal a life as possible, in reality treatment centers relished their growing importance and centrality in the lives of patients and their families.

Although Paul Starr described the "decline of professional sovereignty" in the 1970s, as noted in Chapter 5, there was little evidence that this trend had permeated the hemophilia community.[37] The consumer movement mind-set, questioning a physician's judgment, and the increased tendency of the courts to view the doctor-patient relationship as a partnership in decision making were still alien to most hemophilia families during those years. In general, these families still consisted of young boys and their parents who were grateful to have become recipients of high-quality comprehensive care. Located within the framework of the academic medical center, the HTCs became the place where parents found treatment for their children and guidance for themselves. The locus of hemophilia community identity was shifting from the chapters to the HTCs. Just as the deaf community refers to its schools as a substitute for a geographical identity marker, hemophilia families in the late 1970s and early 1980s often referred to their treatment centers and their medical directors in identifying themselves.[38]

The influence of medical directors was enhanced by their inclusion in a pivotal meeting held by MCH on January 8–10, 1976, in La Jolla, California. The purpose of the gathering was to define the main issues involved in establishing the configuration of the Hemophilia Treatment Center Program.[39] Bringing these physicians in at this early stage reinforced the tone of respect and inclusiveness that MCH had established from the outset of the federally funded program. The substantial representation at this important meeting of HTC medical directors based in academic medical centers reflected the federal government's view that they were becoming important players in shaping health policy and programs.[40] Among the fifteen physicians at the meeting were NHF medical co-directors "Victor" and Gilbert, but they were identified as affiliated with the Mount Sinai Medical School, a clear indication of which of their identities mattered most. There were no other representatives of other provider disciplines or NHF lay leaders present.

During the discussion, lists were compiled of reasons for favoring one treatment over another. In ranking the relative merits of concentrates and cryoprecipitate, the participants considered "the reliable potency" offered by concentrates as the top priority. (Factor concentrates are literally more concentrated than cryo and smaller doses are required. Cryo may also contain impurities.) The "mobility it afforded the patient" was listed as fifth. Once again, as in the 1972 NHLI *Pilot Study*, physician "treaters" were seen as the appropriate participants to decide about and select treatment. The voices not heard at this meeting were those of patients and families, nurses, social workers, and other health care personnel. MCH had taken the initial steps in making hemophilia community planning a participatory process; however, it had not yet reached out beyond considering physicians the appropriate spokespersons and planners in this stage of the process. Terms such as the "desire for freedom" and "not being tethered to a hospital" were not voiced or heard in La Jolla. Parents generally deferred to physicians. The first generation of men with hemophilia had not yet reached sufficient maturity to assert themselves and express their feelings when they differed from those of the treaters. Ancillary personnel were new additions to hemophilia treatment centers. No one from these groups was seated at the table.

CHAPTER 7

The Meanings of the Golden Era

Throughout the 1970s, officials of the Office of Maternal and Child Health (MCH) and directors of hemophilia treatment centers conveyed their optimism to the hemophilia community, especially to new parents whose sons had the condition. These boys, who had access to comprehensive care, including home care education and concentrates, could look forward to a relatively normal childhood and a normal life span. This transformed version of childhood included a relatively pain-free existence, normal school attendance, participation in selected athletic activities, and summer fun and camaraderie at one of the growing number of "hemophilia camps." In the 1970s these camps provided a significant place for bonding with "blood brothers" and for gaining self-esteem.

Other Voices, Other Perspectives

In the absence of a national health insurance program, however, geographic, ethnic, and socioeconomic variations continued and with them glaring inequities in the quality of life in the hemophilia population. Money provided by federal funding was directed initially to treatment centers in academic medical centers and to their associated "affiliates." State-funded programs provided additional care in some geographical areas, but there were gaps where access to high-quality care for hemophilia did not exist. Data generated by the federally funded participating treatment centers failed to reflect the experiences of those outside the funded network.

"Kent H.," an informant with severe hemophilia A born in 1965 in South Carolina, recalled that his memories of growing up with hemophilia were just awful. Because his father was in the navy, "Kent" went to the naval hospital for every bleed. It routinely took a week to control his bleeds, and he remembers considering nurses his "second parents." He was treated with plasma until 1972; after that he received cryoprecipitate, but only because one of the doctors intervened and persuaded the hospital to obtain the equipment to make it. "Kent" became aware that the equipment that they had, "such as old Fenwall filters, which would clog up with cryo, was very primitive."[1] The closest hemophilia treatment center was in Chapel Hill, North Carolina, seven hours away. At that time he did not know that it existed, nor did he know that children his age were being treated entirely differently.

The turning point in his life came when he was twelve, and his parents learned of a hemophilia camp he could attend. He remembers he arrived at camp with a knee bleed, but hadn't told his father for fear he would turn around and go back home. With his splints and crutches, he said, the others looked at him "as if I had come from another century." When the camp director discovered the knee bleed, she treated it as "no big deal." "Kent" received his first infusion of concentrate in the camp clinic. After leaving the clinic, he began to look around at the other children: "I was so amazed, looking around me at the kids who were handling their bleeds much differently. They were playing, they were fighting, they were doing all the things that kids do. No one was taking as much pain medication as I was, and they were having fun. . . . By Monday evening, no crutches. I went ahead and limped, . . . no splints or anything. And the rest of the week was a blast." After he returned from camp, he convinced his parents to bring him to the hemophilia treatment center at Chapel Hill. There it was discovered that he had developed synovitis, an inflammation of the synovial joint of the knee. He believes that if he hadn't been placed on a prophylactic regimen there, he would have lost the joint within a few years.[2]

Another informant also born in the 1960s with severe hemophilia A, "Harold H.," grew up in Oregon. At that time, the nearest NHF chapter was "a fledgling chapter in Seattle." "Harold" noted:

People from the East Coast don't realize this, but Westerners have very little contact with each other out here. You look at the big cities, Seattle, Portland, and then you've got seven hundred miles . . . until you reach the San Francisco–Sacramento area. There's no overlap of television, there's no overlap of radio, or newspapers, nothing like that. We're completely different cultures. . . . We also have demographics that are very representative of the entire U.S., but we are very isolated. It's changing, but it certainly didn't happen in the 60s or the 70s.[3]

During his early years, he went to the University of Oregon Medical School for treatment because it was state-owned and therefore lower in cost than private care, but he referred to it as "the place of last resort," because the treatment offered was unequal and behind the times. Boys with insurance were given plasma; those without received whole blood. "Harold's" mother, whom he described as "very assertive," questioned the use of whole blood when it was known that plasma had a richer concentration of Factor VIII, but was told not to interfere. When she learned that frozen plasma was being used in California, her efforts to obtain it for all patients were actively resisted by the laboratory director. She persisted in asking for plasma, but at that time most doctors in that community "didn't want to deal with the problem," "Harold" said. "You had to find someone with a good heart or an interest in science." Eventually his mother formed a chapter of the NHF and became its first president. As "Harold" described her,

She was the kind of person, . . . when she got a Ford Mustang the first year Ford Mustangs came out and it was defective, she called Mr. Ford, Henry Ford II, and got through. It took her two weeks, but she got through and said, "You're giving me a new car"—and he did. She was an extremely assertive woman, and so she had no problem calling anyone in authority. Because she came off as very intelligent, people would talk with her for a very long time and took her very seriously.[4]

While other boys were benefiting from a more normal childhood in the Golden Era, "Harold" remembered "looking like the Michelin Man" because his mother would sew foam rubber into his clothing to protect his joints. In the 1970s, he recalled, he still had to go to the hospital for infusions and usually experienced long waits. Because he was not given the product to use at home, he once had to go to the hospital at two in the morning for a bleeding emergency.[5]

After he went on home-infusion, at the age of twelve, "Harold" was able to "maintain five paper routes, ride my bicycle, and work in my garden." But he was increasingly plagued by serious problems with one of his knees. Eventually, a severe infection that had gone undetected caused him many months in and out of the hospital, in traction, in a cast, and eventually in rehabilitation. He missed an entire school term in 1977. Fortunately, because the Education of All Handicapped Act included children with hemophilia among those with disabilities, funds were available for a home tutor, and Harold was able to catch up with his studies and graduate on time. By 1979, when he was seventeen years old, he was having "a wonderful time"; it was "phenomenal to be having fun and dating. . . . I was really in my element." Interestingly, he recalled the arrival of federal funding and the formation of a treatment center in his area as the time when the NHF chapter began to fall apart. After that time the members only got together to raise money for the summer camp.[6]

Access to Concentrates

Without exception, informants reported that, once they had access to concentrates, life was "golden." For informants born in the 1950s, initial exposure to comprehensive care and concentrates often came in college or graduate school. "James H." (Dana Kuhn) was born and grew up on Long Island but moved to South Carolina when he went to college. He is considered a mild hemophiliac and wasn't diagnosed with hemophilia until he was seventeen years old, not long before he went to college. He first encountered comprehensive care in Memphis, Tennessee, when he was in Memphis Theological Seminary acquiring a master's degree. He recalled:

They did an excellent job of taking care of me there. They gave me a full evaluation and gave me the Factor that I would need. That's when I first experienced what comprehensive care was. It was excellent. . . . That's when I started to get involved with NHF and the chapter there. . . .

Things really got better when Factor came out. Cryo was good but Factor was, like, *Wow!* We have reached it. It's like hemophiliacs now looking toward gene therapy, looking forward to that. . . . For me to experience Factor was: This is like a miracle drug. We can now be normal. All we have to do when we get hurt . . . or I play soccer and get injured, injure my ankle, is come in and get some Factor infused—be up and around in two days. . . . This is a miracle![7]

"Brett H." grew up in Ohio in the 1950s. His parents were "virtually cofounders of the Northern Ohio NHF chapter." A severe hemophiliac, he recalled that in those days "you did not have a normal childhood, not even a remotely normal childhood"; his sense of life in Ohio at the time was as "barely above the Dark Ages, barely above the level of Rasputin in czarist Russia." He noted that his father's employer agreed not to move him around the country so that they could stay where there was medical care and good insurance coverage. "Brett" was not treated as an outpatient until he went to college. He "discovered the comprehensive care model and Factor" when he went to graduate school in Ann Arbor, Michigan. Liking the "whole team setup" and "all the advantages of rapport," he particularly appreciated being able to get on the phone and talk to the nurse "almost instantly."[8] To him, life was totally transformed at that time.

For "Eugene H.," another member of the 1950s informant cohort, his childhood in the Bronx, New York, was remembered as "an age of misconception about hemophilia, ostracism by your peers, and overprotection by teachers." For him "isolation was the norm until high school." Noting that having "a chronic problem that separates you from your peers can be difficult," he developed a degree of denial that is reflected in the first job he had—bouncer and bartender in a topless bar. "Eugene" also recalled from his younger years that his father, a fireman, ran blood drives. His parents were involved in the local NHF chapter and became acquainted with "the physicians who were the thought leaders of the day."[9] By the time he reached college, "Eugene" was self-infusing Factor on a regular basis and was able to go to school and work full-time. Increasingly self-confident, he was proud of his ability to walk normally as well as his athletic build and growing strength, built up by swimming. A pre-med major, he was unable to gain admission to medical school and so decided to get a second bachelor's degree, in nursing. After graduation, he was employed as the nurse coordinator in a federally funded hemophilia treatment program.

In addition to his own personal sense of "freedom and accomplishment, aided by being on concentrates," "Eugene" recalls a particular work-related experience that emphasized the significance of this mode of treatment:

One of the experiences that was invaluable, I think, was the first time I was asked by "Dr. H." to help her with a new family. It was new parents. This was their first child. He was born with hemophilia, and as with most new parents [they were] having a difficult time coping with that fact and putting it in perspective. . . . "Dr. H." asked me to go and meet the family. As I walked into the room they were there with the baby. I was probably the same age as the parents. I introduced myself, because they were wondering why I was there. I said: "'Dr. H.' asked me to stop by and say that I have hemophilia."

They just looked and looked. Obviously they had this image that hemophiliacs were on crutches or in wheelchairs or they look like they came from a concentration camp. In the brief span of five or ten minutes I accomplished more than anyone else could have.[10]

The Oldest Informants Become Adults

By the late 1970s, the oldest informant cohort, those who had experienced and survived the latter part of the Dismal Era, were "using concentrates and savoring experiencing the American dream."[11] All were employed and married. Two of them, "Adam H." and "Cliff H.," had completed graduate school, had begun to rise in their chosen fields, and were enjoying raising families. Being able to travel for both business and pleasure was one of the best aspects of "life with Factor." Both men had also become active in their local hemophilia chapters. Within the next few years they would emerge as two of the major national leaders of the hemophilia community, representing this first generation of adults with hemophilia who had a sense of their own future. They brought to the NHF an adult consumer perspective and ideas for change.

"Adam H.," an attorney, "got very much involved at the time the American Blood Commission was being formed." He had attended his first national NHF meeting in 1975, as president-elect of his local chapter. By the late 1970s, he recalled, the meetings had become "very large and very hostile." At one meeting, "Adam," who described himself then as "a brash young kid who wasn't easily intimidated," challenged one of the key medical leaders who was, in his opinion, making decisions unilaterally on a number of issues, particularly blood issues. Not long after that the NHF began to establish committees to resolve a number of issues, and "Adam" himself was elected to the NHF board. As a board member he frequently found himself in conflict with "Dr. Marcus Victor" over the medical co-director's presumption of authority and tendency to make decisions without consulting the board.[12]

"Cliff H.," a scientist employed by a large corporation, "was interested in organizational matters." His wife had originally seen something in the paper about an NHF council meeting in Northern Ohio. After he attended one meeting, he said, "It was 'Brett H.'s' mother and dad who convinced me to get involved." His involvement in the Northern Ohio chapter grew after a state program was enacted and an advisory board was established, on which he served. "Cliff" felt that he was able to make a contribution regarding what needed to be done to deliver care and that the Northern Ohio chapter was beginning to develop a cadre of leaders. He described how he began to view both himself and the leaders who would follow:

Unlike the generation of parents of sons with hemophilia, who had to influence providers when there was very limited communication, . . . and when whatever the physician said was the final word, and the only way to break through was for parents to network with each other, . . . I did not have to know other families to make things happen. I think there's another difference too. . . . I have always thought of myself as a scientist, even though I'm in management now.

I've been trained as a scientist, and I'm successful as a scientist. I'm not a physician, but I understand medical sciences. As a result, I've not been intimidated by needing to talk to physicians. There are some physicians who don't care for that attitude, and I've had some difficulty, but that never made me feel bad towards them or vice versa. . . .

I've felt that the control of the disease was in my hands. . . . I think many of the leaders today are of the same bent. . . . Consequently, family linkages become less important, and there are two different eras involved. But we would not be here today if it weren't for the investment these mothers and these fathers made earlier, saying "I may not understand all of this terminology, but I know that I've got to find improved treatment and care."[13]

The NHF in Disarray

By the late 1970s, as energies became focused upon expanding and ameliorating the delivery of comprehensive care, the NHF's internal organizational and fiscal problems took another turn for the worse. By April 30, 1977, the NHF "had slipped into technical bankruptcy again," as a result of mismanagement; in the following year the administrative staff allowed "the unrestricted fund to go negative, and NHF went further and further into debt." Chapters "no longer trusted the executive director, and there was a continuation of juggling of creditors, payments deferred, liabilities, and prepaid expenses."[14] It wasn't only the chapters that were disturbed by the state of finances at NHF. By 1978, there was a clear indication the MCH respected and supported the health care delivery system fortified by and housed within prestigious and reputable academic medical centers, but felt that NHF was not a stable base for health care delivery. When the recently created NHF Nursing Committee submitted a proposal for a nationwide assessment of hemophilia education for patients, families, and health professionals, MCH agreed to fund it only on the condition that funding would be directed to the hemophilia treatment center of the Nursing Committee chairperson. The chairperson was Catherine Mintzer, R.N., nurse coordinator of the New England Hemophilia Treatment Center, of which Peter Levine was medical director.

In February 1979 the executive director of NHF was dismissed. When the NHF Administrative Committee subsequently arrived at the central office, "they opened drawers in desks and found unpaid bills stuffed inside, some as old as two years." A newly appointed acting executive director quit without notice at the end of May, and a replacement, who also "proved to be less than ideal for the role," came aboard. Before the end of the year, he would be terminated and seven other employees let go to reduce payroll costs.[15]

Despite the staff turmoil during the latter part of the 1970s, the medical co-directors, Marvin Gilbert and "Marcus Victor," continued to interact effectively with both the plasma manufacturers and the MCH leadership regarding professional matters (their chief concerns). They helped NHF to survive by acquiring funding from the manufacturers to produce educational publications for both professional and lay audiences and also to support meetings for newly formed professional committees. The Mental Health Committee, the Nursing Committee, and the Social Work Subcommittee were offshoots of the original Medical and Scientific Advisory Council (MASAC). For Gilbert and "Victor" day-to-day administration of NHF was put on the back burner.

Perhaps this is more understandable when we recall that this was a time of hope and good will within the hemophilia community. During those years, the medical co-directors and many of the professionals from hemophilia treatment centers who served on NHF committees, worked without compensation to write NHF publications and to define whatever programs were created, establishing a tradition of professional voluntarism at NHF that still exists today.

These were also the years when sales representatives from the plasma companies became increasingly familiar figures in the hemophilia treatment centers, at the NHF office, and at NHF annual meetings, fostering a flow of informal exchanges and increased communication. Barbara Chang, who began her career as a sales representative with Hyland Laboratories in 1979, recalled:

> I was so impressed and actually surprised that a manufacturer such as Hyland was so closely involved with trying to help meet the needs of the hemophiliac and would be concerned much beyond producing a product and having that product available. What is so unique about the manufacturers, and I think this stands for all manufacturers, is that it is a very special product we make. Our interests go far beyond "Here is the product" and handing it over to the physician and then it is given to the patients. I find all of the manufacturers and representatives of the companies involved in many, many ways. And there is a range of things: participating in summer camps, participating in . . . workshops that the families attend, and trying to help the nurse coordinators. It became immediately evident that one did not just make a product; there was more to it. There was service involved and a concern for how the patient was educated and that grew into the whole aspect of home care.[16]

During this time, MCH encouraged the forging of linkages, holding annual meetings for HTC directors to discuss key issues and delineate future needs and directions. Among the major issues discussed were financing of care, "turf issues," and incorporating psychosocial and vocational personnel into the comprehensive care teams.[17] One important outcome of these discussions was the development of guidelines for the relationship between primary care physicians and the treatment centers. Another was the development of satellite centers, later known as affiliates, which served as a step towards regionalization.

Thus, the progress in hemophilia health care delivery in the late 1970s provided a stark contrast to the continuing downward financial spiral and the deteriorating image of the NHF. Witnessing the growing administrative turmoil, the chapters became increasingly disenchanted with the NHF staff. The relationship between the central office and many chapters had disintegrated markedly. Parents continued to focus on their children's needs at the local level and to become more involved in groups organized by the treatment centers.

Adult Hemophilia
Leadership at the National Level

Change only began to occur at NHF when "Adam H." and several other adults with hemophilia who had all in recent years become involved on the local level decided to become actively involved on the national level as well. Because "Adam H." is an attorney, he was selected for membership on the Bylaws Committee. Another attorney who was asked to be a member of the committee was G. William (Bill) Bissell. Although Bissell does not have hemophilia, he had become involved in hemophilia activities as a philanthropist and board member of a local chapter in Pennsylvania. Despite their very different life experiences, the two men had an instant rapport. Both had the ability to step back and analyze the NHF's current situation from a historical perspective, using an organizational and political framework. They not only agreed about many of the perceived flaws; they also viewed the Bylaws Committee as an appropriate springboard for introducing change and transforming the organizational structure—in "Adam's" words, planning to "create a culture." Adam discussed his perceptions and his involvement:

I probably didn't know a lot of what I should have known, but I wasn't afraid to express my ignorance and ask questions. And Bill Bissell, to a certain extent was the same way. . . . A lot of the problems had to do with blood issues, . . . a lot of it had simply to do with arrogance. It was an arrogant style. . . . I think entrenchment promotes arrogance. As situations continue, people continue. . . . I think it is a thing that historically exists and that is the way institutions tend to operate. What we really tried to deal with on the Bylaws Committee was to develop a constitution for NHF—more than a constitution, a set of procedural rules. And it established a whole new set of power relationships between the chapters and NHF, or at least we intended [it] to.[18]

"Adam" was also concerned that "NHF had a tendency to close people out." Specifically, he recalled not being allowed to attend a Medical and Scientific Advisory Council (MASAC) meeting because he was not a physician, although he had served on a committee that developed policy recommendations to MASAC about blood issues. He described his reaction as "outrage." He felt exclusion from certain board meetings was also a problem and made sure that the new bylaws contained a provision that every chapter had the right to send a representative to every board meeting. With regard to MASAC, he described the solution as "working out some interesting compromises"—such as not informing attendees at the annual NHF meeting of the location of the MASAC meeting but not excluding them if they managed to discover where it was to be held. "Adam's" desire to attend MASAC meetings stemmed from his feeling that they were "very important, because doctors make decisions differently when patients are present. . . . I have always found it important from a policy perspective that patients be present. It reminds physicians that they are dealing with people, not with data."[19]

Bissell became interested in the national NHF problems when he attended his first annual meeting in 1975. He remembered that when he had first become involved with the hemophilia community, "I saw things that made me angry. I thought I saw a bunch of naive, vulnerable people being ripped off." When he was asked to chair the Bylaws Committee, he refused but agreed instead to staff the committee and act as counsel to it. Seeing the "leadership in disarray," he noted:

When I came into NHF it was [supposed to be] a business corporation form of government; but in fact it was a convention form of government. The governing body had a group of about a hundred people. Now, a hundred people cannot conduct business. . . . There's an article by Ted Taft of the Taft family of Ohio. The thesis of the article is that the largest group of people who can really carry on a conversation is seven. There you have one kind of animal, and if you have more than seven you have another kind of animal. The larger the group, the less inclined some people will be to participate. His thesis is that the larger the group, the smaller the group that will control the organization. . . . The larger the outer group, the smaller the inner group—so that is one of the ironies of democracy; and of course you see this in the history of democracies and totalitarian societies.

The NHF body was a hundred people, which means that's not a board of directors. That's a convention. A convention form of government is very common in advocacy organizations. . . . We went from a convention form to a business corporation form, where the governing body is about twenty people, which is still bigger than Mr. Taft says you can have a conversation with. . . .

One of the most significant changes, from my perspective, is the change from a convention form of government to a board of directors, a business form of governance, which I regard as significant because the convention form of government was simply out of control.[20]

Bissell asserted that at NHF in the late 1970s, "there were significant systems failing in the accounting, auditing, and financial reporting, in all of these functions," compounding the need to "improve the level of trust," which is a central issue in the corporate governance model. Bissell maintained that "Part of the corporate governance activity is to put . . . mechanisms into place" that "provide the regular and formal systematic exchange of information from one person to another, from one group to another." He saw himself as a "technician" who was "fixing the engine," noting that after the engine is fixed, "you have to figure out where to drive the car."[21]

In Bissell's view, the 1970s was a time when the nation saw a "series of corporate scandals which brought to the public's attention that we had institutional problems." In particular, he cited the Penn Central bankruptcy, which he considered "a watershed event in American social history," as well as "the Boeing scandal and the Gulf Oil political slush fund scandal."[22] In a personal letter he included voluntary agencies among the institutions having problems by characterizing them with a time-specific reference: "the Richard M. Nixon I-am-not-a-crook model."[23]

Bissell considered the National Hemophilia Foundation a "sick" institution rather than a "corrupt" one but noted that there was "significant denial among the participants as to how sick the organization was." In his view denial may be "an appropriate response in a patient dealing with an illness but [is] inappropriate for professionals." Using the analogy of the institution of the Church, he said that because of the nature of the NHF, many constituents had difficulty accepting the "all too real worldly realities of the organization." He added: "What I'm getting at is that there's something about the hemophilia organization and the degree to which people invested themselves that induced denial. It caused them to think the best of the organization and to refuse to think badly [of it]."[24]

Bissell enjoyed being a party to making a difference within NHF, but considered himself a "community outsider." In reflecting on the changes, he saw the late 1970s as "a period of transition from a private club to a public charity." He considered "the leadership of the new inner circle as 'Cliff H.,' Nathan Smith, 'Adam H.,' and Margaret Hilgartner." He noted that, as the 1980s began, "the leaders were patients."[25] Indeed, the 1979 NHF annual meeting, held in Los Angeles, marked the end of the old regime and the emergence of new leadership. These leaders, the first generation of adults with hemophilia with a vision for the community's future, enacted the new bylaws and acquired the reins of the organization. "Cliff H." was elected president and Nathan Smith, a leader from Texas, became chairman of the board. Neither of them had served on the former executive committee.

"Cliff H." noted that his original "entire motivation" in becoming involved nationally "was to observe—how do you bring all of the systems together, how do you create an atmosphere where you don't have to do it all, but the people you bring in are talented and capable?" He began to realize that the national organization was not working as well as the hemophilia chapters he knew in Ohio. At the 1979 annual meeting "the organization was in such turmoil that I said, 'Enough is enough, we have to make a change.'" He had visualized being nominated as a member of the board, but had instead "been thrust into the presidency."[26]

"Cliff H." created "a kitchen cabinet, a close core of people that I took a risk with that their judgment and character was good." He, "Adam H.," Nathan Smith, and Bill Bissell "spent endless hours, till three or four in the morning, just trying to understand what this was." Within six months he realized they had to "do some drastic things." He asked Bissell to resign from the board because he trusted him and wanted to hire him to go through the office files and "tell me what was going on." "Cliff" added that Bissell uncovered "some very distasteful situations, but it was only through that surgical process, as he and I called it, that we were able to heal the NHF."[27] Bissell recalls that "Cliff H." built trust by both hearing and telling the truth. When unpaid tax liabilities were revealed, he immediately told the Executive Committee and then brought in an accounting firm to check the numbers. Bissell added, "He then sent out a letter telling everybody exactly what the story was and what the figure was."[28]

According to "Cliff H." the question was whether the organization "had any right to survive, and if it was affirmative, could it survive?" Since the NHF was on the brink of full-blown bankruptcy, the Executive Committee decided to "cut back to bare-bones staffing" and make an effort to become solvent within two years. Once that decision was made, "Cliff" began to advocate for the hiring of "a professional executive director," preferably with a background in public health. He created a list of criteria; first on that list was "impeccable honesty and dependability"; specific skills and responsibilities ranked below that. He wanted to put an end to "smoke-screen management" and "an era of a pseudo-professional image." By establishing "participatory management, but with clear objectives in mind and accountability," he hoped to achieve "credibility" and "respect in Washington."[29]

"Cliff" considers one of his "crowning accomplishments" the hiring of "Paul Phillips" as executive director in September 1981. "Phillips" was asked to put management systems in place that would enable NHF to define programs with measurable objectives. "Cliff" felt that going to sponsors with specific programs was preferable to "the tin-cup approach." With the hiring of "Phillips" and the installation of management systems with defined programs and strategic planning, he considered the Foundation too was at last "entering the Golden Era."[30]

The NHF Nursing Committee's Patient/Family Model

One positive discovery "Paul Phillips" made when he arrived at the NHF was a Nursing Committee project that was gaining recognition in U.S. public health circles and in the international hemophilia community. The Educational Resources Project referred to above had begun in 1979, shortly after I was hired by the NHF to assess educational needs of both chapters and treatment centers; my findings led to requesting funding to create an educational tool for "educators and learners" that would serve as a model for dealing with chronic illness. Ultimately published as *The Hemophilia Patient/Family Model* and packaged in a modular format, it was designed to introduce self-care education into comprehensive care. It contained a "basic information" module and six additional modules concerning other aspects of total care, including Factor replacement and home therapy.

After field-testing the teaching modules with families in their treatment centers, the Nursing Committee submitted the drafts to other NHF committees, representing the other disciplines on treatment center teams. This participatory process strengthened the final product and added an emphasis on public health education philosophy and methods. Shortly after the project began, I recruited nationally known health educators to participate on an ad hoc Health Education Advisory Committee, whose contribution went beyond simply giving advice regarding the creation of the guidelines. Committee members became faculty for education workshops for providers, the second phase of the project. They emphasized that adult education views the learner in an egalitarian way, as a partner and an active participant in all phases of the educational process. Thus, the Patient/Family Model cast patients and families in an active rather than a passive role and fostered interdisciplinary collaboration at the treatment center level. This teaching guideline also enhanced the nursing role as nurse-clinician coordinators became the educational pivot of the teams.

The overwhelmingly positive response of the first cohort of nurses who received the guide encouraged the project directors to seek renewed funding from MCH and to launch a collaborative effort with the World Federation of Hemophilia (WFH) to produce the guide in English, Spanish, German, and Japanese. Through the Patient/Family Model other countries could emulate the successes of the United States by providing comprehensive care and enabling patients to actively participate in achieving a more normal life. The decision was also made to collaborate with plasma manufacturers, for the benefit of the hemophilia community. This project was seen as a joint effort that would benefit everyone and harm no one. Everyone agreed that patients and families, health care providers, and any sponsoring manufacturer would all be "winners."

Funding from one plasma manufacturer augmented the MCH moneys and supported the process of developing and translating the guides. Physicians and nurses from abroad traveled to the United States to work on the foreign language versions. Attending WFH meetings and working with nurses from other countries further broadened the horizons for the core group on the Nursing Committee, as well as offering both visibility and prestige. Three of the nurses in this core group, Maribel Clements, Regina Butler, and Karen Meredith, expressed both enthusiasm about participating in the project and satisfaction with their treatment center responsibilities and their sense of the unique role of nursing in hemophilia treatment.

Maribel Clements began working with the Hemophilia Program at the Puget Blood Center in Seattle in 1976. Her earlier experience, as a student nurse, with hemophilia patients had been "very negative," but "in 1976 when a lot of people were on home care, it was a very positive field to be going into." She recalled joining both the Mental Health Committee and the Nursing Committee of the NHF in 1977 and serving as a liaison between them, but what she "remembered best was working on the Patient/Family Model." After using it, she was surprised "by some of the things even experienced patients didn't know." She felt that the treatment center was "a rewarding place to work. . . . After the first year, just about everyone accepted me as someone who was there to help in any way I could." She considered her job during those years "exactly what I wanted as far as long-term involvement with the same families."[31]

Regina Butler had entered the hemophilia community when she was searching for a job and found an opening for a nurse to start a hemophilia program at Children's Hospital in Philadelphia. She recalls:

It wasn't at all difficult to get involved with the families. The families seemed to be really waiting for someone to talk to, to serve as a liaison between themselves, the hospital staff, and the physicians. There was a lot to learn. Hemophilia was in an era when the emphasis was on prevention and infusion programs. . . . I never for a moment felt that it was a difficult time getting involved with the families. . . . I knew all of those thirty-seven families really well. . . . My role was a decision-making role from early on.

She discovered, however, that in a lot of ways being a hemophilia nurse in an outpatient setting was professionally "isolating." She welcomed the chance to join the NHF Nursing Committee "with the possibility of forming a nursing network on the national level." She recalled, "A lot of work began at the World Federation of Hemophilia Meeting in New York"; it was "exciting to see that there were people doing the same things, with the same ideas, and same problems; we could help each other."[32]

When she first started working in hemophilia, "it was the Golden Years and there was hope. . . . It was a time of community acceptance and people accepted people with hemophilia." She adds:

Outside of my day-to-day activities with patients, working on the Educational Resources Project was the highlight of my work with NHF. That was the thing I was proudest of and the thing I had the most fun doing.

It was a great group of nurses, who have remained friends ever since. We got together with our babies and with our cribs and baskets and spent hours and hours, days upon days, developing the educational tool which is called the Patient/Family Model.[33]

Karen Meredith helped to develop the hemophilia program for the state of Wisconsin. She recalls "beating the bushes and making phone calls in the evenings" to find patients and to encourage them to come. She credits the director of the Wisconsin program, a well-known pediatric hematologist, Jack Lazerson, with teaching her about hemophilia and creating the program. She attended the first meeting of the NHF Nursing Committee and also attended a WFH meeting, where she presented a paper in which she proposed developing a "more systematic framework for patient education"—the origin of the Patient/Family Model. Recalling that "The thing that made us kind of an interesting cohort is that many of us were pregnant or having babies at the time," she remembers "the camaraderie and closeness." She had had many different experiences with other chronic diseases before working with hemophilia, but said, "It wasn't until I was working with hemophilia that I actually fell in love; fell in love with the people." Meredith added: "The thing that has been so satisfying about hemophilia nursing after comprehensive care arrived, in the Golden Age, is that you could follow the patients over time. You could see them as babies and as they grow and adjust. . . . We were here to share wonderful knowledge of treatment with this population and there was such tremendous self-satisfaction with it."[34]

Legislative Support for Comprehensive Care

During the "Maternal and Child Health Years," data accumulated on an annual basis revealed the growing successes of comprehensive care in terms of health outcomes and cost efficacy. With Peter Levine's effective presentation of the data and the full support of the NHF's advocacy at all levels, the hemophilia program flourished. A first funding extension, which authorized the expenditure of funds for 1978, went through Congress "with no controversy whatsoever as part of a larger package, Public Law 95-83."[35] On November 10, 1978, Public Law 95-626 was signed, providing funding for fiscal years 1979, 1980, and 1981.

In 1981, the Comprehensive Hemophilia Program was brought under Title V (services for women, children, and families at the state level) of the Social Security Act. As a result of NHF advocacy, hemophilia was also determined to be eligible for Special Programs of Regional and National Significance (SPRANS). Since the new Reagan administration was committed to decreasing the responsibilities of the federal government and assigning greater responsibilities to the states, extensive lobbying was necessary to assure a special "set aside" provision, which conserved the existing configuration of the Hemophilia Treatment Center Program and kept it from falling under individual state block grants, which might have resulted in a substantial decrease in funding.[36] As noted at the end of Chapter 5, data on the hemophilia program inspired the Congressional Record to note that the Hemophilia Treatment Center Program was "one of the chronic illness success stories of the decade."

Other Perspectives and Reflections

In later interviews, some physicians who were HTC directors revealed other facets of the situation not captured in health outcome and cost-efficacy data reports. Describing satisfactions gained in the Golden Era—or as some came to call it, the Golden Interval—one doctor spoke of sharing the "successes of a patient . . . who has a black belt in Kung Fu, another who is a cross-country bicycle rider, and another is a captain of his college swimming team." Another noted a special excitement and bond with "successful athletes" and delighted in the fact that so many patients expressed the idea that "they were grateful."[37]

One medical director, Richard Lipton, director of the Hemophilia Treatment Center Program at Long Island Jewish Medical Center, highlighted the extent to which doctors basked in the glory of their patients' successes—and vice versa—adding another dimension to reflections on this period:

I suppose many people who were involved in hemophilia care in the Golden Age probably made some serious mistakes as health professionals in how we approached patients and how we advocated for these programs, and what I mean by that is that we were all on this gigantic high, and I used to—now in retrospect, in a very arrogant fashion—talk about how we were at the cutting edge of scientific breakthroughs . . . and all we'd have to do is fine tune this system and with this wonderful medication and the right team and the right setup, everything would be wonderful.

To the extent we bought into this, . . . and in an inappropriate way, [that] causes the things that people criticize doctors for all the time, which is sort of God-like and omnipotent.

All of these things fed into that, and it was fed to the patients in that way too, who became linked to us in an inappropriate fashion, so that they were a whole piece of this experiment, which can't help but take on certain elements of your own ego trip. I suppose psychiatrists might describe it in terms of transference relationships. . . . This is fine as long as everything is going all right.

I have never in any of my other practice experiences laid myself so open and been so vulnerable to this kind of thing. . . . I'll never again buy into this kind of business where the patient is in collusion with you to sort of further this gigantic ego trip and scientific breakthrough or whatever you want to call it, known as the hemophilia treatment center. . . . They've become wrapped in the importance of furthering hemophilia as a project, as an activity that needs to be promoted.[38]

This sobering assessment is, of course, retrospective. The momentum at the time embraced the entire community. Hailed as heroes by patients and families and as role models by international doctors at the WFH conferences, the U.S. medical directors of HTCs enjoyed frequent travels to meetings at home and abroad. The men with hemophilia who were the new leaders of the NHF shared in this euphoria, and they, too, became involved actively in the WFH. Frank Schnabel, the founder of the international organization, who was spearheading the development of comprehensive care throughout the world as the means to achieve lives of normality and independence, served as a role model for U.S. leaders.[39] Looking back, Keith Hoots, the director of the Gulf States Hemophilia Treatment Center speaks for the hemophilia community physicians when he says, "We were in the Golden Age, and we were the golden boys."[40]

CHAPTER 8

The AIDS Era Begins

The Years of Confusion and Denial, 1980–82

As the 1980s began, a number of changes greeted the hemophilia community. On the political front, Ronald Reagan assumed the presidency of the United States, vowing to return America to its full glory as a recognized, esteemed leader of the world. His ideology expressed itself through strengthening the military while diminishing the role of government in protecting social welfare and civil rights. The mandate to return to conservatism included reshaping domestic policy so that responsibility for payment of many health and welfare services shifted from government back to the individual.[1] Reagan also sought to eliminate what he called "big government" by "do-nothing" federal government agencies and to return power and responsibility to the state level. He accomplished this primarily by distributing block grants to individual states, leaving it up to them how to spend the money, and by reducing the budgets of federal agencies administering health and welfare programs. There was a climate of anxiety and anger among professionals involved in these arenas—the potential of becoming "losers" as a result of the redistribution of funding and power loomed large.

As part of a campaign to slash funding for the entire U.S. Public Health Service, both the Centers for Disease Control (CDC) and the Division of Maternal and Child Health (MCH) were designated for budget cuts. The CDC anticipated a 15 percent budget reduction.[2]

However, as noted in Chapter 7, intensive lobbying by the NHF and its constituency reinforced Congress's perception of "the uniqueness" of the hemophilia population and its usefulness as a chronic illness model. Both the Hemophilia Treatment Center Program and the level of funding allocated were salvaged.

By the early 1980s, neither outside observers nor community insiders considered hemophilia a dreaded disease, but viewed it instead as a chronic illness that could be managed. In this perception the disease had become inseparable from both its cost-effective service delivery model and treatment with Factor concentrates. As "Paul Phillips," then executive director of the NHF said, "The hemophilia success story is summed up by the following equation: Clotting factor concentrates plus comprehensive care equals home infusion therapy, which in turn equals free, independent lives for people with hemophilia."[3]

As we saw at the conclusion of Chapter 7, this did indeed seem to be a golden time. The euphoria of "being placed on a pedestal" and being involved in treating a "good-news" disease solidified the hemophilia treatment center directors' sense of ownership of both "their centers" and "their patients."[4] The "golden boys" and their "golden patients" were linked in a mutual admiration society in a community turned inward. Nurse coordinators, recognized for their ability as decision makers, educators, and data collectors, derived satisfaction from long-term relationships with parents and their children and the growing population of young adults. Some of the plasma company representatives also felt that they had become part of the community as over time they came to know both hemophilia families and HTC physicians and nurse coordinators.

As the NHF's new lay leadership and executive director established financial accountability and instituted corporate governance practices and procedures, the Foundation achieved greater respect from both community members and outsiders. For the first time, in "Paul Phillips," a public health professional with solid academic and professional credentials, was responsible for developing the Foundation's programs. Drawing on his masters degree in public health and executive experience in other health and social agencies, "Phillips" demonstrated his abilities in both advocacy and community organization. Asserting that the NHF chapters were the Foundation's constituency, he invested his energies in improving the central organization's relationship with them and worked to strengthen them. He also began to develop better channels of communication for rapid dissemination of information to the chapters. The new communication technology of telephone conference calls facilitated ongoing dialogue. Frequent evening "meetings" by phone became a recognized part of the community's culture.

By 1982, the efforts of the Director of Habilitation Services of Maternal and Child Health to promote regionalization of the hemophilia treatment center network came to fruition.[5] She understood that an altered configuration of services with a designated lead grantee in each region would lead to better allocation of resources and improved access to quality care for a greater number of people, especially in outlying areas. Despite some remaining gaps and flaws, considerable progress had been made in achieving a greatly improved quality of life for an increasingly larger number of persons with hemophilia—a term those with the disease now indicated that they preferred to "hemophiliacs."

Scientific Advances

The early 1980s also brought scientific advances. Theodore Zimmerman, M.D., who had discovered the von Willebrand Factor while working with Oscar Ratnoff in Ohio (see Chapter 5), had gone to the Scripps Clinic in La Jolla, California, "where he rose from fellow to staff member." As Ratnoff tells the story, Zimmerman's focus was on

[working] out the chemistry of different varieties of von Willebrand's disease, but from a practical point of view [he] made a quantum leap by figuring out how to purify antihemophilic factor on a column which was constructed by attaching the same kind of antibody which he had made in Cleveland to an insoluble base. He could then trickle plasma or a fraction of the plasma through the column, and then the Factor VIII and its attached von Willebrand's Factor would attach to this antibody. He could wash the column then, and there was nothing left but the column itself and the Factor VIII and the Von Willebrand's Factor attached to the column. Then he'd split off the Factor VIII, so that what you got coming out of the column was essentially pure Factor VIII. This was in 1982. And that's what is used today.[6]

The fractionation of pure Factor VIII provided the basis for the development of monoclonal antibody concentrate products in the mid-1980s. Advances in genetic research technology also contributed to the cloning of Factor VIII and the development of genetically engineered concentrates by the end of the decade. Factor VIII was originally cloned at Genentech in Northern California in 1983. "Adam H." recalled visiting that company with "Cliff H." and "Paul Phillips" to hear a presentation by Gordon Vehar and Dick Laun, the scientists primarily involved in the breakthrough. "Adam" remembered that the visit became a celebration of this special event; they called it "Factor VIII Day," and the company gave everyone beanies with "Factor VIII" written on them. For "Adam H." this breakthrough brought the exhilaration of discovery, which he likened to Columbus: "You're driving across the ocean, and that was the moment that you saw land. It isn't the moment you landed, but it's the moment you saw land and you saw the future and you saw where it was—not that you had gotten there."[7]

These discoveries seemed to signal the beginning of "utopia," the time of the cure. The cloning of Factor VIII suggested a paradigm shift toward viewing hemophilia primarily in terms of genetics, not blood. More sophisticated methods for carrier testing (one of which also grew out of Zimmerman's work) gave genetic counselors a basis upon which to discuss options for the future with female relatives of men and boys with hemophilia. The hemophilia community was unified, both in its optimism about the future and in its enjoyment of the present. Retrospectively, this would be viewed as the golden moment before the tragedy, before AIDS and its invasion of the community were recognized, before that disease became the major concern of involved government agencies, NHF, and hemophilia treatment centers.

The Gay Community: "Before" and the Beginning

While the hemophilia community was savoring its Golden Era, the gay community was also luxuriating in the time "before." In *And the Band Played On,* Randy Shilts wrote that "before" meant "innocence, excess, idealism, and hubris." Promiscuity was central to "the raucous Gay movement of the 70s" and "sex was part of political liberation."[8] The legal climate in those years created "the flowering of the jurisprudence of privacy" and "the freedom of intimate association," which gays interpreted as a validation of their right to pursue their alternate lifestyle.[9] There was a strong sense of "communitas," which fostered intimate bonding, and of connecting, which cut across social classes and races, coupled with growing political activism.[10]

By 1980, San Francisco "was acquiring a legendary quality in political circles providing a blueprint for [gay] political success." Bathhouses and sex clubs "thrived, and so did venereal and enteric diseases." The Gay Freedom Day Parade in that year had more than 30,000 marchers and 200,000 spectators. Tapping into the gay community's desire to achieve "respectability," the local blood bank sent mobile collection vans. According to blood bank officials, between 5 and 7 per cent of the donated blood during that year was collected from the gay community.[11]

But 1980 was also the year that "the first isolated gay men began falling ill from strange and exotic ailments."[12] The official documentation of "the beginning" by the Centers for Disease Control (CDC) was in the summer of 1981, when its *Morbidity and Mortality Weekly Report* (*MMWR*) commented on an "unexpected occurrence in five young homosexual Los Angeles men of an unusual and often lethal type of protozoan infection of the lung (pneumocystis carinii pneumonia)."[13] The newsletter noted that some of the men "had an even rarer form of cancer," skin lesions known as Kaposi's sarcoma.[14] By December 1981 the *New England Journal of Medicine* contained articles from three separate groups of physicians in New York and Los Angeles describing "a variety of serious infections as well as Kaposi's sarcoma in the same homosexual population and in patients who had abused intravenous drugs."[15]

In these early days the media "tended to shy away from AIDS, seeing it as a gay story they shouldn't touch." The early reporting, as it appeared in 1982, set the tone for the social construction of AIDS by the media. The disease was politicized and depicted as "a Gay Plague" by the press: a *Philadelphia Daily News* headline read, "Gay Plague Baffling Medical Detectives"; the *Saturday Evening Post* announced, "Being Gay Is a Health Hazard."[16]

As we have seen, the Reagan years brought with them a combined sense of fiscal austerity, which would cut the services needed by people becoming sick from this new disease, and ideological conservatism, which included condemnation of gays by right-wing moralists. Initially labeled as "Gay Cancer" and then as GRID (gay-related immune deficiency), the new disease arrived at a time when "the old religious, moral, and cultural arguments against homosexuality [had] seemed to be collapsing." But as the spread of this disease became linked in the public imagination to male homosexuals, a group who already "occupied a stigmatized position in our society," the "gay visibility and affirmation of the past decade allowed for some very nasty scapegoating."[17] The Centers for Disease Control did not use the terms "GRID" or "Gay Cancer," but referred to the syndrome as "Kaposi's sarcoma and related opportunistic infections." It is likely that the emergence of gays as a "recognized social, cultural, and political minority during the 1970s," shaped the CDC's responses, which included creating a task force to monitor the condition in 1981 and consistently consulting gay groups.[18]

During these early years, research focused primarily on the "gay lifestyle" rather than on the search for a specific organism. One of the first theories about the cause of the syndrome was the use of "poppers," amyl and butyl nitrites, widely used by gay men during intercourse. In May 1982 the British journal *Lancet* published a paper which concluded that "amyl nitrite exposure and sexual promiscuity were associated with the development of Kaposi's sarcoma, as well as histories of mononucleosis and sexually transmitted diseases." Another theory "expressed by a number of doctors, particularly in New York," concerned "overloading of the immune capacity"—and overload theories were linked to the homosexual lifestyle. A Harvard physician suggested that "overindulgence in sex and drugs and the New York City life-style" were responsible for creating the condition.[19]

The coexistence of the different diseases in the same patient led some researchers to the conclusion that this was a syndrome. The noted AIDS researcher and advocate Dr. Mathilde Krim observed, "It was obvious almost from the start of the epidemic that those cases reported to the CDC and counted as AIDS, defined initially as an acquired immune deficiency associated with Kaposi's sarcoma, were only a more advanced stage of a complex, progressive, and apparently irreversible pathological process." She mentions that, in addition to the investigators who considered it possible that an "overload" of the immune system could impair its function sufficiently to make people vulnerable to opportunistic infections, others suggested a novel viral infection transmitted sexually and through blood.[20]

A strange syndrome that primarily affected male homosexuals did not interest or concern most of American society in 1980 or 1981. The tone of what limited press coverage there was and the prevalence of homophobia caused many people to see this syndrome as an aberration affecting a group defined as "other," not as "us." Few contemplated that they could be vulnerable to the same fate which had befallen these gay men.

NHF's Telephone Rings in the Hemophilia AIDS Era

On July 8, 1982, the executive director of the NHF received a phone call from Bruce Evatt, M.D., then Chief of the Host Factors Division of the Centers of Disease Control. He had called to notify NHF that there were three reported cases of immune dysfunction in hemophiliacs with hemophilia A. As "Paul Phillips" remembered the call,

There was some concern that the source was simply a coincidence, or it might be due to their dependence on blood products and that there was a possibility that AIDS was a blood-borne disease. . . . It was at that point and from that point on that this organization became consumed with AIDS, dealing with AIDS, developing programs directed at AIDS, that caused my attention to be distracted from what I considered to be the primary constituency, the chapters.[21]

Evatt recalls that "Phillips" was very concerned about this and was "certainly pressing for immediate kinds of activities and information." He also vividly remembers thinking by that time that the strange malady that had surfaced in the gay community might also affect the blood supply. Although "in 1982 there were many theories about what was causing AIDS," and "speculations were that it was due to anti-sperm antibody, amyl nitrites, or . . . a number of other kinds of possible causes," two things had happened that influenced Evatt's thinking about the disease.[22]

The first was that "Jim Curran's group, Sexually Transmitted Diseases (STD), then the key group in CDC, began investigating a group of individuals that had come down with HIV infection who were all homosexuals and found that a large proportion of the group had had sex with each other." This began to suggest to him "the possibility that it was an infectious agent." The second was a phone call he received in January 1982 from a Florida physician who treated hemophiliacs. One of the physician's hemophilia patients had died of pneumocystis pneumonia, and he asked whether Factor VIII could have become contaminated with pneumocystis. Since the physician had ordered no lymphocyte counts or immune function test for the patient, it was not possible to say that he had AIDS. However, in conjunction with his CDC work in Atlanta, Evatt had a fifteen-year association with hemophilia patients, and he could not recall ever having seen pneumocysitis carinii pneumonia associated with hemophilia. He validated his personal experience by searching through the literature and consulting the FDA. Since the Division for Host Factors distributed pentamidine, the experimental medication used to treat pneumocystis, he asked the clerk in charge of that file to check whether there had been any prior history of hemophilia patients using it. She found none. He asked her to notify him immediately if any such requests should be made in the future.[23]

Evatt recalls that two requests soon arrived, the first in June from Colorado and the second in early July from Ohio. At that point he requested that Dr. Dale Lawrence investigate what was happening in all three cases.[24] Lawrence, a physician who is both an epidemiologist and a tropical medicine parasitologist, was Chief of the Human Leukocyte Antigen Lab at CDC. Because of his studies in the genetics of human immune responses, he had been brought in by the director of the Division of Immunology to study the outbreak of pneumocystis pneumonia.[25]

Lawrence found that the Florida case "was a bit of an iffy AIDS case," because the person had taken cortical steroids and because no immune function tests had been done. He then flew to Denver and on to Ohio on the Fourth of July weekend. Both those cases proved to have the full-blown immune disorder we now call AIDS, and Lawrence recalled thinking, "That was it"—that there would be an epidemic among hemophiliacs by the end of the summer. His concern at the time was that "There was an organism out there which had already infected undoubtedly large numbers of hemophilia patients."[26]

His thinking was influenced by what he called the key group working on AIDS in CDC at that time, the Sexually Transmitted Diseases (STD) group. He credits their training in epidemiology and infectious diseases, and years of experience with enabling them to quickly perceive that "this had to be an infectious disease, even if we didn't *know* it." Other concurrent events reinforced his judgment. The "legionella epidemic and the laboratory correlates of that and the epidemiological investigations" made the CDC researchers attentive to the "possibility of a new organism." Also, the toxic shock syndrome outbreak was a reminder that there could be "new properties of agents that we hadn't put together as a pattern before." The result was that Lawrence and his colleagues "sort of refreshed our minds that we're not omniscient in this field, and we were convinced that we were seeing a new virus or a new epidemic."[27]

Commending the emphasis on "utter precision" and "absolutely quality work" in the CDC Immunology Division's Epidemic Intelligence Service, Lawrence attributed this orientation to the division's director, Dr. Alexander Langmuir, who instilled a rigorous approach to infectious disease epidemiology and a "real disdain for armchair epidemiology." The idea was "to get out there, evaluate the details for yourself, be utterly scrupulous in getting every shred of information, and then account for every person or case one way or another. . . . You don't say, 'There are about twelve cases'; you say, 'Here's my case definition. There were fifteen provisional cases. I now see that twelve meet the case definition and these [other] three do not, because one didn't have this [defining feature] and two didn't have that [defining feature]." Lawrence added, "There's a quality of 'Here's your suitcase. Here's your hat. Be on the next plane and report back twice a day about what you're finding and analyzing.'" He described his colleagues and himself as "epidemic commandos," or perhaps "firefighters." And backing up these investigative epidemiologists were the CDC's world-class laboratories, which Lawrence called "the Supreme Court" of decision on microbes and their identities.[28]

Lawrence recalled some contacts with hemophilia treaters at this time. One was a medical director of an HTC in New York about the Florida case—by this time designated as Case #1—who was originally from the northeast; he also spoke to the medical director of the Denver Hemophilia Treatment Center Program, about Case #2. Both physicians were concerned. Lawrence sensed that "They didn't know what this meant, they didn't know whether it was serious or not; but they were listening"; they "had their patients' best interests at heart."[29]

Lawrence noted that he was essentially "at the working level" and that it was Evatt who was involved with most of the conference calls and official interactions with the hemophilia community, but he did register an impression of "Paul Phillips" at the time. Recalling that "Phillips" has a Masters of Public Health, "as opposed to an MBA or another degree and that he had an attentiveness to CDC and the epidemic method and the kind of data analysis that they were presenting," Lawrence said "that made it easier for him to see the trends, or at least to accept them." With regard to Evatt and his role in this opening phase of the Hemophilia AIDS Era, he noted that "Dr. Evatt is really a brilliant epidemiologist. He could pick up or sense the validity of one of these epidemic trends very early." Lawrence felt that Evatt understood what was happening without Lawrence's having to present hard documentation.[30]

Following the July 8 phone call to the NHF, Evatt sent a letter to "Marcus Victor" as medical co-director of the NHF, reporting the three cases and suggesting that "it was probably a viral disease being transmitted in blood and in blood products."[31] Regarding this letter "Victor" said: "The trouble was, when did we really think it was going to be a problem for hemophilia? . . . Not for at least a year after the first cases. We thought they were spurious. There was a *Lancet* article showing that little kids [who were leukemics] got T.B. on units [because their immunity was suppressed] . . . There was a whole literature on immunosuppression—we thought this was from the concentrate. We thought it wasn't really AIDS in the same way."[32]

By July 14, 1982, only six days after the initial phone call, the NHF sent out a notice to its chapters in the official newsletter, *Hemophilia Newsnotes,* entitled "Hemophilia Patient Alert #1." It referred to the three cases reported by the CDC, describing them as "rare and unusual infections associated with a condition in which there is a decrease in the body's ability to combat disease." It noted that this condition may have developed "as a result of an unknown potentially immunosuppressive agent. One hypothesis that is being investigated by the CDC is that the agent may be a virus transmitted similarly to the hepatitis virus by blood or blood products." The notice emphasized by the use of italics that "It is important to note at this time the risk of contracting this immunosuppressive agent is *minimal,* and CDC is not recommending any change in blood product use." The message is repeated at the bottom of the page with a heading in bold print saying "IMPORTANT" and the directive "If there are any questions, contact your physician or hemophilia treatment center." Two days later, the CDC's *Morbidity and Mortality Weekly Re-*

port (*MMWR*) published an article reporting the three cases, noting that two of the persons reported had died. It also noted that a process of review had determined that no two of the patients had received concentrate from the same lots.[33]

On July 27, the CDC convened a meeting in Washington, D.C., that brought together representatives of the plasma manufacturers, the NHF, the blood banks, the Red Cross, and the American Society of Hematology to discuss the few hundred total cases of the condition and the three hemophilia cases. The NHF's president and a medical co-director attended. Bruce Evatt recalled:

Obviously there was a tremendous amount of skepticism, especially on the part of the blood banks, that this was even a real disease and that we were alarmist in thinking that three hemophiliacs would be even remotely associated with a blood-borne disease at this point in time. I think that the Hemophilia Foundation at that point became very alarmed about the possibility and began pushing for development. [But] I don't think that the NHF medical leaders were at all convinced, thinking it might not even be a real disease at that point. I think that everybody was demanding that we collect more patients, and so for the rest of 1982 we collected several more hemophilia patients, and we began looking for transfusion-associated cases.[34]

Over the next several months NHF continued to communicate with its constituency about the situation through separately designated mailings: a series of medical bulletins went to treaters and chapter advisories were sent to the chapters, who were asked to communicate the information to their members. In Medical Bulletin #2, dated July 30, the NHF medical leadership advised physicians of the CDC notice urging the report of Kaposi's sarcoma and included "Victor's" promise that "I will keep you posted." They added, "More evidence is needed to determine whether the three cases are part of the AIDS pattern."

Many of the hemophilia treater informants first learned about this developing situation from the *MMWR* and NHF medical bulletins, and the initial stage of communication with patients and their families reflected a traditional medical model. There was skepticism about the true nature of the "disease" on the part of the medical leaders. In addition to this kind of conservatism, "Victor" expressed his feelings about communication at that time: "Until you had to tell them [patients] that it was definitive, that you could say what you could or couldn't do, or that you could offer a therapeutic intervention, I did not feel that we should become a 'ticker tape' operation where every piece of information should be fed, because it would wreak havoc."[35] The Golden Era had established a pattern among the members of the hemophilia community of looking to their medical directors for opinions, particularly in matters defined as "medical." The community rarely brought in outsiders as consultants or speakers at meetings, and the array of physicians who were treaters in the early 1980s was considered "the best and the brightest." The community had a sense of "Victor's" reputation as "brilliant," as a "Renaissance" doctor who looked at the total picture. Did reliance on his judgment initially lull other hemophilia treaters, as well as patients and families, into complacency? If he wasn't alarmed, if he favored the "immune overload theory," why should any drastic actions be taken?

In the past, NHF's medical leadership had demonstrated vision in matters beyond clinical care and research. They had led the community forward by promoting the comprehensive care model and controlling negotiations with plasma manufacturers. However, as specialists, their medical training and clinical research experience were, like that of other specialists, focused on their area of expertise. They did not share the same broad frame of reference as CDC physicians. Few if any would have had a public health perspective or training in depth in epidemiology. They functioned primarily as "treaters," not as "preventers." Also, the expressed attitude about not constantly funneling every new development or smallest piece of information to patients and their families reflects a composite of these physicians' generation-specific training and their life experience in the hemophilia community. Concern about the consequences of revealing every detail when there was still confusion about what to do to ameliorate the situation was not aberrant behavior. This attitude in fact represents what was considered acceptable medical model thinking throughout history, until very recently.

Attitudes about Disease

This long-established attitude of those in positions of medical authority has been mirrored in both nonfiction and fiction, perhaps nowhere more aptly than in *The Plague* by Albert Camus. "The public must not be alarmed" was the official medical stance taken by the physician who is the central character, and he added, "All that can be said at present is that we are dealing with a special type of fever and it's unwise to jump to conclusions." He would not venture to name or to describe the nature of the disease that had suddenly appeared in the little town until he had received "the post postmortem." An older doctor, who had been to China, indicated that he didn't have to wait for "any post postmortem," since he had "seen cases like this twenty years ago." After there were eleven deaths in forty-eight hours in the community, a citizen asked what the name of the disease was. The physician replied, "That I shan't say, and anyhow you wouldn't gain anything by knowing." In the early days of this fictional (and metaphorical) plague, "the townspeople were like everybody else, wrapped up in themselves. . . . They went on doing business, arranged for journeys, and formed views. . . . They fancied themselves free and the dead, fantastically unreal." The physician stated that "a few cases didn't make an epidemic, they merely call for serious precautions."[36]

In these beginning years of the AIDS era, skepticism about the credibility of the blood-borne virus theory promulgated by Evatt, Lawrence, and others at the CDC, was widespread, both inside and outside of the hemophilia community. Evatt and Lawrence encountered this attitude in physicians, blood bankers, microbiologists, and the FDA. Possibly the mistake the CDC had committed several years earlier, with dire predictions of a "Swine Flu" epidemic that never occurred, added to a perception of lack of credibility. Evatt also noted another possibility, that "people thought we were making this disease up just to generate increased funding"; it was general knowledge that the CDC had to cut its budget by 15 percent. He was also aware of the perspective of physicians who were used to thinking about individual patients and had not been trained to think in terms of entire populations, noting that "there was a lack of understanding of epidemiology and its usefulness." Evatt believes that his own background helped him to pick out the trends that were meaningful as they followed developments very closely. In reflecting on the situation, he added: "You have to realize that at that time all infectious diseases had been conquered. There were no more new infectious diseases. To suddenly come up with a devastating disease that was so crazy made it difficult for people to believe."[37]

This was the challenge Evatt and Lawrence faced at a meeting of the NHF's newly reconstituted Medical and Scientific Advisory Council (MASAC) on October 2–3, 1982.[38] MASAC now included the chairpersons of the NHF committees that had arisen in the late 1970s. Regina Butler, chair of the Nursing Committee, cites this meeting as "the exact moment when I thought—'Oh, my God, this is it. This is a horrible thing, and it's going to kill our patients.'" She went on to describe the meeting.

Dr. Evatt came and said, "You know, this is a virus which, although we don't know what it is, we think it's in the blood product and that it causes immune deficiency that cannot be cured. We think it can be transmitted to hemophiliacs through the blood product." And at that moment, at that talk, listening to him, I thought, "This is it. From now on it's never going to be the same." I just had a profound feeling, a sense of doom that this is really major stuff. And, of course, ultimately it turned out to be true.

But the physicians' voices, representing medical authority at that meeting, emphasized gathering more data before drawing conclusions, and Butler did not openly argue against this, feeling, "Well, what do I really know? What can I say?"[39]

Her behavior at her HTC in Philadelphia was more assertive, however. Before the MASAC meeting, before the new disease was called AIDS, and before NHF, MASAC, and CDC went public with any connection between HIV and hemophilia, her center had become involved in a unique program. Since the 1970s the center had sponsored parent groups in conjunction with a local child guidance clinic, at which specific topics of interest were discussed and relaxation techniques were practiced. As a result, Butler notes, "Parents had become so connected and empowered to deal with crisis, . . . when one of the parents read about what was identified in the paper as 'the Gay Plague,' they wondered whether it would affect hemophiliacs, because people get hepatitis [through contaminated blood]. And if gay people have this nebulous virus that is causing them to be sick, [we] wonder if that is in the blood supply and will cause our children to be sick." The parents had called a meeting, to which they invited Butler and the HTC's medical director. They inquired about the possibility of starting a designated donor cryoprecipitate program for children. Butler and the medical director reacted positively: "We don't know enough about it to know if it's true or not, but you're right. Hepatitis is transmitted through the blood, and we don't know. If it's a concern of yours, let's work on trying to do something so that you will feel in control of your blood product." Mobilized by this threat, the families and the treatment center worked together to start a designated-donor cryo program. The results were evident in 1990: Butler reported that the youngest child in their program with HIV infection was fourteen years old and there were eight-year-olds who had never used concentrate.[40]

In October 1982, after the MASAC meeting, Butler and the medical director sent letters to the families requesting informal meetings. Butler said, "We had to honestly tell them that there was a lot that we didn't know, but that we did know [now] about AIDS and hemophilia." Although many of the parents who had not already switched to cryoprecipitate chose to do so now, Butler recalled that it was a time of "a lot of confusion and trying to understand the facts." After so many years of using concentrates, "cryo was like a foreign language to most treaters." Many parents didn't realize that cryo could be used in a home program; it did entail having special frost-free freezers and thawing and "pulling" the cryo, but, Butler said, "it is not that complicated." She recalled that some parents began to restrict their children's activities, feeling that if they didn't bleed, they wouldn't have to be treated. She also noted that, ironically, some of the patients who did not follow the rules, "some of the most noncompliant patients, who never did what they were supposed to do and infused less often—they are the ones who escaped."[41]

After reading the reports in the *MMWR*, one other HTC medical director began a designated-donor cryoprecipitate program, and following the MASAC meeting, several other treatment centers proceeded to offer the alternative of cryoprecipitate, particularly for children. Two programs that had used cryo all along had been the butt of much teasing for being "dinosaurs"—the Seattle program and Oscar Ratnoff's program in Ohio. But through December 1982 most of the treaters continued to treat as usual.

"Adam H." recalls first hearing about hemophilia and AIDS in July 1982, when "Paul Phillips" called him to say that "Cliff H." would be attending the Washington meeting to discuss the topic. "Adam's" reaction was, "It sounds like a medical problem. Let it be referred to the medical director." He noted, "I didn't personalize on it, . . . didn't take it very seriously." He recalls "Cliff" making the decision after the Washington meeting to reconstitute MASAC so that "medical experts" could meet regularly to look at medically relevant issues including, but not solely restricted to, AIDS; genetic engineering was another topic to be discussed. "Adam" asserted that MASAC was established to be advisory only; the ultimate decision maker at NHF remained the board of directors.[42]

Of the informants with hemophilia for this book, all but two continued to treat as usual at this time. "Brett H.," who was from Ohio and was born in the 1950s, had listened to Ratnoff over the years and was already on cryo at that point.[43] "Harold H.," one of the two youngest men, called the CDC directly to inform himself and then sought to persuade his local treatment center to provide cryo. Although initially resistant, the center finally agreed.

In November 1982, NHF sent the plasma manufacturers the MASAC recommendations that the donor pool be restricted. *The NHF Narrative Chronology* noted that "many months before the U.S. Public Health Service, NHF was the first organization to demand donor screening as a preventive method to safeguard the nation's blood supply."[44] Uniting in an effort to make the nation's blood supply safer was something that everyone in the hemophilia community could comfortably promote. There was no confusion about the merits of this stance inside the community. By early December CDC had additional confirmed AIDS cases and one more suspected case among people with hemophilia A, making the total in the hemophilia population now eight confirmed cases, of whom five had died, and two suspected cases. All of these patients had been exposed to Factor VIII concentrates and had not been exposed to the other "groups known to be at risk." At that point CDC recommended that all hemophilia patients be advised of "the risk."[45]

CHAPTER 9

The AIDS Era, 1982–85
Tension Mounts, Conflicts Erupt

Tension mounted in the winter of 1982–83. The CDC sent out messages that conveyed an increasing sense of alarm and concern regarding the hemophilia community and the AIDS epidemic, while the official voice of the NHF, in newsletters and bulletins transmitted to local chapters, continued to be soothing and to advocate watchful waiting. This hesitancy to advise changes in treatment inside the community was in marked contrast to NHF's assertive stance promoting blood donor screening. AIDS cases continued to appear in persons with hemophilia, but the numbers were still very small. In the early 1980s hardly anyone in the community actually knew any individual who had become sick; the threat that this plague would actually touch their lives still did not seem very real.

On December 10, 1982, the CDC recommended that all hemophilia patients be advised of the risk. On December 11, NHF held an executive committee conference call that resulted in the decision to send out Chapter Advisory #5, quoting the *Morbidity and Mortality Weekly Report* (*MMWR*) in reporting "an increased concern that AIDS may be transmitted by blood products."[1] In the advisory NHF advocated "no change in treatment" but suggested that newborns and mild cases should use cryoprecipitate and patients who had not used concentrate before should not begin to use it. The advisory also stated:

It is important to note, that while there is insufficient data to directly link the spread of AIDS to concentrates, there is an increased concern that AIDS may be transmitted through blood products.

It is the NHF's point of view that patients and parents should be aware of the potential risks. If you have any questions regarding this matter, they should be directed to your physician and/or NHF.[2]

As 1983 began, NHF increased its efforts to persuade the Public Health Service to take precautionary measures to safeguard the blood supply and to adapt the MASAC resolutions recommending donor screening.

On January 4, 1983, a meeting of the ad hoc Advisory Committee of the U.S. Public Health Service was held at the CDC in Atlanta. The meeting included the American Red Cross, the American Association of Blood Banks, the National Hemophilia Foundation, the National Gay Task Force, the Pharmaceutical Manufacturers Association, representing the plasma manufacturing companies, and representatives of the NIH and the FDA. Dr. Bruce Evatt of the CDC recalled that he wanted two results to come from that meeting. The first was to "have all the homosexuals screened before giving blood" and the second was "a surrogate test using hepatitis B as a core antibody marker." Instead, he recalled, "The meeting turned into a circus; it was just a zoo."[3] One CDC colleague pounded the table with his fist and asked: "How many people have to die? How many deaths do you need? . . . Give us the threshold of deaths that you need in order to believe that this is happening, and we'll meet at that time and start doing something." But the blood bankers remained skeptical that AIDS could be transmitted through blood; some FDA officials were still unconvinced that AIDS actually existed; and the gay groups called screening out homosexuals "scapegoating." In fact, the San Francisco Coordinating Committee of Gay and Lesbian Services had issued a policy paper asserting that "donor screening was reminiscent of miscegenation blood laws that divided black blood from white blood and was similar in concept to the World War II rounding up of Japanese Americans in the western half of the country to minimize the possibility of espionage."[4]

One of CDC's "top virologists made the case for testing all blood products," stating that since "virtually everyone in AIDS risk groups—by then including hemophilia—had been exposed to hepatitis B, antibodies [to it] remain in the blood." Based on the fact that 88 percent of the blood from gay AIDS patients had hepatitis core antibodies, he argued that testing for these antibodies might not screen out all AIDS carriers, but it would reduce the threat of transmission of AIDS through transfusions. Rather than discussing this issue, the blood bankers continued to ridicule the CDC representatives for "overstating the facts." The president of the New York Blood Center spoke of the evidence being "very soft" and noted, "There are only a handful of cases among hemophiliacs." The director of the blood bank at Yale University Hospital, who was chairing the FDA's Advisory Committee on Blood Safety, said: "We are contemplating all these wide-ranging measures because one baby got AIDS from a person who later came down with AIDS and there may be a few other cases." The CDC group was enraged. An assistant CDC director said, "To bury our heads in the sand and say 'Let's wait for more cases' is not an adequate public health measure." At that point Evatt restated the hemophilia data and pointed out that there had never before been an incident of this nature in the hemophilia population.[5]

In the end, each group stood by its own agenda, no agreements were reached, and nothing changed. The blood bankers were concerned about attracting new donors, the FDA was smarting from "their turf being so brazenly invaded by the epidemiologists from Atlanta," and the gay groups were concerned about their fight for respectability being undermined. The hemophilia community persisted in looking outward rather than inward and focused on screening out the "groups at risk." Each group was firmly entrenched in preserving its self-interest and unable to believe that it might have made a tremendous mistake. Evatt was dismayed; he had not anticipated that the CDC would be unable to influence public policy and would have to stand alone.[6]

Two days after the CDC meeting, the American Association of Blood Banks (AABB) held a meeting in Washington. Attendees included the blood banking group, government agencies, the National Gay Task Force, and the National Hemophilia Foundation. After the meeting the Gay Task Force and the blood banking industry issued the statement that "Direct or indirect questions about a donor's sexual preference are inappropriate." Gay groups cheered "the preservation of gay rights" and "the human right to privacy and individual choice."[7] NHF, however, continued to press for donor screening and the introduction of surrogate testing for hepatitis B. Dissatisfied with the inaction of the group that had met at the CDC and disturbed by the statement issued by the AABB, NHF's MASAC issued a comprehensive statement to the plasma fractionation and blood-banking industries as well as to the government agencies, outlining steps to safeguard the blood supply.[8] On January 17, NHF issued a combined medical bulletin and a chapter advisory including the specific MASAC recommendations.[9] NHF then contacted the media to state its case. This stance created what Executive Director "Paul Phillips" recalled as

a pretty rough time, where they [the media] called it the "hemo-homo wars." They tried to pit hemophiliacs against homosexuals. We were then approached by . . . right-wing groups to engage the National Hemophilia Foundation in this war against "sin." . . . I'm really proud of the role of the hemophilia community in resisting these demagogues in trying to exploit this horrible situation.

As the organized world of hemophilia, we will not cast stigma on anyone. That was a very firm position. That was strongly adhered to and promoted by our president, "Cliff H." The chairman of our AIDS Task Force for the next three or four years is a religious fundamentalist Christian and he would not buy into that. . . . I have great respect for "Cliff H." in going beyond and appreciating what NHF's role should be, that we should not cross social value boundaries. I think it was very important to have his leadership in this regard.[10]

"Adam H." recalled that exactly at this time the NHF received a confidential status report that, "in retrospect, confirm[ed] the Golden Era." Ultimately published as a journal article, the report showed that in the years before AIDS, "liver disease, next to bleeding, was the leading cause of death among persons with hemophilia and that when you do age adjustment, the expected life span of a person with hemophilia was essentially the same as the nonhemophiliac population."[11]

Diverging Opinions

Another important event took place in January 1983, signaling the first solid indication that the views of the NHF's medical leadership would be challenged and that other perspectives would begin to emerge. At the NHF Executive Committee meeting held on January 21, "Adam H." insisted on being the one to take the minutes. He recalled thinking, "as a lawyer, from a litigation perspective and from various other perspectives," that these minutes would eventually be some of the most important in NHF history, in relation to AIDS and HIV infection. He emphasized that the minutes, as he wrote them, stated the agenda was to be limited to AIDS and related topics. He noted that the view expressed by two physician leaders was that "NHF was devoting too much of its time and energy to AIDS and neglecting other areas" and that "our AIDS advisories were heightening the fear of the community."[12] Other physicians argued that the NHF was pursuing an appropriate level of activity. In fact, most attendees supported the NHF's approach. This difference of opinions marked the initial split both within the medical community and between some lay and medical leaders.

The NHF Executive Committee approved and endorsed the general approach of the AIDS Task Force and the MASAC recommendations of January 14, stating that "the NHF should continue to provide credible, accurate information and not try to alarm patients or to shield them in a paternalistic fashion." Noting that this decision was unanimous, "Adam H." confirmed that this meeting "was the first step along the road of clear, very gut-level policy disagreement between the direction that the patients and NHF wanted to go in contrast with the direction that some of the medical leadership wanted to go"; it stated "the underlying philosophical perspective as to how we approached problems over the ensuing period of time."[13] The subsequent resignation of "Dr. Marcus Victor" as medical co-director was the beginning of a redistribution of power and a diminishing of medical sovereignty that would continue in the 1980s and rise to a crescendo by the early 1990s.[14]

In other ways, however, the medical and lay leadership remained united. One 1983 decision not to act reveals the continuation of a value system long shared by both treaters and patients: an emphasis on keeping down the cost of blood products. When a plasma manufacturer revealed the development of a heat-treated blood product, "Adam H." noted that the cost was "twice the price of their non-heat-treated product." At that time he felt

There was no economic justification for doubling that price. They did so, I believe, on the marketing expectation that the fear of AIDS would drive the demand, stampede its use. Price would be no object and they would make a killing. [But] there was a clear rejection of the product on two grounds: (1) its efficacy had not been proven, and (2) there was insufficient data as to whether or not heat treatment of the product would cause molecular changes to the protein, thereby causing more problems and perhaps increasing the incidence of inhibitors.

In my judgment, had the pricing been different, the opposition to the product on scientific grounds would not have occurred. A whole lot of history that happened thereafter was frozen in by those initial positions that were very difficult to change.

. . . Six months later another plasma manufacturer came out with a product. The price got reduced so there was a one- or two-cent differential between heat-treated and non-heat-treated product. But now the doctors were stuck with their scientific opposition.[15]

In fact, several informants who are treaters stressed that they based their opposition on the grounds that in trials the heating process had not been able to kill the hepatitis virus in the blood products. Several other informants who were not treaters, including those from the CDC, mentioned the probability that the product's high cost may have been the chief motivation in NHF's not endorsing purchasing it. For himself, "Adam" noted that this was "the one occasion in which I decided to do personally what was not reflected in what I chose to advocate on behalf of NHF." He switched to the heat-treated product based on "a gut feeling, not having to do with the rationale" and on the encouragement of "Eugene H.," who had been a former nurse coordinator and who at about this time "became a salesperson for a plasma company."[16]

"Eugene H." recalled that the decision of the NHF medical leaders not to endorse the new product helped to motivate him to take a job with the manufacturing company that was producing it. He felt that heat-treating the product made sense and that striving for safer products was important. He also acknowledged that joining the company enabled him to afford to use the product.[17] During that time, other persons with hemophilia also began to work as representatives of plasma manufacturing companies. No longer solely dependent upon the policies of their local treatment center directors, they became enmeshed with industry. By late 1983 four of the twelve hemophilia informants had personally chosen not to continue the use of the regular concentrates: two had previously elected to use cryo, and two were already using the new heat-treated products. "Adam" mused, "The problem with the application for heat-treated product was that when it was filed with the FDA, it was designed to treat hepatitis, and the problem was it probably didn't work. But the problem also was: 'Who in their right mind would not have pasteurized milk over raw milk?'"[18]

In *And the Band Played On,* Randy Shilts refers to 1983 as a "year of denial" of the gravity of the problem in all quarters. It was also a year of adherence to values that were inappropriate for the situation at hand. The U.S. hemophilia community leadership would continue to make decisions about the merits of a life-sustaining treatment based upon knee-jerk reactions to cost. The context of the academic medical center, within which most of the key medical decision makers worked, fostered a persistent belief in the importance of maintaining low costs while maximizing bringing in funding to support the personnel involved in running the HTCs. In addition, by 1983, viewing blood as "a product" within an economic framework was a given. Neither the professionals working at treatment centers and at the NHF nor the younger persons with hemophilia had paused to reflect upon how this commodification of blood and the intertwining of a commercial product and health care delivery had come about. The first generation of men with hemophilia who were now in leadership positions initially avoided thinking about the threat of AIDS touching them or their brothers personally; it was too awful to face. Therefore, they allowed the question of how to respond to AIDS to be cast as a medical decision, deferring once again to the medical leadership of NHF and its familiar ways of doing business.

Dr. Oscar Ratnoff, who since the mid-1960s had persisted in advocating the use of cryoprecipitate while warning of the dangers of bloodborne disease in pooled products, had attended the initial meeting called by the CDC in July 1982. He recalls "sitting in the back of the room and saying, 'Gee, if they're debating whether this is infectious or not—and that's what they're doing—I have the perfect set-up.'" Back in Cleveland he had two groups: the adult patients he had treated with cryoprecipitate and the pediatric patients who had been treated with concentrates. He went home and enlisted a colleague to study "small groups of patients with classical hemophilia treated in the two different ways." He found "that those treated with the lyophilized concentrate material had severe impairment of their immune systems and those treated with the cryoprecipitate were okay." Ratnoff published these findings in an article that appeared in the *New England Journal of Medicine* in 1983. He described his impression of "the resistance of the hemophilia community" as "unbelievable to me." In particular, he recalled an encounter he had with a man from Northern Ohio: "He didn't care what I found. He wasn't going to advise anybody to stop using the commercial material." Even a year later the "medical advisors of the National Hemophilia Foundation said this was ridiculous and that there wasn't any difference between the immune status of people on cryoprecipitate vs. concentrates." Ratnoff also recalled reading in an NHF publication that there were "doctors who were hysterical about AIDS," which he felt was "a direct barb" intended for him. He said that he didn't mind these attitudes in "a lay person" but found them disturbing in scientifically trained people.[19]

Hemophilia Informants Face HIV and AIDS

As mentioned above, "Eugene H." left his position as a nurse coordinator in a treatment center to work for the plasma industry. He described a concern that provided the impetus for him to leave in 1983, when heat-treated concentrate first came out:

Hemophilia treaters from academic institutions did not for the most part switch to using heat-treated products in the beginning because there was not enough research information that it was safer. I'm more a "shoot from the hip" kind of clinician and the theoretical basis for the product being safer was there, in my estimation. There were pioneers around the country who started using it right away. Obviously history has shown that heat kills the AIDS virus. But there were a lot of people in a lot of centers who were slow getting on it.[20]

"Irwin H.," one of the older group of informants, recalls that at his treatment center "they seem[ed] to keep hemophiliacs somewhat isolated, . . . very much separated and mis[informed] or not informed at all." In the early 1980s "Irwin H." said the information he received was that "there was a disease going around in the blood that was very unlikely to affect any hemophiliacs, but we should know about it." He went on to say

They said they had just found out about it and were letting us know that it could be in the blood, but to have a bleed and not treat it was more serious than being treated for the bleed and that the chance of getting HIV and AIDS wasn't that large. It was such a small chance that you should go ahead and treat [as usual].

Now by my being a heavy user of product, I'm supposed to have contracted it [HIV] in '84. . . . At the time that I was informed about the product having AIDS, I was never given a chance or told that I would have an option [for treatment]. There were options that I could have taken a look at . . . like taking cryo versus the concentrate. At the time . . . I was just told to keep treating; the treatment wasn't as bad as what would happen if I did not treat.[21]

"Irwin H." also remembered these years as the time of product recalls. He used to buy a large supply of product to keep at home. On one occasion he was called by the treatment center and alerted that others who had used product with the same lot numbers as what he then had had come down with "full-blown AIDS." After the phone call, a man from the hospital came to his house and brought his supply of product back to the hospital; Johnson was told not to even touch it. The gravity of the situation reached him at that moment: "It really hit me with a thrust which was like a bullet in the chest, because I came through all these negative things and restrictions and all, and here I am where I am free, and to say now that the thing that freed me is going to kill me was just overwhelming."[22]

Another informant, "Daniel H.," remembered that up to this time he had not been secretive about having hemophilia. However, when HIV became connected with hemophilia, he "went completely private"; by 1984 "HIV phobia" was rampant in the community where he lived. At this time he also sometimes "began to let a bleed go and to treat myself with small doses of concentrates." He noted that this was not what was being advocated by "national leadership," but "every person is different." He reflected on the role of denial in his life in a 1990 interview: "Denial still occupies the majority of my waking hours with hemophilia. With regard to HIV infection, I guess I'm at a stage where I was with hemophilia before, where I tried to use denial 99 percent of the time."[23] "Gregory H." recalled that he first became aware of AIDS in 1982 after the CDC discovered the earliest cases of Kaposi's sarcoma, but at that time "AIDS was like a small dark cloud on the horizon." He was "vaguely aware, but it didn't seem to have much bearing on us."[24]

Then came "the traumatic learning period," for physicians as well as patients—which ultimately included having to become aware of recommendations regarding having children.[25] During these first years the responses of most treaters reflected their medical training and the impact of the contexts within which they worked. They did not think that the first hemophilia patients who came down with pneumocystis pneumonia represented the beginning of an epidemic. Dr. Frederick Rickles, one of the leaders of the NHF's MASAC, recalls:

I think it was part denial and part the natural skepticism that all physicians are taught in medical school to develop. I think that part of the natural history of what others have called neglect on the part of the medical community of this epidemic is really an outgrowth of the skepticism that this was real. Until you see sufficient data, people tend not to change treatment programs that are making a difference.[26]

Rickles went on to say that he was "so happy," that "everyone was so happy with how efficacious concentrate therapy was in keeping people working, in school, and leading normal lives, . . . that nobody wanted to change what was a very effective program." Although he was aware that "Dr. Ratnoff and others were opposed to the use of concentrates," he noted "the trade-off was made by many." He went on to say, "since cryo was not easy to use, people weren't going to treat themselves as much, and they were going to get joint disease. So that is the bargain with the devil, if you will; in retrospect, that is what was done." Rickles, who teaches courses in medical ethics and legal ethics in medicine, believes in "the principle of 'over-truth'"—he has always told patients everything he knows. He found the years between 1982 and 1985 "a very difficult time, particularly because there wasn't good information out yet." He said it remains to be seen whether there are geographic differences in the incidence of AIDS and noted that "no one really knew what to tell patients." He repeated that "doctors are slow to change standard treatment, and clearly we were guilty of being too slow, but MASAC, as early as 1982, began to consider this and certainly by 1983 was active in pursuing better approaches to treatment."[27]

Dr. Shelby Dietrich had gone to "the famous meeting of the CDC in Atlanta" in January 1983, flying overnight from the West Coast because she had "some kind of subconscious idea that this must be awfully important." The first California meeting about AIDS was held for patients in 1983. The main speaker was a physician who had worked with AIDS patients from the earliest recognition of the condition. He talked about the disease and "scared everybody to death"—but "it was in gay men." Dietrich recalls feeling that

We really didn't have evidence specifically that it was transmitted through concentrate. There was a suspicion. No one knew what the agent was. I think 1983 was one of the most difficult years I've ever spent, due to the uncertainty and the tension. We had no ill patients. We simply had all these people we were trying to reassure.

We were being reassuring, and I think, unfortunately, some people feel betrayed by that. I don't feel that we betrayed anyone. I think we did our very best with the information that we had. I don't know any group that worked harder or worried more than we did.[28]

When Dr. Craig Kessler entered the world of hemophilia as a young medical director of an HTC on the East Coast, he had what he describes as "a stroke of luck." He was interested in "some of the newer concentrates that had been developed using heat treatment as a technique to get rid of hepatitis," so in 1982 he started a study at his treatment center. He calls this "a stroke of luck" because many of the patients who were randomized and received the heat-treated product are still HIV negative.[29]

David Agle, M.D., a psychiatrist who had worked with Oscar Ratnoff since "I was a fledgling house officer" and had been a pioneer in integrating a mental health component into comprehensive care for hemophilia, views the situation slightly differently.

One of Dr. Ratnoff's opinions was that while cryoprecipitate is excellent stuff, the lyophilized plasma products [concentrate] . . . he considered a "cesspool" of whatever goes into them. Unhappily he had been proven right, of course, with AIDS, but even before that with hepatitis. Dr. Ratnoff became somewhat of a controversial figure, because he would stand up—it was sort of like it was against motherhood. Some people thought because he said, "You've got to be careful with this stuff, it's not necessarily so wonderful"—many in the hemophilia community and care providers saw him as being too conservative and [were] saying, "You're against us taking care of ourselves; you're too paternalistic," and so on. The home care movement was made possible by lyophilized products, because otherwise you couldn't do much self-treatment. Unhappily it got us into the AIDS Era. Of course, if the product had been cleaned up to begin with, none of this would have happened. In other words, there's obviously nothing wrong with the home care movement and with the comprehensive care that has promoted it. It's the medication, the product itself, that technology didn't advance enough in the beginning to clean up.[30]

The decision of government regulators not to intervene early on and the increasingly held view of blood as a product to be purchased as inexpensively as possible were both well within the mainstream of the

American culture and value system and were certainly embedded within the hemophilia community. The contentious gap between the perspective of the epidemiologists at the CDC and that of clinician decision makers in the hemophilia community prolonged the status quo. The first generation of adult hemophilia leaders, who had gained so much as a result of life with concentrates, were equally reluctant to give up what had given them the American dream and what they perceived would give their blood brothers the same opportunities.

Fortunately, the impasse was broken by Bruce Evatt's persistence in getting the CDC to support testing of the heat-treated product and the resultant finding in 1984 that heat *did* in fact kill the AIDS virus. In August 1984, Evatt presented his research and discussed "preliminary virus inactivation reports." By September he reported, "Heat treatment was effective in killing or destroying the HIV virus that was present in 'HIV spiked' clotting Factor."[31] Subsequently, in October 1984, NHF's MASAC recommended the use of heat-treated Factor, a stance that was bolstered by the CDC's citing the MASAC recommendation in the *MMWR* and supporting NHF's position. Within eight months the FDA licensed the enzyme-linked immunosorbent assay or ELISA test, which could detect the presence of HIV antibodies. The NHF considered that at last a "safety net was in place," consisting of donor deferral, virus inactivation, and HIV antibody testing. In April 1985 the Western Blot Test was developed, and by May both the ELISA and Western Blot Tests were in use to test all antibodies for HIV. This would require a new set of decisions and new policies from the government and the NHF leadership.

CHAPTER 10

The AIDS Era, 1985–88

The Hemophilia Community
Rises to the Challenge

Availability of heat-treated blood products and testing technologies ushered in the next phase of the hemophilia AIDS era. Rather than resulting in a sense of progress and comfort, however, testing resurrected old fears associated with discrimination. Many men with hemophilia hesitated to be tested for HIV, worrying that confidentiality might not be preserved and job discrimination and social ostracism might result. Ever responsive to its vocal constituency, the National Hemophilia Foundation did not advocate the necessity of testing at this stage. Many men who had been open about having hemophilia began to retreat, as "Daniel H." reported he did (see Chapter 9), into a private world of their blood brothers and their families.

In 1985 denial and confusion still persisted, shaping the behavior of both treaters and patients. As "Lloyd H." recalled,

In 1984 everyone was still optimistic. They thought that once there was a test, in six to twelve months or something like that, there would be a cure for this. No problem. . . . Even after people with hemophilia were tested, they still did not understand [whether] the fact that people had antibodies meant that they had an active infection or not. . . . There was still debate among the hemophilia treaters as to whether having the antibody was even good or not good and whether there was an active infection or not.

"Lloyd" recalled that his treater in fact said it might be good to have antibodies.[1] Some treaters said the opposite, while still others said that "not to treat a bleed was more serious than being treated for the bleed and the chance of getting HIV and AIDS wasn't that large, so go ahead and treat."[2]

The Ascendancy of Mental Health Professionals

Many patients lost confidence in the judgment of their treaters. Some felt they had been told only partial truths initially, and as ever-changing information and advice followed, the effect was devastating. As a result of the confusion and lack of consistency among physician treaters, the special relationships forged between them and their patients with hemophilia were severely tested and often began to erode. Mental health professionals within the hemophilia community expressed concern over this deterioration in physician-patient relationships and about the increasing evidence of anxiety and frustration among both patients and treaters. In particular, the NHF Mental Health Committee was a welcome resource for direction, strength, and support as it highlighted the need for special HIV counseling at the treatment center level for both families and center staff.

The NHF strongly advocated additional federal funding specifically for HIV for both the treatment centers and its own programs and galvanized the local chapters to support this effort. In response to the demand for a clearinghouse for HIV information requests, it also proposed the creation of an NHF-based National Resource and Consultation Center (NRCC), for which the NHF sought and obtained funding from the Maternal and Child Health Bureau (MCH). At the same time the Director of Habilitative Medicine of MCH contacted the Foundation and the medical directors of treatment centers in order to include their perceptions in shaping an MCH response to the impact of AIDS on the hemophilia community. At that point, in the absence of clinical advances in HIV treatment technology, the vacuum would be filled with support and counseling. Psychiatrists, psychologists, and social workers already provided mental health services at the treatment-center level, and many participated in the national NHF Mental Health Committee. Their high visibility in these roles hastened the application of funding to serve the needs they had identified. Since the psychosocial component of care was already in place to some extent, it was both comfortable and familiar for the medical directors and the NHF leadership to rely on the Mental Health Committee's guidance in these matters. Going outside of the hemophilia community to seek other kinds of expertise was not the way things were done. This was still a community turned inward.

Although the initial concept of the NRCC was to offer information and support, it became evident that it was important to respond to the emotional needs of people as well. Because they were helping to define the emotional needs of the community as it began to face AIDS as well as the measures to address those needs, the visibility and status of the psychiatrists, psychologists, and social workers involved in hemophilia care increased considerably during the mid-1980s. For the first time, several were included as principal investigators in seeking funding for research. In harmony with this shift, Peggy Heine, a social worker from the Denver HTC team who had assumed a leadership role and actively been involved in the NHF Mental Health Committee, was selected as the director of the NRCC.

Since most physician treaters were experiencing a loss of confidence in their ability to guide or treat their patients with regard to HIV and AIDS, they, too, felt the need for counseling and support. Richard Lipton, M.D., medical director of a treatment center in the northeast, recalls approaching the chief of Consultant Liaison Psychiatry at his institution to ask about obtaining therapy for his team of providers. Comparing the need to that of "ballplayers who can't win a game," he said, "We were used to playing a high-speed passing game. Now we have to slug it out on the ground yard for yard. We're a bunch of talented players, but we're not having any fun and we're losing." The team met with a psychiatrist once a week for ten weeks. As a result of these sessions, Lipton felt they gained new insights into the situation. Fostering patient denial had been "healthy when things were going well." Now, however, the situation was different:

[We'd say,] "Don't worry, just take your clotting factor and you can be an astronaut." That has now come back to haunt us, given the response of this whole community to the issues of testing and counseling and the hemophilia stereotype. This is the old "denial daredevil" stereotype back here again.

. . . We fed this denial, of course. "You can play ball; of course you can go to camp." They didn't want to hear about this stuff [HIV and AIDS]. It is now that people are getting sick—it takes time for people to face reality and to plow through the denial.[3]

Despite the efforts to address the emotional impact of HIV and AIDS, denial continued to manifest itself in a variety of attitudes and behaviors on the part of both providers and consumers. The realization that there was a strong possibility of transmission through heterosexual intercourse was not discussed in NHF mailings until 1985. Once again, this lack of communication was within the context of our entire society and was not solely confined to the hemophilia community. In the mid-1980s most people still viewed AIDS as a gay disease and were not prepared to deal personally with steps that might need to be taken to prevent the spread of the disease. The likelihood of heterosexual transmission at first was downplayed by many hemophilia treaters. For both treaters and patients the implications of this idea were overwhelming. Having to abide by instructions regarding "safe sex" was viewed by many persons with hemophilia as an unnecessary and unwanted intrusion. Sexual prowess was frequently part of the hemophilia male's self-image. "Mindy H.," the wife of an older man with hemophilia, spoke glowingly of his "being a wonderful, sexy lover"[4] and reported that many wives had confided that their husbands were also. Initially, neither treaters nor patients wanted to intrude into this personal area of male self-confidence and strength.

In addition to the issue of heterosexual transmission, the possibility of pregnancies resulting in the birth of an infected child was not widely discussed during these initial years, although "Diane H." (Bea Pierce, the wife of "Daniel H.," or Glenn Pierce) recalls that the first time she heard of a child born HIV-positive was in 1984.[5] Having to grapple with this possibility in planning a family became the next hurdle for many young couples. There was confusion about both the likelihood of transmission and the mechanism and time frame of transmission of the virus to the baby. Decisions to have children were made for a variety of reasons, including the hope that transmission was unlikely and the wish to leave a living legacy behind. As "Adam H." has been previously quoted as saying, couples with hemophilia often had incurred criticism in the past about having children, before the advent of AIDS, so they had learned to live with what people thought and to ignore it.

A Paradigm Emerges:
The Tri-Agency Leadership Model

Sharon Barrett was hired by MCH in 1986 as the new Hemophilia Program Director. With her interest in program development and her background in community organization and social work administration, she took a leading role in shaping the Hemophilia Program. Her vision and style were to play a significant part in the development over the next few years of a new, cooperative approach to hemophilia care in the AIDS era, a model that transcended the limits of traditional bureaucracy and wove together the concerns of several differing constituencies.

When Barrett came on board twenty-five hemophilia treatment centers were MCH grantees. Information providing guidance in applying for supplemental grants had been sent out, and the beginnings of the NHF's NRCC were in place. She recalled quickly learning that "if you shared a thought with one person in the hemophilia community, it was across the country in seconds" and added:

It was the first time that any person within a community had my home phone number. . . . The telephone thing is an anomaly that exists, I think, solely within the hemophilia community. In hemophilia it is not uncommon for anyone to ask for your home phone number. It is not uncommon for anyone to call you at 10, 11, or 12 at night, . . . be it the executive director of the National Hemophilia Foundation or someone working with you on a project.

. . . There was too much to be done at work, so in order for us to really sit down, think, and accomplish something, we had to talk on the telephone. . . . And conference calls too—it all fits into a philosophy which I endorse, participatory management. It is a much slower process. Sometimes you feel defensive and you set yourself up for this particular role, but what happens is you understand the true feelings of the players. You get input from them and move forward. It's not you sitting in your ivory tower making bureaucratic decisions about program and policy.[6]

Barrett's view of the hemophilia constituency included "not just the docs; it's the consumers, it's the nurses, the social workers, who make up this community." She realized that before she assumed the directorship of the program, there was more of an adherence to "the traditional medical model, where nurses and social workers weren't included in the decision making."[7] The circle of participants had begun to enlarge when adults with hemophilia assumed leadership roles within the Foundation. However, the advent of AIDS had, as noted, raised the profile of professionals involved with the psychosocial aspects of care, even as the medical treaters faltered.

Although Barrett's previous experience in community organization meshed with NHF Executive Director "Paul Phillips's" background and philosophy to a large degree, they did differ, initially, in how they defined who comprised the hemophilia constituency. Realizing that the central organization's resources were not sufficient to reach everyone, "Phillips" considered the NHF chapters to be the Foundation's primary constituency, its "arms and legs." Barrett, however, viewed all individual consumers and potential consumers as her constituency.

The changing concerns of patients and their families were also an important issue facing Barrett. The influence of the men with hemophilia who were in leadership positions within the Foundation, coupled with chapter leadership, led to the Foundation's stance of maintaining a low profile and avoiding measures that could further jeopardize the lifestyle and positions that they had acquired. Unfortunately, widespread ignorance about AIDS led to incidents that legitimized hemophiliacs' fears of being stigmatized or isolated. Perhaps the most notorious of such incidents involved Ryan White, who had contracted AIDS from a blood transfusion and was "picketed by schoolmates' parents, shunned by his classmates, driven by fear and hatred from his school and town in Indiana," and the Ray family, described by Dr. C. Everett Koop as "three little hemophiliac boys—infected with HIV through no decision of their own" who "not only suffered humiliating discrimination, but also saw their house burned down by arsonists."[8] In response to such prejudice and violence, hemophilia families reached out to support each other, and many withdrew from the larger community.

From the early years of the epidemic, however, the NHF had played an important role in confronting prejudice in Congress and in paving the way for Congressional support for AIDS research and education. "Paul Phillips" noted that "Many members of Congress told hemophilia representatives that they opposed funding for AIDS because of the populations that were affected. For these members of Congress, people with hemophilia were seen as innocent victims and thus engaged a great deal of sympathy and support for AIDS research. Although NHF did not exploit those social value judgments, they were able to lay a proactive role . . . partially due to these perceptions." Perhaps the most important example involved the scheduling of Senate Health Committee hearings on AIDS. "Phillips" recalls, "Senator Orrin Hatch of Utah was the chair of the [committee]. Given his state and constituency, it was not surprising that he did not (initially) place a high priority on AIDS. Through NHF, however, he was introduced to Nathan Smith, a Mormon and former resident of Utah, who had acquired AIDS through his use of blood products. This was in important factor in motivating Senator Hatch to convene the first Senate hearing in 1985, with Nathan Smith as the opening witness."[9]

Following that hearing and a major lobbying campaign by the NHF, Congress appropriated supplemental funding for "risk reduction" in the hemophilia community to the Centers for Disease Control (CDC), with the understanding that funds would be distributed to the treatment centers through Maternal and Child Health's Hemophilia Program. However, the CDC had its own agenda in confronting AIDS. In its view epidemiological data collection, case finding, and education leading to behavior change were all necessary components of a primary prevention approach to halt the further spread of the disease. The hemophilia community's emphasis on psychological support and counseling, coupled with their insistence on maintaining a low profile by avoidance of testing, did not mesh with the CDC's concerns.[10] In addition, promoting education for "safe sex" to the men with hemophilia and reaching out to locate and educate their sexual partners were high on the CDC's list of priorities but not part of the NHF's agenda. Since the CDC now received and distributed funds, it began to gain greater clout in deciding how moneys should be spent.

Another issue that surfaced in the late 1980s revolved around the lack of clarity about the content of education in HIV risk reduction at the treatment centers and about the role of the risk-reduction personnel. Initially, new staff hired at the treatment center level to counsel and educate patients and families were viewed by many as a separate entity. Integration and acceptance by the other team members was a slow process. In fact, at one treatment center people referred to "the old team and the new team."[11] The same kind of initial thinking had influenced the NHF's creating the NRCC as a separate unit within the organization.

The reality that AIDS would not go away, would ultimately affect over half of the patient population, and would become relevant to everyone in the community was not yet understood or accepted.

Most of the HTC medical directors were clinicians, used to thinking in terms of treating their individual patients, not in terms of watching trends affecting a population. They wrote grants using the term "family-centered care" but, for the most part, applied that term to parents and young children. With their adult patients, they limited their focus to the males whom they treated. The idea of considering their patients' wives also as potential patients was hard for them to fathom. They did not approach the situation with the philosophy, tools, or skills of public health or health policy makers; nor were they comfortable wearing the hat of either an infectious disease specialist or a health educator. As a result, the initial dollars allocated for risk reduction were spent in a variety of ways throughout the treatment center network. Few established programs even set goals and objectives, and in those that did, they weren't standardized or evaluated.

The NRCC had jumped into the vacuum when there was a need to do something. Its educational role, however, was limited to producing a question-and-answer sheet about hemophilia and AIDS, incorporating a newly created AIDS module into ongoing provider training sessions that focused on the Patient/Family Model, and sending out materials on the topic when requested. Boxes filled with samples of pamphlets about AIDS developed by other organizations were housed in the office, but there was no system in place to provide appropriate materials to various subgroups of the community. By trying to be all things to all constituencies, the NRCC soon became the lightning rod for criticism from providers and consumers alike. By establishing itself as a resource center, it drew requests for every kind of assistance imaginable.[12] Lacking the tools and expertise to serve as a professional clearinghouse, it created frustration among those who ran it and those who sought its assistance. A dedicated staff wasn't enough to do what needed to be done.

By the end of 1987, both the CDC and MCH expressed a desire to maximize the quality of hemophilia risk reduction efforts. MCH decided to hire an outside group to evaluate the program and awarded the contract to a consulting firm directed by J. William Flynt, M.D., a pediatrician and epidemiologist who had been a private practitioner and had directed programs on birth defects and diabetes at the CDC before moving into the private sector. Flynt's group immediately realized that there would be great difficulty in evaluating the program because "there weren't any real stated objectives or goals that had been articulated." In discussions with Barrett, the consultants agreed to modify the contract to begin by identifying what the goals ought to be. After visiting treatment centers and the NHF headquarters and interviewing staff in both locations, Flynt's group issued a report in July 1988. They had found widespread frustration among treatment center staff members, which was attributed both to the increasing amount of illness among their patients and to increasing levels of anger among patients as a result of their situation. There also was discomfort with receiving "mixed messages" from MCH, NHF, and CDC.[13]

In fact, these three agencies had never consolidated their ideas concerning goals for a risk reduction program. Further, they had not delineated their own roles or those of the treatment centers in enabling the hemophilia community to achieve the general goal of risk reduction. The consultants recommended that one of the first steps should be a meeting of the leadership of the three agencies to begin to resolve these matters and to establish strategies. They also developed a diagrammatic representation of a functional model for the risk reduction program, which would assist the planning process. The model assumed that efforts to prevent transmission of HIV would be undertaken and identified functions necessary to accomplish this in the areas of leadership, education, training, dissemination of information, data collection, and evaluation. As Flynt described it:

We explained how we could help to continue the process, and one of the things I personally felt quite keenly about was that there really needed to be some high level discussions between the Foundation, CDC, and MCH. Having worked at CDC, I appreciated the fact that there were two different parts of the Centers for Disease Control who were involved in the project. [Bruce] Evatt, who is a hematologist and somebody who has been interested in hemophilia for a long time, had one perspective of hemophilia. But the reality was that the funds that Congress had appropriated came through another segment of CDC. . . . Part of what we were doing in establishing a leadership model was establishing a forum where the two sides of CDC could get together, where MCH could understand who the actors were at CDC, and they could meet with the Foundation.

These meetings took place in September of 1988. They [the NHF, CDC, and MCH] agreed that there should be continued planning and a continuing process to help develop goals and objectives that everyone could agree to. . . . There would be clarification of who was doing what in the functional areas.

Out of those agreements, we formed a committee made up of treatment center staff representing various disciplines, trying to make it as broad-based as possible. This committee was given the charge to develop the goals, the objectives, and the various activities that should take place. The committee set out to establish a frame of reference for the treatment centers where they could begin setting their own goals and objectives.[14]

Rising to the challenge, the committee worked hard during the last months of 1988 to prepare a manual that would provide guidance to the treatment centers. A meeting, which became known as "Las Vegas II" (there had been an earlier meeting in that city on related issues) was planned for January 1989 to introduce the guide and articulate the three agencies' expectations of the treatment centers. These expectations were a marked departure from the past. There would have to be consistency in terms of grant applications and in developing a minimum data set, or list of data to be collected.[15] Emphasis on the importance of outreach to female sexual partners and to minorities would lay the groundwork for future funded programs that would focus on these two underserved segments of the community.

The Tri-Agency Leadership Model, as it became known, established a new paradigm. Working together, two government agencies and a voluntary, not-for-profit health agency would systematically assume the responsibility for leadership of risk reduction efforts for the community, with each agency taking on a leadership role in specifically defined areas. Continually meeting to share perceptions and to eventually achieve consensus, the leadership of the three agencies would communicate with one voice, offering a clear road map for the treatment centers and chapters. Their discussions resulted in strengthening the NHF chapters and fostering their collaboration with the treatment centers in outreach and education—a by-product welcomed by the Foundation and its executive director.

The model also led to a more democratized hemophilia community by including a wide range of providers and consumers, both as reviewers of treatment center grant proposals and planning and as MCH conference presenters. Participatory democracy would be further reflected in the early 1990s as the Maternal and Child Health Bureau sponsored town meetings and conference planning for the next decade of hemophilia care.

The new process of planning also resulted in the transformation of the NHF's NRCC. The need for a high-quality clearinghouse for HIV- and AIDS-related information that could respond to its constituency in an effective and timely manner led to the creation of the Hemophilia and AIDS/HIV Network for the Dissemination of Information (HANDI), which was staffed with trained and experienced personnel. NRCC shifted its focus from being primarily psychosocial to educational, reflecting the CDC's interest in promoting behavior change that would lead to risk reduction. Increased levels of funding from a variety of sources facilitated the expansion of the staff and enabled the Foundation to expand its office space at this time.

The Hemophilia Community: Opening a Window into the Future

By the end of 1988, the data showed that 90 percent of the severe hemophilia population were HIV positive.[16] Informants recall that it was a time when everyone began to know someone who was sick. (See Appendix G.) It was a time of other changes in the hemophilia community as well. One of the most significant was in its role in confronting AIDS as it moved beyond concerns about the nation's blood supply and found it had valuable experience to contribute to society. The community was now viewed as a living laboratory for observing the effects of coping with HIV and AIDS. As Dr. C. Everett Koop, who served as the U.S. Surgeon General from 1981 through 1989, observed: "The experience of hemophiliacs who had become infected with AIDS by a transfusion before the blood test had become available or by injection with clotting factors before heat treatment made them safe made a major contribution to our understanding of the disease. From hemophiliacs we also learned about the strength of young people who now had to live with two diseases as well as the fear of discrimination."[17]

Since the mid-1980s the NHF had become increasingly involved in research projects related to HIV and AIDS. Many of these were clinical research projects, coordinated by people with nursing backgrounds. The first project to achieve recognition was known internally as "the household study." According to Dr. Koop,

information provided by the National Hemophilia Foundation through this study was critical. . . . The experience of hemophiliacs nailed down the evidence that AIDS was not spread by casual contact. Six hundred families of hemophiliacs were studied. Families who lived with an HIV-positive male touched each other, used the same utensils, kissed each other, and shared razors without passing the virus. Even the 7 percent who shared toothbrushes (I was surprised by that figure!) did not transmit the virus to their toothbrush partners. This and a number of other studies confirmed that most Americans were not at risk if they did not engage in high-risk behavior with sex and drugs.[18]

Although the strength of the formal and informal support systems in the hemophilia community was enhanced by the more uniform information provided through the framework of the Tri-Agency Model, cracks were forming in the once cohesive community, foreshadowing a major earthquake. Perceptions of what had happened and who was to blame increasingly reflected the age of the informants. The youngest men, who had not lived through "the bad old days," were particularly enraged. They had been raised with the expectation of living life to the fullest and of having a normal life span. Now, for many, this promise was gone. They had not experienced the endless pain, isolation, absences from school, and expectation of living only until their teens that characterized the early life experience of the oldest informants. They found it incomprehensible that keeping a low profile was more important than joining other at-risk groups to demand financial compensation and to gain immediate access to drugs to treat opportunistic infections. Because they had not witnessed the earliest days, when doctors they knew of as medical leaders spent endless voluntary hours advocating for insurance coverage for their patients, they viewed the behavior exhibited by some of these leaders as totally unacceptable and inexcusable. They felt they were being abandoned, cynically written off as physicians planned for the future that was in store for the next generation of healthy, uninfected "virgin" babies.

By the late 1980s, in fact, some of the medical leaders were focusing on the hopeful future for hemophilia care generated by new patients, the young boys who would receive either heat-treated, solvent-detergent-treated, or new genetically engineered blood products. Some expressed a wistful yearning to return to the golden days, a wish to be in control again. Several became conspicuously absent from their hemophilia clinics, immersed in new high-level jobs at their academic medical centers. Yet they remained actively involved in the international hemophilia arena, if away from the devastation occurring on a daily basis. Many, however, fought their anxiety and frustration to stay the course and remain at the treatment centers to offer care and support, working within the community to maximize the quality of life for all.

The courage of the families coping with the specter of AIDS or with the actual illness was complemented by the dedication of care providers from all professional groups. Often relating to patients in a more egalitarian fashion than did medical directors, many members of the provider staff stayed to support the families who were suffering and to reach out to educate the new families with young children. Nurses who had reveled in sharing birthday parties with the families of young patients reported that they were now attending a growing number of these same patients' funerals; they accepted sharing the families' pain as they had shared their joy. Informants often mentioned their appreciation of the nurses who remained involved. At the Mount Sinai Hospital Hemophilia Treatment Center in New York City, patients compiled a scrapbook dedicated to "Alice," the nurse whom they consider a "hero."[19] Growing recognition of the nursing profession's strengths led to the selection of nurses to fill major jobs at the CDC and NHF.

As 1988 drew to a close, the tri-agency leadership recognized the tensions and new divisions within the community as well as its role in meeting this challenge by promoting collaboration and participation.

CHAPTER 11

"A Vote for the Status Quo," 1988–92

In 1988, George Bush and Dan Quayle ran against and triumphed over Michael Dukakis and Lloyd Bentsen in the national election. The media interpreted this choice of Ronald Reagan's vice president to be his successor as a vote for continuity. The *New York Times* declared, "People are satisfied with the way the country is—a vote for the status quo."[1] There were signs, however, that all was not well, that segments of society were not satisfied, particularly with the Reagan administration's approach to health-related matters. On July 19, 1988, delegates to the Democratic Party National Convention had passed the Jesse Jackson amendment to the party platform, calling for the establishment of a National Health Program (NHP) that would guarantee comprehensive health benefits coverage to all Americans.

By the autumn of 1988, another sign of discontent focused specifically on AIDS research. Members of the Boston chapter of the activist group ACT UP (the AIDS Coalition To Unleash Power) came to Harvard University on the first day of classes at the medical school, wearing hospital gowns, blindfolds, and chains and chanting, "We're here to show defiance / for what Harvard calls 'good science.'" While some demonstrators poured fake blood on the sidewalk, others gave students "a course outline for AIDS 101." The outline included titles such as: "PWAs—People With AIDS: Human Beings or Laboratory Rats?" and "Medical Elitism—Is the Pursuit of Elegant Science Leading to the De-

150

struction of Our Community?" Steven Epstein's book *Impure Science,* which describes this scene, examines how certainty is constructed and deconstructed and analyzes what expertise means, showing how accepted knowledge emerges out of credibility strategies. Epstein contrasts the real complexity and depth of the "course outline" with the shock value of the ACT UP activists' theatrics and protest symbols. ACT UP used "in-your-face politics" to promote a sense of urgency as they criticized the quality of scientific practice. At bottom, they framed the Republican administration's inaction and lack of appropriate response to the epidemic as genocide by neglect.[2]

Discontent over the nation's response to AIDS was not limited to the more radical groups. Initially, the mainstream national gay rights organizations had focused on issues of discrimination against people with AIDS and budget appropriations to fund research into the disease. By the late 1980s, gaining immediate access to HIV-fighting drugs and to clinical trials became the top priority. The Food and Drug Administration (FDA) and the National Institute of Allergy and Infectious Diseases (NIAID) became their targets, as they disputed the necessity of maintaining the government's lengthy scientific process for testing drugs, which required three sequential phases of randomized clinical trials before a new drug could be approved for use. Armed with scientific language, newly acquired expertise, and cultural competency, they fought to streamline what would have been a six-to-eight-year-long time frame before new AIDS drugs were available. They successfully established working relationships with FDA and NIAID officials, supplementing street activism with meeting room intelligence.

Treatment activism began in gay communities because gays had felt the need to assert ownership of the social problem and because they had the resources to organize themselves in confronting opposition. Epstein asserts that the AIDS Movement also expresses "social movement spillover," having been built upon the foundation of both the gay movement and the feminist health movement.[3] Gay men had previously worked to "demedicalize" their identity, eliminating it as a listed form of mental pathology, and gay women, many of whom had been active in the feminist health movement of the 1970s, were striving for autonomy in health decision making while protesting against the medical establishment's paternalism and lack of access to clinical trials. By 1988, the Women's Caucus of ACT UP began to confront obstacles preventing women from receiving health and disability benefits that were based on the CDC's definition of AIDS. Symptoms manifested by women did not mimic the male pattern. Often they developed pelvic inflammatory disease, not a part of the original list of AIDS defining symptoms. Activists pointed out that, because of the fear of harming fetuses, women of childbearing age were excluded from the very clinical trials that would have collected the required data. Women were defined as "vectors" or "vessels" by the medical and scientific establishment—viewed as transmission routes to men or babies or as carriers of fetuses. Their protests eventually led to the CDC's augmenting the defining criteria for AIDS.

Another aspect of the AIDS Movement involved shifting the balance of power in doctor/patient relationships. In 1985, groups of patients issued a "Founding Statement of People with AIDS/ARC [AIDS-Related Complex]" and a "Patient's Bill of Rights." In their statement, People with AIDS (PWAs) proclaimed, "We condemn attempts to label us as 'victims,' which implies defeat, and we are only occasionally 'patients,' which implies passivity, helplessness, and dependence on others. We are 'people with AIDS.'" They further insisted not only on the right to self-representation but also on the right to full and total explanations from health professionals, the right to anonymity and confidentiality, and the right to refuse treatment.[4] This assertiveness did not stem from the tendency of outcasts to practice rebellion; many PWAs came from the same social and financial strata as their physicians. They were not intimidated by medical authority. While activists employed newly acquired expertise and language to effectively participate in choices about making and doing science, PWAs employed medical terminology in conversing with health providers, striving for a more egalitarian relationship and control over management of their disease.

While PWAs wrestled with illness and discrimination, other gay men, women, and health providers focused on preventing the further spread of the disease. Health education became the major strategy for promotion of behavior change on both coasts. In New York City, the Gay Men's Health Crisis began support groups and emphasized peer education. This organization produced visually appealing educational books, pamphlets, and videos promoting "safer sex," stressing the use of condoms. Since sexual freedom of expression had become a hallmark of the gay lifestyle, many members of the community were initially angered by what they felt were efforts to invade their privacy and inhibit their behavior. As time passed and more men became ill, however, safer sex, which avoided exchange of body fluids but incorporated alternative means of sensual sharing, became widely accepted, in large part because the emphasis was placed on pleasure and enjoyment rather than on deprivation.

Staying in the Medical Closet

In 1988, regular, ongoing contact between the gay community and the hemophilia community, particularly at the local chapter level, was far from the accepted norm. Several NHF staff members in the National Resource and Consultation Center (NRCC) were members of the gay activist community and introduced some of their health education material to chapters and treatment centers; they also promoted the idea of greater interaction with gay organizations. For the most part, however, the hemophilia community, particularly on the local level, retained an inward-turned posture. Most men with hemophilia did not become involved with AIDS task forces at the local level, and NHF continued to maintain a low profile rather than embracing activism as a member organization in the AIDS community. The hemophilia community had asserted a modicum of control over their right to know the full story and to have options presented. Although they had promoted the resignation of the NHF medical co-director who symbolized the medical paternalism of the early 1980s, many individuals in the community had not joined AIDS movement protest demonstrations. Association with the AIDS epidemic—and the gay community—still raised fears of potential discrimination in workplaces, schools, and local communities.

Michael Davidson captures the plight of persons with hemophilia during the AIDS era in the poignant description and analysis of his "Strange Blood: Hemophobia and the Unexplored Boundaries of Queer Nation." Davidson speaks of persons with hemophilia as "nominal queers": although they had acquired AIDS "iatrogenically," through medical treatments, certain features of social "others" were now ascribed to them. Noting the harassment many suffered—citing in particular the Ray family, whose sons were taunted at school and whose Florida home was burned down, forcing them to relocate to another city—Davidson writes: "With the entry of AIDS into their community, many hemophiliacs closed the door to their medical closets in order not to be associated with gays or not to be subject to the same prohibition that gay people with AIDS were facing. Many were resentful of gay men whose sexual liberation had transformed their medical liberation into a nightmare." He also offers a personal view of what happened beginning in the mid-1980s:

Since I have a rather moderate form of Factor IX hemophilia, I never had to use the concentrate during the years it was contaminated, but visits to the clinic in the mid-1980s revealed a profound change in the hemophilia community. Now in addition to the more recognizably crippled hemophiliacs, one saw patients . . . who were emaciated by various opportunistic diseases characteristic of persons with AIDS. Mailings from the organizations changed from being about new blood products and treatment to information about HIV infection, AZT, hospice networks, AIDS hotlines, and invariably memorial services. Persons with hemophilia who had been medically integrated into "normal" life were now ostracized from schools and businesses, their already fragile insurance policies canceled and their access to life-sustaining blood products profoundly altered.[5]

An important source of information for the years since 1988, Glenn Pierce (formerly identified as "Daniel H.") who had earned a joint Ph.D.-M.D., discussed other dimensions of the situation. He became chairman of NHF's AIDS Task Force in 1988 when his mentor, "Cliff H.," left to become president of the World Federation of Hemophilia. Pierce had played a variety of roles within the organization since 1984, when he had joined the Board of Directors. He described this task force, which developed AIDS policy for the Foundation, as quite insular in its makeup, a small group of people who were very conservative regarding AIDS policy. Community members, including himself, continued to keep their heads in the sand. The period from 1988 to 1992 was a time of continuous and strong disagreement within the community about how public to go with AIDS. "Paul Phillips" recalled that in an effort to overcome the reluctance to be more open about AIDS and hemophilia, he had gathered some communications experts and members of the hemophilia community over a weekend "to lay the groundwork in a sensitive but forceful way for communication to the public about how the hemophilia population had been infected with the AIDS virus."[6] This meeting paved the way for the AIDS Task Force to develop a White Paper, discussing the fact that AIDS infected people with hemophilia. Although this was an important PR message that could have been used to increase awareness for fund-raising, for access to treatment, and for many good purposes that would benefit the community as a whole, the NHF Board and chapters voted it down:

The chapters just got up in arms and said, "You can't do this; we have people living in this community. If they're exposed, their house could be destroyed, this will happen, they'll be kicked out of school." . . . So this White Paper never saw the light of day. It's important to point out, because that was really the mentality of our grassroots community. When the behavior of the NHF is criticized today, in retrospect, NHF's behavior as an organization was consistent with what its constituents wanted. It's revisionist history, and the people who are the loudest critics of what the organization was doing in the 1980s were as deep in the closet as you can get. In fact, in many cases their chapters didn't even know about them. . . . I can remember a number of instances where some of the guys were asked to get involved with AIDS task forces on the local level and they would refuse. It wasn't until the reality set in—in one case, Jonathan Wadleigh, the person who founded the Committee of Ten Thousand [COTT], had refused to get involved with the New England Hemophilia Association AIDS Task Force. Well, in 1988 or so, his brother died, and that was the beginning of his awakening.[7]

"Phillips" noted that "others report that Wadleigh had some good ideas regarding AIDS education with the [NEHA], but he would never deliver, so NEHA proceeded without AIDS education programs and was an active participant in community-wide AIDS walks that were organized by the gay community in Boston."[8] Steven Epstein offers another view of Jonathan Wadleigh, based on a 1994 interview. Wadleigh told Epstein that he had felt the New England Hemophilia Foundation was not taking sufficient action, so as a result, he began to associate with the gay community and to relate to the activism going on there. He began to attend meetings of ACT UP/Boston in the late 1980s, soon realizing that he was the only straight person, as well as the only person with hemophilia, in the room. Recognizing that there was a paucity of information about AIDS treatments in the hemophilia publications, he started a treatment newsletter for the hemophilia community, summarizing articles from established grassroots publications. He also became involved in debates about the inclusion criteria for AIDS trials. Trial protocols routinely excluded persons with elevated liver enzymes, but since people with hemophilia often develop liver disease, many have elevated liver enzyme levels. Wadleigh asserted that he successfully fought to liberalize the entry criteria, which provided access to the trials for people with hemophilia.[9]

The First Steps toward
AIDS Community Involvement

Nineteen eighty-nine marked "Paul Phillips's" ninth year as executive director of NHF. Mirroring our societal climate, the organization's annual report described a community apparently satisfied with its leadership and its mission, which was stated as "working to increase understanding and assistance to the entire community." The report went on to announce that as of June 30, 1989, 600 members of the hemophilia community had died of AIDS. (See Appendix G.) There was also some good news to report amidst the horrors of the period. Beginning in 1985, a number of broadly applied viral inactivation techniques came into use, making the blood products needed by persons with hemophilia "virtually safe," and clinical trials of recombinant Factor VIII were under way.[10] However, there was still a crisis in both supply and cost of the products. One effort to address these issues was the Compassionate Care Program, through which fourteen NHF chapters received either clotting factor or $50,000 for health insurance premiums for those who were underinsured or uninsured. Another aspect of the cost problem was the new limitations on insurance coverage imposed by the insurance companies' Diagnostic-Related Groups (DRGs), which defined how much would be paid for a given condition or treatment. NHF effectively lobbied to have the cost of clotting factor fully reimbursed under Medicare Part A DRG diagnostic codes.

The NHF annual report also noted involvement in AIDS-related research protocols. Funding sources included the CDC, the NIAID, and the FDA. One important study (known as Protocol 36) was to evaluate the use of AZT as treatment for HIV-positive asymptomatic men. Several men with hemophilia who were research subjects became representatives on advisory committees. As a result, they were introduced to their counterparts from the gay activist community. Other opportunities to interact with a diverse group of people outside of the hemophilia community came in 1989 when "Adam H." was appointed to the National AIDS Commission. In addition, on Surgeon General C. Everett Koop's "Day of Recognition of Gratitude" both the Ray family of Florida and the White family of Indiana were among those honored.[11]

As noted in Chapter 10, this was a time in which differing constituencies and agendas began to come together, ultimately leading to the Tri-Agency Model. In 1989, NHF's stated goal was to provide support and assistance to the hemophilia community. The CDC, however, emphasized the urgency of halting the AIDS epidemic. Both the CDC and MCH encouraged the hemophilia community to expand their horizons by considering strategies in use outside of the hemophilia community that were designed to halt the spread of AIDS by changing behavior. It was at this time that MCH contracted with Dr. J. William Flynt to initiate a study evaluating the risk reduction measures in the hemophilia treatment centers and at the NHF. In addition to the aspects of this report discussed in Chapter 10, one of the major findings of Flynt's study was that many HTC directors resented the direction that these activities were taking. Having run the show for many years, they chafed at having to tailor their grant renewal applications to conform to standardized measurements determined by government agencies. Also, they were uncomfortable with stated goals and objectives written in unfamiliar terms—"public healthese." (In fact, more stringent guidelines for grant renewals would soon contain a section with uniform measures. These would become known as the minimal data set, a source of pride for the CDC in at last achieving more refined, appropriate measures.) Other areas of discomfort at the HTCs related to clinical practice. As the CDC began to place emphasis on outreach to women who were sexual partners, many physicians expressed resentment at having to deal with people they did not perceive as "their patients."

In retrospect, Dr. Bruce Evatt, Director of Host Factors at the CDC at that time, recalled:

There were several issues. First of all, until that time, the funding that had been supplied by HRSA [Health Resources and Services Administration] was really designed to deliver care rather than prevention. . . . They were not funding research, and they did not want the program to appear as research. . . . I think that the CDC's [mission] was one of prevention, and for adequate prevention, we needed outcome studies. We needed to know what the problem was. And so to find out what effect the HRSA programs were having on the community necessitated instituting the collection of data in terms of a minimal data set and a different approach to problems—one that hemophilia treatment centers had not thought of, that is, prevention and a lot of education in terms of behavior modification. I think that there was a fair amount of resistance because, one, they didn't think they had the skills and, two, it was a different approach to hemophilia than they had thought about. . . . They thought they just didn't have the time to do that as well as their regular duties.[12]

Sowing the Seeds of Grassroots Leadership: Peer Outreach

Between 1989 and 1990 the NHF sponsored three new peer outreach programs, all of which became fertile fields for developing new leadership in the hemophilia community and which also succeeded in contributing to reducing the spread of AIDS. The first came about as the CDC and MCH recognized that there were segments of the U.S. hemophilia population that did not receive health care within the HTC network but represented an important piece of prevention strategy. Locating and contacting them in order to insure that they would not contribute to the further spread of AIDS became a priority. The first NHF program formally instituting outreach to these underserved segments of the hemophilia population (for reasons described as "due to geographic or ethnic circumstances") began in ten NHF chapters in 1989 and was called the Chapter Outreach Demonstration Project (CODP).

Richard Johnson (formerly identified as "Irwin H."), who has become a forceful spokesperson and leader of CODP and also of MANN, which is described below, became involved with CODP from the outset. His initial project was a rap (support) group in North Philadelphia, an area that is predominantly African American and Hispanic. He described what happened in the group:

The experience we all shared was that we came up through some pretty rough times, rough neighborhoods, gang wars, drugs, and everything else. And a lot of us kept ourselves on the straight and narrow and tried to do the best we could because of our bleeding disorder. And then to be given a death sentence, after you worked so hard to try to . . . keep yourself healthy and to educate yourself because you couldn't use your brawn, you had to use your brain. You know, it was kind of deflating as far as emotions and so forth. I think that was the magnet that actually drew about twelve to fifteen guys together on a weekly basis. . . . These were people who at one time were considered in denial and noncompliant to what the treatment centers wanted, but they all found that they couldn't identify with the people at the treatment center. . . . Some people who [the] psychosocial people [said] wouldn't talk—we couldn't shut them up. They had so much to talk about, so much pent up inside. . . . I just presented myself as nonjudgmental. In other words, whatever you decide is your decision; I just want you to know what is available to you. And whatever a person decides, I'm not saying what's right and what's wrong, or what you should do or should not do. I'm just letting the person know their options and educating them as much as I could as far as the disease is concerned or their HIV status, or how to spread it. And then they have to make decisions.[13]

The second outreach group arose out of the self-organizing efforts made by another underserved group, the wives of adult men with hemophilia. Bea Pierce (formerly identified as "Diane H.") recalled that when she began working with the local NHF Ohio chapter, she was known as "Mrs. Glenn Pierce" on chapter stationary and in the minutes of the meetings. During this initial stage, when she entered the hemophilia world by marrying Glenn, there was no defined role for her, unlike mothers of sons with hemophilia, who had historically played a major role. By the mid 1980s, things began to change, as formal risk reduction programs sent out the message: "'Don't have unprotected sex'; or even the message came out truthfully as 'no intercourse—period' and that became a big issue."[14]

At the NHF annual meeting in Houston, Texas, in the fall of 1985, a discussion session for women—both consumers and providers—focused on AIDS and risk reduction. Carol Weisman, a former hemophilia treatment center social worker, and Bea Pierce were asked to be co-facilitators. Bea recalled that there was a room filled with health providers—and only four women, who were all wives of men with hemophilia: herself, Kathy McAdam, Linda Smith (the wife of Nathan Smith), and Patsy Carman (the wife of Charles Carman, formerly identified as "Cliff H.").[15] At that time Linda Smith's husband, who was then one of the main leaders in the hemophilia community, was so ill and fatigued that he could hardly go to the various sessions. (Even though he had manifested a multitude of health problems, he was not officially diagnosed with AIDS until after this meeting, at Thanksgiving time in 1985; he died at Thanksgiving, 1986). Frustrated with the focus on "passing out condoms," she jumped into the discussion: "What about my needs? I have issues that no one is addressing."[16] McAdam, Smith, and Pierce have all reported that this changed the direction of the meeting toward something that was relevant for them. They decided to continue talking in one of their rooms in the hotel afterwards. Linda Smith recalled a lot of talking and hugging as they collaborated in documenting their needs and concerns and agreed to continue the communication and bonding that had just begun. After they returned home, Pierce initiated "round-robin" letters that circulated among them during the following years, between getting together for support sessions at annual meetings. Beginning in 1986, McAdam and Pierce co-facilitated these sessions.[17] According to Bea Pierce:

We wanted to prevent any more transmissions than were possible, but telling people to take precautions was just not the way to do it. There are so many issues. It is an area that is so close to people. It is a very private area, and here you are discussing it in public and it's all over. One of the things I used to tell Glenn and some other people was, here I was this quiet little wallflower that didn't speak up much, and all of a sudden, there I am talking about sex, in these big groups. It was private stuff. . . . But with the peer programs, there were people who were in the same situation. We really worked with each other and were able to get rid of a lot of issues, because even though safe sex was a core issue, there were a lot of surrounding issues to get through first. And that included helping women just to figure out that they would be able to take care of themselves. . . . In the early years, there were a number of women within the support group that had received AIDS transmitted through sex before a lot of the issues were known and before prevention techniques were really out there.[18]

In January 1989, when Dr. Dale Lawrence was invited to speak at an NHF meeting about the AIDS epidemic, he began to think about reaching his audience and to consider delivering a message that would go beyond reporting the CDC's statistics. He recalled Eleanor Roosevelt's philosophy of making a difference by addressing problems affecting society and about the potential of women to do just that.[19] He began his speech by saying he hoped that this audience would no longer consider hemophilia a disease affecting only 20,000 mostly male people, but would begin to view it and the associated AIDS epidemic as a situation affecting at least 40,000 people. He said that HIV would also affect hemophiliacs' wives, partners, and children, families comprising the community. He displayed a chart illustrating the sharp upward epidemiological curve of the incidence of HIV for men with hemophilia—then stated that there was an expectation that, absent intervention, the women's curve would undoubtedly replicate it.

I was a member of that audience and recall sensing the urgency of maximizing all opportunities to reach women directly and immediately. During a break, Ashaki Taha-Cissé, an NRCC colleague, and I shared our similar reactions. We felt that we were working within a community culture shaped by the sensibilities of males with hemophilia, which had resulted in a climate of denial. In an organization where chapters were still considered the constituency and wives were all but invisible, there were no educational outreach programs planned specifically for women and no communication links directly to women. Fortunately, the assistant director of the Foundation and the director of the NRCC responded positively to our request to explore the possibility of creating a national program focusing on women in the hemophilia community. We connected with Bea Pierce and Kathy McAdam, who are themselves health care professionals—Pierce a nurse and McAdam a social worker. In reaching out to women through their rap or support groups, they had since 1986 gathered considerable data regarding women's expressed concerns. These included use of condoms, eroticizing safer sex, interference with emotional and sexual intimacy, abstinence, stress, anxiety and fatigue, the decision to postpone pregnancy, death and dying of the husband, long-term effects of HIV infection, the uncertainty of the future, requirements for HIV testing, the loss of insurance, disruption of family life if the parent has AIDS, and discrimination.[20]

There was a synergistic effect as we collaborated with Pierce and McAdam, which led us to approach Sharon Barrett, director of the MCH Hemophilia Program, to seek funding. She appreciated both the documented need and the concept of an NHF model for a national network of women leaders who would organize and implement local AIDS/HIV peer risk reduction education and support groups. From the beginning, we all visualized a peer-led program that would utilize health educators and other health trainers as resources to provide technical assistance and share their skills and information with the women who would lead the program. We selected an advisory committee, comprising wives, mothers, a social scientist, and health educators. After an initial meeting in June 1989, a workshop was planned to be held in Minnesota in the fall of 1989. This was the official beginning of the Women's Outreach Network of the National Hemophilia Foundation (WONN), which became an ongoing training ground for women leaders.

During its initial period, WONN encountered resistance from some of the male community members, who questioned the need for women to have their own program. Kathy Gerus, immediate past vice president of NHF in 1998, recalled her experience with this on a local level. In Michigan, she and several other women had started a support group early in 1989, before the first WONN meeting. Seventeen women had come, most of whom had never spoken to anyone about their situation or concerns before that time. She recalls how powerful the experience was for all of them—and also remembers that her husband, who was usually very supportive of her involvements, questioned the value of the women's support group and made it clear that he didn't want her talking about him. Many other wives received the same response. Gerus wonders now whether men were worried that women getting together would complain and perhaps decide that they wanted divorces.[21]

After the successful WONN Minnesota conference, Dana Kuhn (formerly identified as "James H.") approached Sharon Barrett, urging her to fund a similar group for men. After an initial planning meeting, a third model program was developed, which became known as the Men's Advocacy Network of the National Hemophilia Foundation (MANN). The tone of its initial meetings was entirely different from that at the women's meetings, which had focused on empathy, support, and empowerment needs. The men shared hemophilia "war stories" and anger. Clearly, having a structure to encompass their needs was as important as it was for the women.

Val Bias, who has since become the face and the voice of the hemophilia community on the Hill in Washington, D.C, was living with his wife Katie in San Francisco in the late 1980s. Both Val and Katie (who has since died) had tested HIV positive, and both were concerned about repercussions if this came to light. He worked closely with children as director of a popular YMCA program, and she worked in retailing. For Bias the MANN program offered the relief of an outlet and a safe place away from his job and local setting to share feelings and concerns about his infection. He quickly became involved at the national level and remembers of this initial stage of MANN, "When it came time to pick a leader for the MANN group, I remember several discussions about it. I think our choice was Dana Kuhn, because of his great charisma. He's a very attractive person with great charisma, but he could not appeal to everyone. He was just another white male hemophiliac, and that's not what they wanted, so they asked him and me to do it together."[22]

Bias and Kuhn did share the first chairmanship of MANN, working together with the other members of the executive committee to develop goals, objectives, and a mission statement. With this, the third branch of hemophilia peer education programs was in place. The three have not only flourished in educating and nurturing their constituents; they have also fostered the development of new community leadership, reflecting both increasing democratization and diversification of the hemophilia community as it entered the 1990s.

A New Era of Hope, a New Decade of Challenge

The upbeat message delivered by NHF's Annual Report in 1990 foresaw a new era of hope, a new decade of challenge. It said: "For the first time we can truly glimpse the day when there will be a cure for hemophilia and related disorders. Never before have members of the hemophilia community—families, doctors and other health care professionals, researchers, and the tens of thousands of volunteers—been so united and enlightened to conquer all these conditions."[23]

For the first time since the AIDS era began, the scientific aspects of hemophilia itself emerged in the forefront of the report, with the promise of "a cure for hemophilia by the year 2000" as a result of major advances in organ transplantation and genetic manipulation of various cell types. As a physician with hemophilia Glenn Pierce had been urging a high priority for gene therapy throughout most of the 1980s. Once Factor VIII and Factor IX were cloned, it was a short leap to realize that putting this genetic material back into a person with hemophilia would cure the disease. Although this kind of thinking was considered very much on the fringe in the mid-1980s, by the late 1980s it was being promoted by scientists at the cutting edge of gene therapy research. Pierce noted, however, that some of the hemophilia doctors ridiculed it as something out of science fiction when he started talking about it at NHF chapter meetings in 1985 or 1986. As he continued to promote the idea, making three or four talks a year about it, he found consumers receptive and slowly gained a modicum of tolerance from physicians. A turning point came toward the end of 1989, when he was in a San Francisco restaurant with a group of NHF MASAC physicians and suddenly some of the doctors realized that gene therapy was "a viable idea and a route that this community was going to take whether they were involved in the study or not."[24]

By 1990, other scientists were also expressing a sense of hope about the potential for successful gene insertion therapy in treating people born with genetic defects. Inder M. Verma, professor of molecular biology and virology at the Salk Institute in La Jolla, California, wrote:

Advances in recombinant DNA technology, which have made possible the isolation of many genes, and new insights into gene regulation are beginning to make this once impossible notion seem feasible. Indeed the first federally approved clinical trial of a gene therapy for a genetic disease began this past September [1989]. . . . The current trial could represent the start of a new era in medicine. The current pace of research suggests that by the turn of the next century clinical trials of gene therapies may be under way for any number of diseases—inherited and otherwise.[25]

Frederick Rickles, M.D., who was Vice President for Medical and Scientific Affairs of the National Hemophilia Foundation from 1987 to 1993, recalls that 1990 ushered in "the recombinant era," which will provide two pathways for improved care for patients with hemophilia, both in products and in somatic cell gene insertion therapy.

The ability to clone genes and grow genes synthetically either in bacteria [in culture] or in mammalian tissue culture systems in cells like Chinese hamster ovary cells or baby hamster kidney cells . . . has permitted the development of large-scale production of recombinant clotting factors—first Factor VIII and later Factor IX. So now [in 1997] we have commercially available two different preparations of Factor VIII and one of Factor IX. The same technology . . . has also provided increasing competence in handling those same genes and being able to ultimately "transfect" or "infect" human cells in such a way that one can envision the potential for gene therapy in the near future.[26]

By the late 1980s, there was increasing community pressure to progress beyond using plasma-based blood products that were "virtually" safe, as a result of ever-improving viral inactivation technology, to recombinant products that would totally eliminate the risk of human-blood-borne viruses. This hope was realized when a three-stage, multi-center investigation of a recombinant Factor VIII product produced positive results. In 1990, the Recombinant Factor VIII Study Group published an article in the *New England Journal of Medicine* reporting a phase III (testing in humans) study of Recombinant Factor VIII in 107 patients, 20 of whom had not been treated previously, comparing the efficacy and safety of the new product with standard therapy. The study concluded that the recombinant product "has biologic activity comparable to plasma Factor VIII and is safe and efficacious for the treatment of hemophilia A."[27] So the door was opened to the "recombinant era" for the hemophilia community.

Spreading the News: More Grass Roots

Publication of that article made it official, but it became important to disseminate the results of the study beyond medical journals. Spreading the news and assessing what it would mean, in particular for new parents with young, previously untreated children, became part of the mission for Laureen Kelley, the mother of a young son with hemophilia and author of a "Dr. Spock"–type book for hemophilia parents. Kelley's son was born in September 1987. She had no history of hemophilia in her family, so when the infant bled continuously after being circumcised, the physician did not initially suspect hemophilia. Not until a month later, following another bout of bleeding, did she and her husband receive the diagnosis. They immediately became involved with the local hemophilia treatment center and were pleased with the nurse's care and comforting manner. They also called the NHF and received some pamphlets from them. Kelley notes that her husband Kevin was very competent and calm during this difficult time.

They also went to a local support group but found, in a scenario that had hardly changed since the bad old days, that the parents of older children "sometimes delighted in providing horror stories." In addition,

October 1987 was International AIDS Month. Kelley spoke of that difficult period:

The month after my son was born, October of 1987, is the month that the home of the Ray family was bombed. . . . I know it was in *People Magazine* in October, that they portrayed them on the cover. . . . So it hit us that this was very serious, but I think the more we read, the more we became confident that although there are no guarantees in life, or in products, or in medicine, that we felt pretty comfortable giving him what we were giving him [monoclonal product].[28]

The idea of writing a book for parents surfaced when her son was six months old.

He was just learning to pull himself up to stand. He was pulling himself up and chewing on the crib rail and he cut his gum a little bit, just the tiniest slice on his gum, just enough to make him cry. We checked it out. He was bleeding. We called the treatment center. By the time we called, it had stopped, it was clotting, which is not abnormal, sometimes he does clot. But the problem with children who have moderate hemophilia like Tommy is that they clot but the clot does not hold fast. It dissolves. When it clotted, the doctor said, "He's fine. Put him back to bed." But sometime during the night, the clot dislodged, because the mouth is a very slippery, wet place and not a very good place to keep a clot. It continued to bleed, so the next morning when I went to get him, he was bouncing up and down in bed and was covered with blood from his head to his waist. All you could see were little white eyes staring out at you. His sheets were filled with blood. Luckily we didn't panic, because we knew what the cause was. . . . After that, I related the story to a friend of mine who I've gotten to know through our nurse [and] who has a son the same age as Tommy, and she said, "Haven't you heard of Amicar® [a drug that helps prevent the breakdown of clots in the mouth]? You should have given it to him when he had his initial clot." . . . And then I said, "Why didn't anyone prepare us?"[29]

Kelley recalls that "a kind of light dawned on me." She remembers thinking that often doctors are too stretched for time, so she could probably actually get more information from parents. She began to jot down notes, listing topics that she would bring to the attention of a mother with a newly diagnosed child, in order to help others avoid what she had just experienced—among the items she listed were teething and table corners. At the suggestion of their nurse that she make a story out of it, Kelley wrote what ultimately became two chapters of her book, *Raising a Child with Hemophilia.*

In 1989, when her son was two, the family began infusing him at home, which brought them a tremendous sense of freedom, completely changing their lives. It also gave Kelley the time to organize her efforts into a book. She compiled a questionnaire and sent it out to parents and set about obtaining funding for further research. Basing her focus on the concerns expressed in the approximately 130 responses she received to a questionnaire, she completed a draft for the book in eight months, wrapping it up the night before she went into labor with her next child, a daughter. Dr. Peter Levine reviewed the book for medical accuracy— and wrote the foreword. The initial printing of ten thousand copies sold out within three years, and a second printing was ordered.

Not long after the book came out Kelley received a call from a North Carolina mother, suggesting that she establish an 800-number telephone line and a newsletter to help parents communicate and share ideas. A short time later, a home care company that delivers Factor products to patients contacted her to congratulate her on her book and to inform her that they were distributing it to customers. The representative asked if there was anything else that they might do for her. She immediately explained her plans for a newsletter, and the company agreed to fund it without restrictions on its content. Kelley maintains that they have kept their word. The *Parent Exchange Newsletter* (*PEN*) began in 1991 with a circulation of fifty; it is now distributed in forty-five countries to a circulation of about six thousand. An early issue featured an article entitled "Is Recombinant Better?" written by Kevin Kelley, who is a scientist at a biotech company. Kelley notes that her husband has both the scientific ability to understand the research and the ability to translate the material into a coherent article for lay readers. Meanwhile, she has gone on to found two more newsletters and to produce several illustrated books for children.

Her voice and perspective would become a mainstay of the constituency of new parents of children with hemophilia in the 1990s. Communicating through her publications, she has reached family households directly, not going through the NHF chapter structure alone. She does, however, also share channels of communication with the Foundation, sending newsletters that can be distributed when people request information she has covered. Although she primarily represents the needs of the non-HIV-infected segment of the hemophilia community, she realizes that had her son been born only two years earlier, he too might have been infected. It wasn't until 1993 that she became acutely aware of the need for her to bridge both parts of the community. She has since added HIV and AIDS information to her book and newsletter and has actively supported efforts to obtain financial compensation for those who had contracted HIV through the blood supply.

Currents Beneath the Surface

The 1991 NHF Annual Report continued the theme of community unity and strength, but this masked a growing uneasiness that was surfacing, primarily in MANN discussion groups. "They" became "us" as the number of sick and dying increased. Men began to express frustration and to question NHF's nonconfrontational posture and lack of support for and involvement in government compensation and litigation. As frustration grew, decisions made in the early 1980s began to be questioned and challenged.

CHAPTER 12

Approaching the Biotech Century
Out with the Old, In with the New, 1992–98

Bill and Hillary Clinton and Al and Tipper Gore swayed to the music of the Fleetwood Mac song "Don't Stop Thinking about Tomorrow" as they swept into office, supported by new and old coalitions—baby boomers, minorities, the elderly, the gay community, the disenfranchised, the frustrated, and the hopeful. Bill Clinton made it clear that by electing him, the American public had acquired a special bonus. Not only did we have a dynamic new president but also a highly competent, professional first lady who would make a significant contribution to our society. Since health care reform was a centerpiece of the campaign, Clinton established a Health Reform Task Force in 1993, appointing Hillary Rodham Clinton as chair.[1] Ira Magaziner, an old friend of the president's, was appointed executive director.

In a critical review of proposals to reform the U.S. health care system, Susan Browning suggests that a number of factors seemed to indicate in 1992 that fundamental reform could be implemented in the near future. The general public, including various mainstream groups, such as organized medicine, business, and labor, had become vocal advocates for reform, and the media increasingly focused on the topic. At least five reform proposals purporting to offer health care for all Americans had been developed by the time the Clinton administration took office. Browning notes that criticisms of the health care system were based on two perceived deficiencies: first, total health care spending was commanding an ever-increasing share of the nation's resources—11.6 percent of the GNP in 1989, despite cost containment measures taken in the 1980s—and, second, a growing number of Americans had limited financial access to health care.[2]

In a thoughtful comparison between the enactment of Medicare during the Johnson administration and the reform efforts of the Clinton years, David Blumenthal suggests that health care reform must involve a "federal legislative initiative that provides all Americans financial protection against the cost of illness and that also contains a coherent approach to reducing the growth in health care expenditures." With this as a goal, the new administration forged ahead, gaining momentum from the perception that the election had revealed widespread support. The Task Force visualized themselves orchestrating a successful outcome, perhaps seeing an analogy to the climate in the mid-1960s, when a political team consisting of President Lyndon Johnson and Assistant Secretary of Health, Education, and Welfare Wilbur Cohen championed the Medicare program. As Blumenthal points out, however, there were vast differences between the two situations. Cohen had worked for decades in the Social Security Administration and was known and trusted by both Democrats and Republicans. Lyndon Johnson had been Senate majority leader and "a legendary Congressional tactician who had few peers before or since as a master of the congressional process." Together, they oversaw the enactment of Medicare legislation, which Blumenthal describes as "the most successful effort in history to revamp the American health care system." But unlike the Johnson team, the Clinton team took nearly a year to draft The Health Security Act, with the result that it became a victim of pressures at the end of the Congressional session. Whether or not the bill was technically sound, it was politically unsuccessful. Hillary Clinton's group was perceived by legislators as a group of outsiders, academics who were out of touch with the real world—"academically talented but politically naïve."[3] The lengthy process was seen as not including or welcoming of congressional input in its formative stages.

One proposal, which had originated early in this round of reform discussions, was the Enthoven-Kronick plan, crafted by Alain Enthoven and Richard Kronick, two experienced health strategists. Its appeal for the Clinton administration lay in the philosophy of managed competition. The proposal envisioned government-mandated changes in the structure of medical practice that would enhance the performance of the health care sector. Its two primary goals were to insure that all individuals would have financial protection against the costs of health care and to reduce health costs overall. Although the theoretical framework for the administration's bill began with this "purest form of managed competition," the plan that resulted was perceived as overly complex and detailed, with layers of bureaucracy. A negative media blitz ensued. The Health Insurance Association of America's famously effective "Harry and Louise" advertisements promoted the idea that this health care proposal would insert government into our daily private lives. In addition to the fear of government intrusion and bureaucratic mismanagement, the bill failed to overcome the sense that "universal access issues" related not to the majority of citizens but to an underclass. Medicare, by contrast, was viewed as something that would eventually touch everyone's life—we all eventually grow old. Congress's failure to bring the administration's proposal to a vote marked the indefinite postponement of government-directed health reform and the beginning of a private-sector managed-care movement that would take on a life of its own, changing health care delivery dramatically by the mid-1990s.

The Hemophilia Community:
A Dim View of Managed Care

Although, as we have seen, the early and mid-1990s continued the erosion in trust between hemophilia community doctors and patients that began in the AIDS Era, the idea of replacing the national network of hemophilia treatment centers by managed care providers would be vehemently opposed by most of the community. Just as the packaged freeze-dried plasma products had become an expected part of daily life, meeting most health care needs through the treatment centers had become the norm. Patients feared cost-driven reduction in the quantity and quality of care and were reluctant to adjust to a situation without a familiar team of multidisciplinary care providers who understood hemophilia and who knew them. Although elements of health reform had some appeal, managed care, with new health providers, had little.

By the mid-1990s MCH organized forums of consumers and medical directors to plan "Hemophilia Care for the Year 2000." Some of the medical directors conceived of the treatment center network becoming a health maintenance organization (HMO) of sorts. In California in particular the hemophilia treatment centers decided to collaborate in new ways. Recognizing—however grudgingly—that managed care plans were proliferating, treatment center directors wanted to promote the HTCs as primary providers for persons with hemophilia and their families. At the very least, they wanted the HTCs to be included in the network of listed providers so that consumers could have "unfettered access" to high-quality hemophilia care.[4]

The concerns of the hemophilia community for its special needs in the face of "managed care" had a voice in Washington, D.C. Marc Associates, a consulting firm headed by Daniel Maldonado, was the successor to John Grupenhoff and Grupenhoff and Endicott Associates as the community's advocacy arm. In 1994 Val Bias, an articulate spokesperson for people with hemophilia who is both HIV-positive and African American, joined the firm to become legislative coordinator for the NHF. Maldonado maintained that the hemophilia system of comprehensive care should be viewed as a model for health reform. He said:

It contains all the right ingredients. We have regional treatment networks, we have chapters and peer support, and we even have a research base and epidemiological and clinical trials. The principal of consumer-based comprehensive care has been an essential building block in many of the public health initiatives Congress has appropriated support for. It has allowed us to educate a larger number of people about insurance reform concerns related to patient access, so that the care for hemophilia and other bleeding disorders is not stopped at the gatekeeper level. We will continue to advocate for preservation of the hemophilia system of comprehensive care including recognition of the treatment centers as essential community providers.

Bias added that because states were being aggressive in cost-cutting measures, advocates for the hemophilia community were also trying to make the case for specialized care for persons with chronic conditions.[5]

Dr. Shelby Dietrich, the innovative designer of the hemophilia multidisciplinary treatment center model, who has remained an HTC medical director and caregiver throughout all of these years, described her sense of recent developments and her feeling that it may be time for a new approach to hemophilia care:

When the Clinton administration took office after the election of 1992, I felt that with the president's obvious support, proposals for health reform would take place. And, obviously, they didn't. But . . . whether we like it or not, hemophilia is a terribly expensive disease, and I think it can be managed more efficiently and with higher quality if there is management of care. I don't think comprehensive care is antithetical to managed care at all. There are big wastes in the system. There are inefficiencies. The largest inefficiency obviously relates to the use of concentrate—because concentrate accounts for 75 to 85 percent of the cost of care. So I became interested in joining forces, so to speak, with the company that was terribly aggressive in signing up clients for home care. Again, I think that we have to recognize—we don't have to like it, but we have to recognize—that we operate in a market economy. And until we have some sort of national health reform, the profit motive will drive the market. And I don't think recognizing that makes one sort of evil. I think it's simply reality. There are realities in life—death, taxes—and maybe managed care is one of them. And change is certainly one of the realities to add to death and taxes. I would rather lead change than have to react to it.

. . . But having said managed care is the wave of the future, we come to yet another horn in the dilemma, and that is the role of the primary physician versus the super-specialist role of the hematologist. In this case, I believe and recommend the hematologist assume the dual role of primary physician and specialist for the patient with hemophilia. However, I have to qualify that by saying the hematologist needs a considerable amount of experience, too, in the care of people with hemophilia. And a community hematologist who may have seen only one or two patients in his or her career will not be any more skilled actually than will the usual generalist or primary physician. The system of hemophilia treatment centers, federally funded to some degree, was set up approximately twenty years ago in response to this very need . . . to have a center with a qualified, experienced staff who would see patients with such a rare disorder. However, the hemophilia treatment centers are of very questionable economic viability. They are, in many cases, understaffed with overworked personnel who have a great deal of expertise and are also in the position to carry out research studies where one has to aggregate a certain critical number of patients.

She added that since many HTCs are in academic medical centers, they are also feeling the crunch of funding those centers face. Admitting to mixed feelings about the HTCs, she went on to say:

It's a wonderful concept, and it certainly has worked, but I just wonder if we shouldn't devote some more creative thinking to having a few centers of excellence. By few, I mean on a national basis, probably regionally distributed. No more than three or four in regions and even less in some of the less densely populated regions. And then developing a better secondary system of generalists or specialists, making sure there is always adequate follow-up and adequate communication and transportation in case of emergencies.[6]

The Pot Boils Over: Rage and Rebellion Surface

By 1992, outbursts of anger and signs of splintering within the hemophilia community disrupted business as usual, as AIDS deaths continued to rise. Rage initially began to surface within the structure of MANN, which, as noted, provided a setting for men to bond and to share feelings of frustration and anger. Men were not only becoming sicker; some also had to witness AIDS infecting and killing their wives and children—and deal with the fact that they themselves were the source of the disease. Trying to channel their rage and frustration into action, they began to pay more attention to both AIDS movement activists within the United States and the quest for compensation, which had an international context. In Canada in 1989 the federal government had awarded all groups infected with HIV via blood transfusions the equivalent of $88,000 per person over three years.[7] Events in France, which led in 1992 to the indictment of those individuals considered responsible for not having tested blood products sooner plus the awarding of compensation to infected persons with hemophilia (providing a lump sum of up to 2 million francs, or U.S.$300,000), fueled the growing momentum to seek assistance for themselves and their families.[8] They were also aware of the U.S. Vaccine Injury Compensation Fund, established by an act of Congress to compensate families of children who were injured by childhood vaccinations, and of the alternative resolution dispute model as an alternative to litigation.

Meanwhile the NHF continued its advocacy and its programs, while the organizational leadership went along with what they still perceived to be the community's desire to keep a low profile. At the same time social activists from within the community began to stir the pot.[9] The key radical leaders who emerged would eventually break away from the NHF structure. They were Jonathan Wadleigh, who founded the Committee of Ten Thousand (COTT), and Michael Rosenberg, who began the California-based American H/HIV/PEER Association (commonly known as HIV/PEER). As mentioned in Chapter 11, Wadleigh's association with Boston ACT UP most likely shaped his tactics and philosophy. The activist tactics of ACT UP appealed to the younger men, who must have felt a surge of power and bonding as they united in protest

and in a quest for compensation and revenge. COTT gained a following through its newsletter, *The Common Factor,* which Wadleigh began
publishing in April 1992 and which sought to raise the awareness of the
hemophilia community about AIDS community activism. Rosenberg
was a featured "guest columnist" in the first edition of COTT's newsletter, in which he called for an "organization that militantly addresses
the economic needs of HIV-ravaged families." His solution was to "roll
up our organizational sleeves and fight."[10]

MANN produced leaders from within the community who sought
to reconfigure NHF rather than breaking away. They developed the
goals, objectives, and mission statement. For Val Bias one critical event
became a springboard for the upheaval within the NHF structure: the
NHF refused to let the Men's Executive Committee (MEC) meet without a staff person in the room. This "paternalistic view" inspired them
to meet away from the NHF office. From this meeting came a political
platform that included encouraging NHF to explore more aggressively
issues of compensation and health care reform, promoting a congressional investigation into the infection with HIV of people with hemophilia through the blood supply, and improving HTC care for HIV.[11]

MANN also engineered the outcome of the election of officers at the
NHF annual meeting in Atlanta, Georgia, in November 1992. Initially,
Glenn Pierce and Val Bias were running against each other for president,
but they chose to collaborate, with Pierce becoming president and Bias
chairman of the board. Pierce made it clear that Bias was to be a full
partner and in his message to the hemophilia community, published in
Newsnotes, he stated:

In reviewing the past year it is clear that the NHF ship needs to be turned—and
not just five or ten degrees, but 45 degrees. Our goal is to turn it during this
next year. We must examine all the issues facing NHF in being advocates for the
people with hemophilia, people with hemophilia and HIV. . . . We need to build
on our strengths. Grassroots activism is important. Several years ago the
Women's Outreach Network of NHF (WONN) was created, and last year the
Men's Advocacy Network of NHF (MANN) joined it. These programs are a
tribute to their members, making their presence felt at every level. Similarly the
Chapter Outreach Demonstration Project (CODP), funded by the Maternal
and Child Health Bureau, has been extremely successful in bringing previously
underserved populations within the purview of chapters and treatment centers,
and is bringing creative individuals into positions of leadership.[12]

Among the several key developments at the 1992 Atlanta meeting, two were of particular importance. First was the formation of a Special Assistance Council (SAC), which was to pursue the campaign for special assistance (meaning compensation for the families of those infected with HIV), with both government and industry initiatives. Marc Associates began discussions with supportive Congressional staff, and eventually Val Bias became their NHF coordinator. The second, and more explosive, was the adoption by the Medical and Scientific Advisory Council (MASAC) of a resolution stating that physicians and others associated with NHF should not testify as expert witnesses on behalf of clotting factor concentrate manufacturers and/or distributors. In fact some physicians had already served as "expert witnesses," testifying about the state of knowledge in the early 1980s. These initial litigations sparked a second wave of erosion of trust and inflamed an already combustible situation. The perception spread like wildfire throughout the hemophilia community that not only had their physicians withheld information and not presented treatment options, but they were now testifying against their patients. The MASAC resolution was drafted in response to these concerns; in the understated terms of the report of the annual meeting, "it may be perceived by some that we may be impairing the ability of individuals or families to obtain fair legal judgment."[13]

The day after MASAC adopted the resolution, it was approved by the NHF Board. That afternoon, Peter Levine, M.D., a former NHF Medical Director and a MASAC member, read the draft resolution during a contentious town meeting. Patients and families who had brought suit against concentrate manufacturers expressed considerable frustration with legal proceedings. A lawyer on the panel suggested that because of the "blood shield laws," which made it difficult if not impossible to gain compensation by bringing suit, legislative action might be a more appropriate avenue for redress.[14] Several speakers gave Michael Rosenberg (who has since died) credit for bringing the issue of compensation to the foreground. Rosenberg had earlier asserted that there was a "vast paper trail" that revealed the process by which he felt the hemophilia community was knowingly infected with AIDS, although he added that the most important issue to him was not compensation but "knowing the truth."[15] Jonathan Wadleigh reiterated Rosenberg's concerns and argued that the success of the alternative dispute resolution process

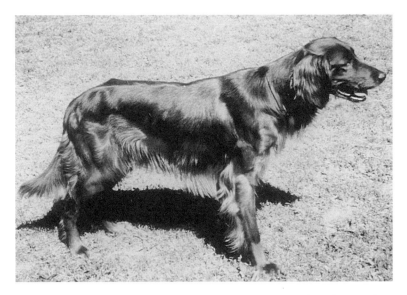

Irish setter with hemophilia A (Factor VIII deficient), one of the dogs in the Chapel Hill colony that were used for both laboratory and clinical work in coagulation research by Kenneth Brinkhous, M.D., and his colleagues at the University of North Carolina. This photograph dates from the mid-1950s when a program for preventing hemophilic arthropathy—or joint disease—was in place. (Courtesy Francis Owen Blood Research Laboratory, Chapel Hill, N.C.)

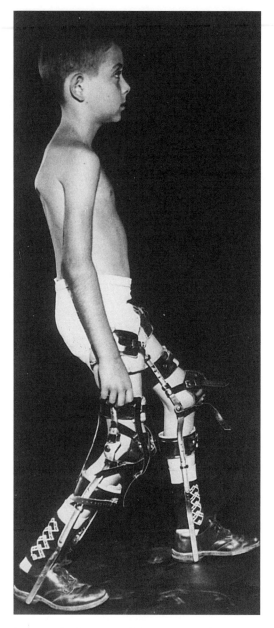

A patient in the Hemophilia Program, directed by
Shelby Dietrich, M.D. This photo, taken in 1959 at
the Baby Clinic of the California Hospital in Los
Angeles (before the Hemophilia Program moved
to the Los Angeles Orthopaedic Hospital), illus-
trates the severe damage to the joints that was
common among hemophilia patients before the
use of home infusion therapy. (Photograph by Alfred Benjamin; courtesy Shelby Dietrich, M.D.)

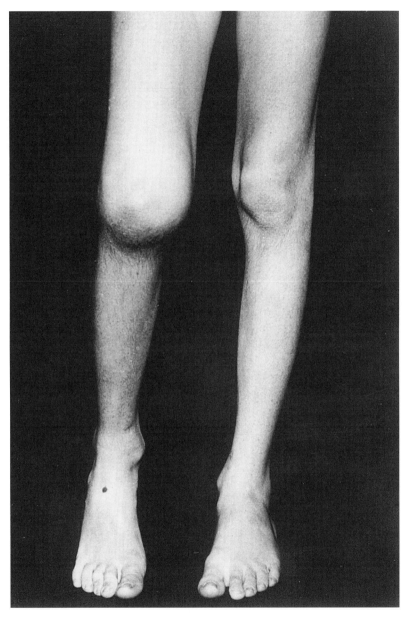

A knee bleed in a patient in the Hemophilia Program, directed by Shelby Dietrich, M.D. Also taken in 1959, this photo shows the extensive damage that occurred in hemophilia patients as a result of such bleeding into the joints. (Photograph by Alfred Benjamin; courtesy Shelby Dietrich, M.D.)

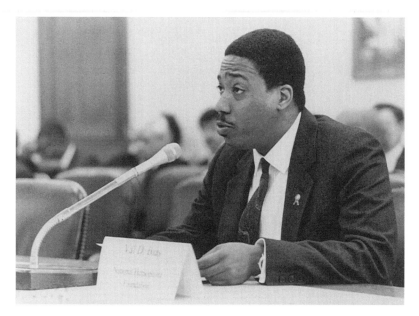

Val Bias of MARC Associates, testifying on behalf of the hemophilia community before the U.S. House of Representatives Appropriations Subcommittee on January 31, 1995. (Photograph by Cable Risdon; courtesy National Hemophilia Foundation)

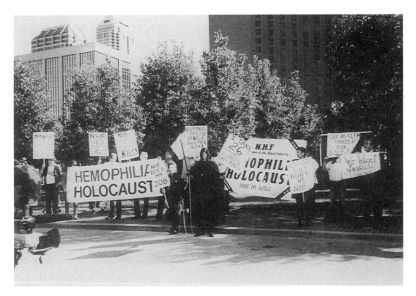

Protestors representing hemophilia activist groups demonstrating outside the Westin Hotel in Indianapolis, Indiana, during the annual meeting of the National Hemophilia Association in October 1993. (Photograph by Eunice Heredia, Southern California Hemophilia Chapter, Los Angeles)

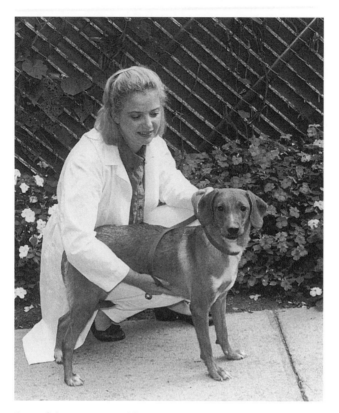

One of the two original hemophilia B (Factor IX deficient) dogs in the Chapel Hill, North Carolina, colony to receive FIX gene therapy, with technician Pamela McElveen. This photo was featured in the report on this research that appeared in *Science* in October 1993. (Photograph by William Brinkhous; courtesy Francis Owen Blood Research Laboratory, Chapel Hill, N.C.)

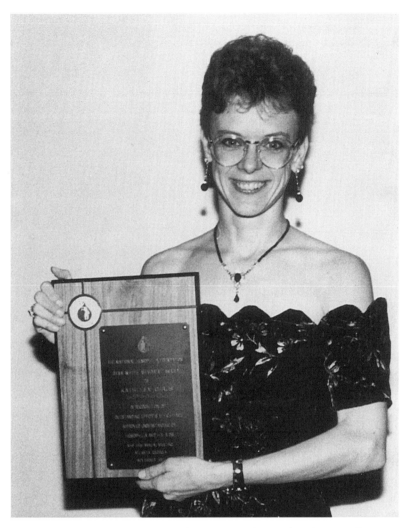

Kathy Gerus, receiving the Ryan White Memorial Award at the annual meeting of the National Hemophilia Foundation in Atlanta, Georgia, in November 1992. The award recognizes outstanding individuals for their contributions to education about hemophilia and HIV. (Courtesy National Hemophilia Foundation)

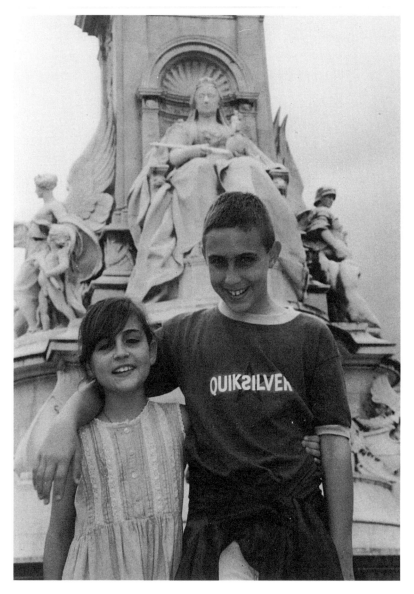

The children of a person with hemophilia, representing the future of hemophilia families as they stand before a statue of Queen Victoria, the most famous carrier of hemophilia in the past; London, 1997.

would be determined by whether the major pharmaceutical companies took part in the discussion.[16] Mark Faitek, president of the Minnesota chapter, praised Rosenberg for accelerating the idea of compensation but also requested that he bring an end to accusations that had begun to split the hemophilia community apart.

Remarking that "'92 was a year of change," Glenn Pierce vividly remembered the polarization and the "heavy-duty reactionaries" at the Atlanta meeting:

For me personally, this was a very rough meeting. We had protesters, we had the splinter groups that came into our board meeting and challenged us for the right to lead NHF. They demanded our resignations. They demanded our accountability, and it was very difficult to have the weight of the past fifteen years of NHF actions upon our shoulders, which is exactly what we had. So though we weren't the people making the decisions fifteen years ago, we were the people running the organization, [and they saw us as] responsible for making those decisions. That was pretty tough, and at a certain point you ask, well, can we get through this or would it have been better to just scrap the NHF, disband it, start a whole new organization? I think in retrospect we did the right thing, which was to try to steer NHF to become an organization that would respond to the needs of the community.

He noted that he and Bias, as newly elected president and board chairman, immediately fulfilled their promise to improve communication to the entire community through a series of frequent bulletins sent to all individuals affiliated with NHF. These bulletins were eventually called the *Community Alert* and had a newsletter flavor, not just the "organizational tidbits" of *Hemophilia Newsnotes*. "Paul Phillips" recalled that Pierce had become increasingly concerned that the AIDS Task Force and the NHF should be more aggressive about assuring that all persons with hemophilia receive bulletins and advisories rather than relying on chapters. Pierce wanted to get information out directly about clinical trials and complimentary medicines and to reach sexual partners.[17] *Community Alert* included information from both industry and splinter groups, and there was a real effort to make the newsletter, which started with a mailing list of 4,000 and now has about 20,000, responsive to the community. Pierce mentioned that during this period COTT began publishing its own newsletter, *The Common Factor*, which he believed had put a lot of "mistruths . . . —about Val, myself, about the previous leadership of NHF." *Community Alert* was the vehicle through which they could point out what the NHF was and be sure that people would get the message, since it bypassed the chapter structure and went directly to families. An important component of this to Pierce was what he says was a misconception about who was running NHF at the time decisions were made in the early 1980s. He encountered people thinking that "NHF was not an organization run by people with hemophilia. Nobody with hemophilia was on the board." He and Bias released the names of everybody on the board in 1982 and 1983 to reveal that over half "had a direct connection with hemophilia." He said that the executive committee, the top leadership of the organization, had a person with hemophilia at the helm throughout this time, and two past presidents had died of AIDS—Nathan Smith and Charles Carman. He added that "it wasn't as if they were making decisions based upon facts that they weren't following themselves."[18]

The Common Factor described itself as a forum for discussion of HIV treatment strategies; ways to stay healthy; the science, politics, and business of HIV; methods of coping with HIV infection and AIDS; and how HIV affects love and sexuality.[19] The initial issue, dated April 1992, included articles by the cofounders of COTT, Jonathan Wadleigh and Tom Fahey, and guest columnist Michael Rosenberg. Although Rosenberg spoke of "constructive dialogue" in his article, he depicted the situation as a great wave of alienation within the hemophilia community between persons with hemophilia and their families, on one hand, and, on the other hand, the hemophilia institutional structure—including the National Hemophilia Foundation, the chapters, the other grant-based or publicly funded organizations presumably providing services to persons with hemophilia, and the personnel of the hemophilia treatment centers. Rosenberg described himself as a person with Factor VIII hemophilia, who was diagnosed as HIV-positive in 1985 and who lost his hemophilic brother to AIDS in 1991. He asserted that "it is still generally the case that persons with HIV—whether it be related to hemophilia or another source—are likely to find better sources of HIV treatment and treatment information, more accessible emotional support, and stronger political and economic advocacy outside the hemophilia establishment than in it," that "the hemophilia institutions are still in denial about the extent of the phenomenon before us." He used the term "we, the alienated," saying that "we do not identify with the hemophilia institutions" and do not need "an organization that cozies up to the corporate factor-makers, that can be bought off cheaply with small grants and PR gimmicks." He called for seeking major financial relief in the form of "a serious class action suit against the pharmaceutical giants for guaranteed comprehensive health coverage, or government subsidies like those granted to hemophilia families in Canada and in more than twenty other countries, or some combination." He went on to describe the hemophilia organizations as working in "splendid isolation," in particular with regard to the gay community.[20]

In addition to presenting the combination of a militant stance and "an opportunity to become wiser, deeper, and more loving," *The Common Factor* included up-to-date treatment information and a listing of buyers' clubs for medications for PWAs (persons with AIDS). It became a conduit for rapid dissemination of information already circulating in the gay community and the AIDS community at large. The editors acknowledged their debt to "Project Inform," *AIDS Treatment News,* the *Bulletin of Experimental Treatments for AIDS* (*BETA*), and many other publications. Wadleigh quoted Ralph Waldo Emerson in the first issue: "Fear always springs from ignorance; . . . knowledge is the antidote to fear."[21] Despite assessing blame with a very broad brush, these splinter groups clearly brought new and useful information to the hemophilia community. They also contributed to creating a bridge between the AIDS community and the hemophilia community.

Glenn Pierce remembered that for the most part 1992 and 1993 were difficult years. Some of the difficulties pertained to "Paul Phillips," because he was the last remaining leader from the early 1980s and because the AIDS disaster struck "on his watch." Although he "tried to diffuse the situation," Pierce found, as he traveled with "Phillips" and Bias, that local chapter meetings and regional meetings became "yelling matches," where they all underwent a great deal of criticism, with "Phillips" as a focal point. Attendees would yell, "Why did you infect me?" For the most part, these men were young; they had been children or teenagers in the early 1980s, when their parents made treatment decisions. Pierce notes that "It's revisionist history, because the son doesn't want to blame the mom, so they say they never received any warnings, any information about the AIDS crisis at all." They all asked him why the NHF hadn't warned them. He remarked that chapters had refused to give NHF their mailing lists so all that NHF could do was to send mail to chapters, not directly to patients and families. This weak link in communications between NHF and the chapters was the first deficiency Pierce and Bias strove to correct with the *Community Alert*. Pierce tried to shift the focus to NHF's current actions—trying to gain assistance for its constituency while striving for a safe blood supply and seeking a cure and sending information directly to individual families. He would refer to SAC as visible evidence that grassroots leaders were involved directly in meeting with the manufacturers.[22]

Amidst the difficulties, Pierce also recalled a very positive scientific event that took place in March 1992, well before the organizational upheavals of the annual meeting in the fall of that year. It was the workshop entitled Gene Therapy for Hemophilia, convened by the National Heart, Lung, and Blood Institute (NHLBI). Having the federal government's official acknowledgment that hemophilia is a particularly suitable target for gene therapy was a big step on the journey to a cure. Indeed, the director of NHLBI, Claude Lenfant, M.D., stated, "Great strides have been made in hemophilia research, and the time may not be far off when genetic therapy for hemophilia becomes the accepted mode of treatment."[23] Glenn Pierce, as both a physician and a person with hemophilia, played a unique leadership role at the conference.

Seeking Compensation: A Journey from Collaborative Resolution to Litigation and Legislation

To enable the Special Assistance Council (SAC) to accomplish its mission, NHF established a fund to support costs involved in seeking compensation, and the board passed a resolution to aggressively pursue a campaign for special assistance. The Hemophilia and AIDS/HIV Network for the Dissemination of Information (HANDI) had become a major resource and was now used to help consumers gain access to information on compensation. HANDI would continue to play an increasingly important role. In 1992 it began publishing *HIV Treatment Information Exchange (HTIE)*, which described treatment options. At first the SAC fostered a process of collaboration, involving an industry and government initiative that would focus on providing special assistance to meet the needs of persons with hemophilia, to be administered by a nonprofit organization. Discussions with pharmaceutical companies began in the fall of 1993. But when SAC proposed that the industry establish a $1.5 billion humanitarian fund, the proposal was rejected as "unwarranted and unrealistic."

According to Glenn Pierce, COTT was initially involved in the negotiations, and then "one day COTT turned around and filed a lawsuit against all industry as well as the NHF." He recalled this as typical of the sort of turmoil that was going on at that time and felt that "it's a very unethical way to do it—to negotiate in partnership with NHF, lead us along, and then turn around and file a class action suit against us." He was totally taken by surprise. He recalled going to the October 1993 NHF annual meeting in Indianapolis, Indiana, with his "stomach churning, more than it was churning in Atlanta," fearing that COTT might serve NHF with papers at the meeting, but they did not. Instead, he experienced personally and directly the faces and voices of rage.

The leader of the HIV/PEER Association, Michael Rosenberg, came up to me in the NHF office, grabbed my tie around my neck and pulled it. He was very upset because he didn't get quite the booth space that he wanted to display his materials. He was definitely out of control. In addition, at the board meeting COTT came in and demanded that the entire board resign. They would come in and pick up the pieces. One of the leadership of COTT, in the hallway, privately threatened me with the lives of my family and told me that I was responsible for killing his son—who was not dead yet. . . . Because of what I did and because of my actions, my family would die too."[24]

Pierce found this attack so traumatizing that he spent a large part of 1994 recuperating from it. Meanwhile, Corey Dubin, another person with hemophilia who took an activist stance, emerged as a spokesperson for HIV/Peer Association. HIV/PEER and COTT joined forces to file the class action lawsuit Pierce referred to, in Chicago on September 30, 1993; Dubin and Wadleigh framed their suit as "on behalf of American hemophiliacs." Dubin in particular became associated with the litigation by writing about it in *The Common Factor* and by appearing in the media in news stories and on television programs. For the next four years, the ongoing drama of litigation played out with heightened media attention, primarily to COTT and HIV/PEER. Early in 1995 the original class action suit was "thrown out because the class was not uniform enough to be considered representative."[25] According to Pierce, the manufacturers then came back to the table, and the way was once again opened for a compensation payment from the pharmaceutical companies. But new conflicts followed. On, June 11, 1996, the Business Day section of the *New York Times* featured a photo of Corey Dubin, labeled "the activist," in an article entitled "Blood, Money, and AIDS: Hemophiliacs Are Split." The article described the latest schism: Dubin, dissatisfied with the way key plaintiff's lawyers were handling the litigation, had gone on a "stealth mission" to negotiate his own deal with the pharmaceutical manufacturers without the knowledge of key plaintiff's lawyers.[26] The article further noted, however, that although the lead lawyer, David Shrager, had initially battled with Dubin, as of that date they had taken a united stand. By June 1997, although two members of the settlement class had filed an appeal, a settlement went through—the U.S. hemophilia community would finally begin to receive some compensation for the tragedy it was enduring. On June 8, 1997, the first page of the *San Francisco Examiner* featured the headline "BLOOD MONEY" and a color photo of "one of the 6,200 HIV-infected hemophiliacs and their survivors who are finally getting money for their pain: $100,000 per person."[27]

An Investigation Begins: The IOM Report

In addition to litigation, hemophilia community activists pursued other avenues. In April of 1993, Representative Porter J. Goss (R-Fla.) and Senators Edward Kennedy (D-Mass.) and Bob Graham (D-Fla.), in response to requests from and information furnished by the hemophilia community, requested that the Secretary of Health and Human Services open an investigation into the events leading to the transmission of HIV to individuals with hemophilia. Secretary Donna Shalala agreed that such an investigation was important and that it would be useful to gain a more complete understanding of the use of blood and blood products for the treatment of those with hemophilia and those who received transfusions in the early years of the AIDS epidemic.[28] She requested that the Institute of Medicine (IOM) establish a committee to conduct a historical analysis that would help both public policy and decision making with regard to our blood supply in the future. The IOM

Committee was to examine decision making in the early 1980s, before testing of blood and viral inactivation procedures were instituted. To do this it would gather testimony from consumers, providers, industry, government, and academia, hold hearings and write a report discussing their findings, and make recommendations. The IOM report, *HIV and the Blood Supply: An Analysis of Crisis Decision Making*, emanated from a process that established an opportunity for grassroots leadership from the hemophilia community to be truly heard and acknowledged. As a provider of information, sharing my doctoral dissertation—the basis for this book—with the IOM Committee, I attended the hearings on September 12, 1994. I recall the heart-wrenching testimony and the intensity of the anger expressed by HIV-infected persons with hemophilia and their families. And most of all, particularly from the women who spoke, I remember the pleas to find out how this came about so that it would never happen again. The tragedy loomed large, affecting the committee members and all others present. The parade of presenters made it clear that the hemophilia community could no longer be viewed only as parents and young poster boys. The once invisible members of the community had come out of their medical closets for the IOM hearings, showing diversity in race, age, gender, and ethnicity.

When the committee issued its report, its conclusions and recommendations included finding that no person or agency had taken the responsibility to coordinate all of the organizations sharing the public health responsibility for achieving a safe blood supply. Recommendations, several of which have since been enacted, included the designation of a Blood Safety Director to be responsible for the federal government's efforts to maintain the safety of the blood supply, establishment of a Public Health Service Blood Safety Council to assess current and future threats to the blood supply, consideration of a no-fault compensation system for individuals suffering adverse consequences from the use of blood or blood products, and the requirement that the composition of the Food and Drug Administration (FDA) Blood Products Advisory Committee reflect a proper balance between members who are connected with the blood industry and members who are independent of the industry. It was also recommended that the FDA should tell its advisory committees what it expects of them and should independently evaluate their agendas and performances. In addition, the FDA should develop reliable sources of information regarding the blood supply and should have its own capacity to analyze and predict the effects of regulatory decisions.[29]

The report also reached conclusions regarding communication between clinicians and patients. Emphasizing the importance of informed consent and autonomy of patients in decision making involving their own health, the report described the NHF's strategy for providing information as "seriously flawed." The committee concluded that "Hemophilia patients did not have the basis for informed choice about a difficult treatment decision. . . . The NHF focused on practice [clinical] recommendations rather than giving complete information about risks and options." Noting that there are both public health and clinical approaches to reducing the risk of blood-borne diseases, the IOM committee recommended the creation of an expert panel to inform the providers of care and the public about the risks associated with blood and blood products and to provide the clinical information that physicians and their patients need to guide health choices. Finally, the committee noted that "voluntary organizations, such as the NHF, that make recommendations about the use of commercial products, must avoid conflict of interest, maintain independent judgment, and otherwise act to earn the confidence of the public and the patients"; this last recommendation is crucial in maintaining "the fabric of trust that holds our society together."[30]

Secretary Shalala's responsiveness to the report and support for its recommendations assured rapid progress in guaranteeing blood safety. The role played by the hemophilia community in safeguarding the blood supply has continued to increase. But none of this could diminish the importance of attending to the tragic loss of life for young boys and the suffering of their families. It did not obliterate the horrors suffered by the White family, the Ray family, and many others. Louise Ray had only begun her public participation by speaking at the IOM hearing, for by the next year she would be spearheading another community initiative, the introduction of legislation in her son's name, the Ricky Ray Act.

In 1995 Representative Porter Goss and Senator Mike deWine (R-Ohio) introduced the Ricky Ray Hemophilia Relief Fund Act of 1995. Goss, in speaking before the Subcommittee on Immigration and Claims on September 19, 1996, said that he had known the Ray family since 1989 and that Louise Ray would later share her story. Another effective spokesperson who has become an increasingly visible activist, Dana Kuhn, a former minister, described his situation, saying that he was never given options for treatment or counseled to use safe sex practices until he was tested in 1986. By then both he and his wife were infected; she died in 1987, leaving him as the sole parent of two young children. Kuhn related the earlier history of the government's willingness to consider it an acceptable risk for hemophiliacs to be exposed to hepatitis in the blood supply. Louise Ray then recounted her tragedy: all three of her sons were infected, her children were denied public education, and her home was burned to the ground by an arsonist. The Ricky Ray Bill would authorize a government compensation trust fund from which each of the victims infected with HIV through the use of contaminated blood products would receive $100,000 in compassionate assistance. The bill was passed by the House in May 1998, and on Thursday, November 12, 1998, as the National Hemophilia Foundation celebrated its golden anniversary at the annual meeting in Orlando, Florida, President Bill Clinton signed the Ricky Ray Act into law, bringing the NHF's first fifty years to a close with a dramatic promise of hope.

Transformations: Healing, Preventing, and Curing

The tides of rage had begun to ebb by 1994. Many factors have combined in the ensuing years to help calm the waters. Most exciting is the gene insertion therapy cure, which now seems within reach by the beginning of the next century. Trials have already shown promise with dogs and were tentatively scheduled to begin on human beings in 1998.[31] In addition to the gaining of compensation for infected members of the community, other conditions and events have also contributed to the sense of transformation. When "Paul Phillips" decided to resign from his position as executive director of NHF in 1994, he said, "As the last remaining leadership figure from the early 1980s, it is my greatest hope that my departure will enable NHF's current peer [grassroots] leadership and all members of the hemophilia community—parents, health care professionals, and NHF staff—to begin to sharpen their focus on the future."[32] Ever-increasing participation and leadership among women and minorities bring new perspectives and dimensions to the fore, broadening and reshaping the formerly male culture. And the interactive electronic communication technology of the 1990s has given the hemophilia community a virtual worldwide village. Chat rooms have removed the need to travel by air or to converse by conference call. The FDA has an Internet Web page where information about withdrawals and recalls of pooled plasma products that may be contaminated can be accessed by an entire community, bypassing bureaucracy to communicate directly with families.

With blood safety now officially on the front burner, the hemophilia community is no longer the "canary in the mine shaft," signaling danger in the blood supply by its demise. Instead it has become the town crier, vigilant in preventing further tragedy. Bea Pierce is a vocal representative for the hemophilia community and served on the FDA's Blood Products Advisory Committee from 1995 to 1997. Indeed, caution has become the watchword, as concerns about hepatitis C and Creutzfeldt-Jakob disease have further changed the "business as usual" mentality. When there is uncertainty about the safety of blood or blood products now, they are withdrawn. Mark Weinstein, chief of the Division of Hematology at the Center for Biologics Evaluation Research at the FDA, makes himself accessible to consumers and listens carefully. He participated in the NHF annual meeting held in San Diego in 1996, mingling with inquisitive consumers in the hallways, responding thoughtfully to their inquiries. He interacts with Bruce Evatt and the other CDC leaders frequently, transforming what was once a nonproductive relationship into a cooperative quest to guarantee the safety of blood products in our nation.

The CDC has assumed a higher profile and become a powerful player since the IOM hearings. Under director Bruce Evatt and assistant director Frederick Rickles, the CDC's Hematologic Diseases Branch now controls funding to the hemophilia treatment centers directly, rather than subcontracting to MCH. CDC-sponsored efforts are framed as prevention, in terms of both blood safety and prevention of joint damage. Dr. Evatt notes that WONN, MANN, and CODP, as models of peer education, outreach, and support, have earned the CDC's respect for demonstrating that this is the effective way to reach more people and to transform a community's tragedy into a renewed desire to forge ahead. He also expresses great admiration for the women of WONN, who helped to stop the spread of the AIDS epidemic. Sally Crudder, R.N., who brings the philosophy, knowledge, and perspectives of both nursing and administration to the hemophilia community and who was initially a nurse coordinator and then the director of the Michigan NHF chapter, is now based at the CDC as director of the Hemophilia Program. She is excited about combining CDC's expertise in research, which can lead to higher quality data collection and approaches to prevention, with the peer outreach models. She particularly hopes that hidden segments of the population will be revealed and reached.

The CDC has undertaken a new initiative to collect information pertaining to blood safety. As Mike Soucie, an epidemiologist in the CDC's Hematologic Disease Branch, notes, given that the safety of the national blood supply is an issue of great public health importance, then from a practical standpoint, when considering how best to monitor the safety of the blood supply, it makes sense to concentrate on a small group of persons with high use, such as the hemophilia population. However, although 60–70 percent of the hemophilia population receive treatment at HTCs, the remainder do not. The population is also geographically dispersed and is clinically diverse in terms of levels of disease severity and resource utilization. Therefore information is to be gathered through two different surveillance systems. The Hemophilia Surveillance System, already in place in six states, identifies all persons with hemophilia, both inside and outside HTCs, using a variety of resources, including HTCs, Factor concentrate suppliers, hospital discharge records, local NHF chapters, and clinical laboratories. Trained data abstractors then collect a wide variety of clinical and treatment information from medical and clinic records including the results of testing for infectious diseases. The results of this testing will be monitored, and other data collected by this system, including hospitalizations, will be examined to search for illnesses that might be missed by systems that do not include all persons with hemophilia. Because this is a retrospective study, collecting what is, in effect, historical data, this system is not useful in identifying acute outbreaks. However, the second surveillance system of the CDC initiative addresses this matter. The Universal Data Collection System is a prospective, or ongoing, system designed to provide a uniform set of data on all persons with hemophilia who use HTCs for at least some of their care. Once a year, during an HTC visit, each person will have a uniform set of data collected by HTC staff and will provide a blood specimen that will be sent to the CDC for free viral testing and storage. The individual results of viral testing will be returned to the HTC, and local and regional rates of positive tests will be monitored and reported in a format similar to the way national rates of infectious diseases are reported in the *Morbidity and Mortality Weekly Report*. This system will be supplemented by direct reporting of acute illnesses that occur among patients with hemophilia. HTC physicians can do this reporting in an easy and timely manner. Personnel at CDC will be specifically assigned to monitor the national data and to conduct investigations as needed. These two surveillance systems will form the backbone of the blood safety monitoring system.[33]

A recent book reminds us both of the urgency of achieving a safer blood supply and of the anger—and divisions—that still remain in the hemophilia community. In *Cry Bloody Murder: A Tale of Tainted Blood*, published in 1997, Elaine De Prince effectively combines the story of her family's personal tragedy in losing two hemophilic sons to HIV and witnessing a third son fight to survive the infection by using the new medications available with a thoroughly researched discussion of what led to the AIDS tragedy. De Prince, who has been an activist in seeking legal reparation from the pharmaceutical companies and an advocate for safety of the blood supply in her home state of New Jersey, says up front that she is angry and proceeds to present a description of horrendous mishaps, cronyism, and illegal and unethical behaviors on the part of many of the players involved in either collecting, safeguarding, manufacturing, or distributing pooled plasma components to the hemophilia community. Separating the wheat from the chaff is not within the purview of this chapter or this book, but respectful listening and acknowledgment is. Not everyone is comfortable with De Prince's continuing anger, but clearly, she has a voice that should be heard, and she contributes new information that deserves to be read. Whatever the allocation of blame, it is important that we remember and learn from this disaster.

Other women's voices are also being heard. Since WONN changed the landscape of the community, women's health concerns are no longer an alien topic. In addition to representing wives and mothers of men with hemophilia, the group encompasses women with non–hemophilia bleeding disorders. Both Jeanne Lusher, M.D., co-chair of MASAC, who has long been a progressive and supportive hemophilia medical leader, and Renee Paper, R.N., a woman who has a bleeding disorder herself, have provided leadership in raising awareness among both providers and consumers about this once hidden segment of the community and about von Willebrand's disease in particular. WONN also initially provided a haven, and then eventually a platform, for Kathy Gerus, who is a widow, a mother, and an infected person. As noted previously, her activism began locally in Michigan, where her husband was a patient in Lusher's hemophilia treatment center. She has emerged as an expressive, forceful leader who served as vice president of NHF and sits on President Clinton's HIV Advisory Council. She does not believe in holding on to anger and has transcended that stage to put all of her positive energies into her work with both the hemophilia and AIDS communities. Bea Pierce is now vice president of NHF. Together she and president Kate Muir, the mother of a thirteen-year-old boy with hemophilia, form the first female leadership team in the history of NHF.

Laureen Kelley, who both represents and reaches out to new families and uninfected children, gained a greater understanding about the importance of the compensation issue in 1993 while attending the Indianapolis meeting. She began to explain the importance of pursuing compensation to her audience and to build a bridge between the infected and uninfected. She stresses the common concern of blood safety for the entire community and for society. She also has featured critical discussions of new techniques and products, such as a review of the strengths and weaknesses of prophylaxis, or treatment designed to prevent bleeds through regular infusion. She is a model for proactive consumer behavior, trying to gather extensive information and stressing that families must decide on their course of action. Through her widely disseminated newsletters, she reaches a broad audience and contributes a valuable perspective.

As the century ends, the medical treatment options for HIV-positive persons are far more promising than several years ago. Many hemophilia community members who have managed to survive until now report that with the new regimens of medications including protease inhibitors they are gaining back weight previously lost and seeing an improvement in their T cell counts and in their overall sense of well-being. Some speak of making future plans, a very different scenario from three years ago.

However, realists remain guarded in their optimism, aware that the virus might mutate, hide, and/or become resistant to current therapies.

Health providers vary in the feelings they express about the hemophilia community of the 1990s. Most of the doctors who have stayed the course, listening to their patients and their families, being there for them during this past decade, feel gratified with that choice. Shelby Dietrich was touched when the mother of a young man who was then dying of AIDS said with tears, "You didn't desert us." Dietrich found that the most magnanimous statement she had ever heard. Regarding the doctor-patient relationship, she said:

I think change has already occurred. Although patients and doctors are always going to be a little bit different in their attitudes and in their modus operandi, there will always be patients and families who, for one reason or another, implicitly trust the doctor and [believe] that the doctor will make the best decision for that patient, and that is the old fashioned paternalistic model . . . at least the one I practiced under most of my career. Then, with the rise of consumerism and the movement of the 1960s, came the informed patient who wants to be involved in the decision. I actually suggested to a research group that we advance to the point where the patient makes the decision as to what concentrate to use, based on risk analysis and cost, since there are very definite available figures now. . . . The doctor will never again be seen, probably rightfully so, as the fount of all wisdom, although I would always hope that patients would have trust in their physician, that the physician had a fiduciary responsibility and is acting in their best interest.[34]

Keith Hoots, M.D., the director of the Gulf States Hemophilia Program and an associate director of MASAC, feels that this is a time for bridge building. As a doctor who has weathered the storm of the AIDS Era by surrounding himself with others who share his sense of commitment, devotion, and determination, coupled with adaptability, he says it's time to build bridges to managed care and to patients. It's not easy, according to Hoots and other physicians interviewed, to attract young doctors to hemophilia today. There is a wariness about the field, perhaps because of the loss of power and the expression of community anger, but it's a good time to look to the future—as Glenn Pierce has said, the gene insertion therapy train is moving forward. He feels that the community will continue to heal its wounds, and respectfully continue to come together, maintaining flexibility and resiliency as we enter the biotech century.

1998 and Beyond: Building Bridges
to the Biotech Century and to Each Other

President Clinton campaigned for reelection on the theme of building a bridge to the twenty-first century. But as we face the new century, whose voices should be heeded? Who represents the hemophilia community? Listening to all voices is important for policy makers and agency directors, but my bias is to work with those who are, in fact, bridge builders—those who are in "the construction business" rather than the "demolition business." The current leaders in the hemophilia community are such bridge builders, both among members of the community and to the future. They are people who respect others' perspectives, who strive to open communication and disseminate information, and who have a vision for the future. They are transforming a community and contributing to our society as guardians of our blood supply and pioneers in gene insertion therapy. They have emerged from their medical closet and approach the biotech century determined to overcome a painful past and savor a bright future.

CHAPTER 13

Conclusion

Lessons to Be Learned

If one advances confidently in the direction of his dreams, and endeavors to live a life which he has imagined, he will meet with a success unexpected in common hours.

Henry David Thoreau, *Walden*

As we approach the twenty-first century, the biotech century, hemophilia is on the verge of being cured and reframed as a genetic disease. This book has presented the history of hemophilia as a history shared by those who have this disease and those who treat it, the hemophilia community. It is a participatory history, told in their voices. It is also a story that has important lessons for society as a whole. In the community's emergence, adaptation, and empowerment we can see successful models worth emulating and pitfalls to be avoided.

The Doctor-Patient Relationship

As recently as fifty years ago, medical ethics was, as it had been for centuries, solely the domain of the medical profession. Today, this ancient medical framework is under great strain. Both the advent of AIDS and the development of many new medical technologies have made medical ethics a subject of broad public awareness and concern. In an important article that appeared in the *Journal of the American Medical Association*, Dr. Edmund Pellegrino describes the metamorphosis in medical ethics. The Hippocratic Oath established the fundamental ethical precepts that governed medical conduct in the Western world for almost 2,500 years: the obligations of beneficence, nonmaleficence, and confidentiality, as well as prohibitions against abortion, euthanasia, surgery, and sexual relationships with patients.[1]

Beginning in the mid-1960s, these precepts began to be challenged, as a result of social change and an "upheaval in moral values" that were part of the era of the civil rights movement, feminism, and consumer activism. Simultaneous with the distrust of authority and the growing demand for participatory democracy that these movements engendered, the medical world was experiencing increased specialization and institutionalization and the burgeoning of new technologies. All of these forces combined to create a demand for alternative models of practicing and teaching medical ethics. According to Pellegrino, "A tetrad of principles emerged at that time, nonmaleficence, beneficence, autonomy, and justice." Two of these—beneficence and nonmaleficence—were the same as those in the Hippocratic Oath; the other two were unfamiliar. Of interest to us is that one of them, the principle of autonomy, directly contradicts the traditional authoritarianism and paternalism of the Hippocratic ethic, but, says Pellegrino, it was the social force of autonomy, which is congruent with American values of individualism, privacy, and self-determination, that set the metamorphosis of medical ethics in motion. He also notes, however, that physicians had a very difficult time accepting it; it is only recently that it is coming to be fully accepted, largely because it is a basic component of informed consent.[2]

Many physicians who were trained before role models, either in medical schools or in practice settings, had shifted from paternalism to autonomy continued to hold to the original Hippocratic framework in exercising judgments and making decisions for their patients, feeling that they knew best. In the early 1980s, as HIV infection began to appear in persons with hemophilia, it is likely that the community's medical leadership reflected these older ways of thinking, making decisions, and exercising judgments, not only in regard to their own patients in their local settings but in the treating of an entire national population, the U.S.

hemophilia community. In 1983, this paternalism was recognized, and the lay leadership of the National Hemophilia Foundation, tacitly supported by other medical providers who shared their mind-set, requested the resignation of its medical co-director. Such paternalistic thinking—deciding that too much information would be frightening or confusing for patients—meant that options and issues were not fully presented in many hemophilia treatment centers. This scenario offers a vitally important case study for medical educators, medical students, and practicing physicians. The end result of not treating patients as autonomous, not sharing the whole picture with them, not updating that picture clearly and completely as information became available, was not only an immense tragedy in terms of lives forever changed, but also an erosion of trust, a breakdown in doctor-patient relationships in the hemophilia community throughout most of the United States.

Some hematologists have reported to me that, today, medical students aren't coming into their field because they have observed the rage and blame directed against hemophilia physician leaders and fear being put in that kind of position. It is important for medical educators to analyze both the ethical decision-making frameworks that were operating in the early 1980s and the nature of the communication. It is also important to look at exceptions to the established patterns. One such exception was the case at Children's Hospital in Philadelphia, described in Chapter 8, where both the nurse coordinator and the medical director validated parents' perceptions of imminent danger and worked with them, in a shared decision-making framework. The Children's Hospital case also shows that the medical profession can benefit from becoming more aware of the priorities and philosophies of nursing. In contrast to the vilification being visited upon physicians, many hemophilia nurses are seen today as "heroes." The partnership they fostered with families in giving care and in their patient and family education sessions strengthened the bond of trust throughout these difficult years.

Also underlying the doctor-patient communication disaster in the early years of the AIDS Era was the sense among physicians, particularly older physicians, that they had suddenly been thrust into a return of the Dismal Era. Once again they were dealing with a problem that had little data to describe it and no known technology to fix it or cure it. Rather than leaping into unfamiliar territory, they recommended staying the course until more was "known." As I mentioned earlier, the depictions of dire consequences coming from epidemiologists were most likely not clearly understood by many clinicians, who dismissed them in favor of the statements from "real doctors"—blood-bank physicians who argued that evidence was very soft and that the CDC interpretation was wrong.

All of this physician posturing took place within the context of the Reagan Era, when the threat of cutbacks to the CDC even seemed to some to lend credence to the idea that it was "inventing" a disease to justify its existence. Since these communication problems took place on a variety of levels and in a variety of settings, they provide a valuable case study for acquainting medical students with the potential role of the physician as decision maker and policy maker, both in the context of a health care setting and in a larger organizational or government domain.

Conflict of Interest: NHF and Its Relationship with the Pharmaceutical Industry

In its study *HIV and the Blood Supply,* the IOM committee addressed the question of conflict of interests between NHF and the blood product manufacturers. With the continuing reduction of government funding in the last twenty years, however, academic institutions and nonprofit agencies have turned more and more to support from private industry in order to survive. Rather than simply painting the consequences of NHF's involvement with specific pharmaceutical company support with a broad and damaging brush, I feel there is a need for a thorough examination and analysis of the situation. To assume that industry could use its clout to control all NHF policies and/or programs is blatantly wrong. As a health professional, I worked within the NHF organization on a specific project with the NHF Nursing Committee that initially received government funding and later derived funding from a manufacturer. I recall the care that was taken by the company representative not only to keep its support low-profile, but never to insert ideas or inject influence in any way. For myself and the nurses on the committee, who were involved in the production of the teaching modules for the Patient/Family Model, there was never a sense of having to compromise our material or adhere to any terminology or format proposed by the manufacturer. During the early 1980s, industry's funding of NHF programs amounted to approximately 20 percent of the organization's budget. Nonetheless, I realize that there are consequences that should be discussed. By promoting an educational guide that contained a self-infusion home therapy module, we inadvertently produced a marketing tool, one that was, furthermore, translated into several languages and used in many other countries.

As a health educator, I would now do two things differently. I would be sure to ask what were the downside and any possible side effects of the treatment being promoted and to ascertain whether the educational materials being provided could serve a commercial marketing function. Neither the nursing leaders nor I thought about these matters ahead of time. Faced with a similar situation now, I would hope to contribute to my profession's ethical standards by raising these specific types of questions—and our general level of ethical awareness.

Costs vs. Safety: The Role of Government

In addition to telling the story of the U.S. hemophilia community, this book has shown how scientific breakthroughs became intertwined with industry and academic medical centers that in effect made up a national health care delivery system. But the primary concern of this system was costs, as attested by all my informants and by the minutes of important meetings. When physicians were surveyed during the Nixon era about hemophilia and their concerns, the matter of costs loomed large. Concerns about safety did not fully emerge. A desensitization about the threat of blood-borne infection with hepatitis was part of the hemophilia culture at that time. Both providers and patients either totally ignored it or chalked it up as part of the landscape. It took the AIDS tragedy to make safety an up-front priority.

The Clinton administration has been particularly responsive to the hemophilia community. It not only listened, it reacted systematically by creating the IOM committee to study HIV and the blood supply. Since the IOM hearings, not only have the CDC and the FDA begun to collaborate in a totally new way, but both are also involved on an ongoing basis with grassroots-level hemophilia community members, including women and minorities. Some of these community members act as advisors for the FDA; among them was Bea Pierce, who served as NHF's representative to the FDA Blood Products Advisory Committee (1995–97). Others serve as education extenders for CDC's preventive outreach programs. A major new challenge for the streamlined FDA is to respond directly and in a timely fashion to a larger consumer constituency, sorting through various voices purporting to represent the hemophilia community. No longer is it only the manufacturer or physician who learns about problems in the blood supply; it is the end user who is to be fully informed and continuously updated. Also, the watchword of caution is fully operative. The old theme heard in the late 1970s and early 1980s, "When in doubt, infuse," has been replaced by the new credo "Please be careful." A new paradigm in the use of plasma products has emerged as a result of advocacy by the hemophilia community. Instead of using "suspect" products until they are proven safe, the community now refuses to use any product whose safety has not already been proven.

The role of government and other outside agencies in insuring not only quality of care but also safety continues to be essential in a time when managed care plans are proliferating and the credo of keeping costs down threatens to become paramount.

The World Ahead

In this book I focus on the U.S. hemophilia community, but it is of vital importance to place this discussion within an international context as we approach the next century. Increasingly, we are becoming aware that our nation is part of an interdependent global village. In the September-October 1997 issue of *Foreign Affairs,* which bore the subtitle *The World Ahead,* Peter F. Drucker points out that in the global economy, businesses are increasingly forced to shift from being multinational to being transnational; for the transnational company there is only one economic unit, the world. Selling, servicing, public relations, and legal affairs are local, but parts, machinery, research, finance, marketing, and managing are conducted with the world market in mind. The transnational company is not totally beyond the control of national governments, but the adaptations it must make to them are exceptions to its overall plans. Successful transnational companies see themselves as separate nonnational entities. Drucker notes that the U.S. government is trying to counteract this trend by extending American legal concepts and legislation beyond its shores, but he feels the attempt to mold the world economy to American moral, legal, and economic concepts is futile. There is, however, a need for moral, legal, and economic rules, and so a central challenge is the development of international law and supranational organizations that can make and enforce rules for the global economy.[3]

Instead of approaching the next century primarily as an advocate of an even more intense entrepreneurialism, it would be incumbent upon us to instead be part of a nation that places a priority on model standards for these supranational organizations (be they here or beyond our shores) that emphasize caring about the end users of products we manufacture and export. As I have mentioned, there has been considerable progress during the Clinton years in government responding to these concerns and taking on the responsibility to safeguard against and prevent further tragedy within our country. How to reconcile giving priority to "commercial diplomacy"[4] —making the promotion of American exports a foreign policy objective—and being a moral world leader is yet another challenge for the twenty-first century.

Glossary of Terms and Acronyms

In addition to terms and acronyms used in the text of this book, this Glossary contains a number of more technical terms pertaining to hemophilia, hepatitis, and AIDS that may be useful to readers seeking additional information. Terms in italics within definitions are themselves defined in the Glossary.

AABB: American Association of Blood Banks.

ABO blood group: The major human blood type determined by the presence or absence of two antigenic structures, A and B, on *red blood cells*, resulting in four blood types (A, B, AB [both structures present], and O [neither structure present]).

Acquired immunodeficiency syndrome (AIDS):   An acquired—as opposed to inherited or congenital—disease characterized by the progressive deterioration of host immune defenses, rendering the affected individual susceptible to an array of infectious and malignant disorders that do not normally afflict persons with intact *immune systems*. AIDS results from infection with *human immunodeficiency virus* (HIV, either type 1 or type 2) and is formally defined by a case definition issued by the *Centers for Disease Control and Prevention* (CDC).

ACTG: AIDS Clinical Trials Group, clinical trials sponsored by *NIAID*.

Activated prothrombin complex concentrate (APCC):   Special *prothrombin-complex concentrate* (*PCC*) used to overcome *inhibitors*. APPC is activated to start the clotting process before being infused, thus bypassing inhibitors to either *Factor VIII* or *IX*.

Active immunity: Protection against an infectious disease that results from induction of host immune defense mechanisms including *B lymphocytes* that produce *antibodies* (*humoral* immunity) and *T lymphocytes* (cellular immunity). These host immune effectors are specifically induced by exposure to constituents of the infectious pathogen as a result of prior infection or immunization. (Compare with *Passive immunity*.)

Acute infection: A suddenly occurring infection, which can end quickly or turn into a chronic (prolonged) infection, as often happens in *hepatitis C*.

ADA: American Diabetes Association.

AEPS: AIDS Education and Preventive Services, *CDC*.

AHF: See *Antihemophilic factor*.

AIDS: See *Acquired immunodeficiency syndrome*.

AIDS-related complex (ARC):   A term formerly used to describe the various signs and symptoms that characterized the early stages of AIDS, including *lymphadenopathy syndrome*, unexplained fevers, weight loss, and specific infections. Initially it was not known whether ARC represented a precursor to full-blown AIDS or a separate, less severe form of the disease. Because history has since shown that persons who manifest these early signs and symptoms will ultimately progress to AIDS, *HIV*-associated disease is now recognized as a continuum spanning asymptomatic infection, mild to moderate symptomatology, and ultimately the profound immunodeficiency of AIDS.

AIDS-related retrovirus (ARV):   A *retrovirus* isolated from an individual with AIDS by Dr. Jay Levy's laboratory at the University of California, San Francisco.

Albumin: A small protein, synthesized in the liver, which is the principal protein in *plasma* and is important in maintaining plasma volume by regulating an osmotic gradient between plasma in the blood vessels and fluids in the surrounding tissues. Albumin also serves as the carrier molecule for fatty acids and other small molecules in plasma.

AmFAR: American Foundation for AIDS Research.

Amicar® (Epsilon aminocaproic acid, EACA):   A drug that prevents the breakdown of newly formed clots by the *enzyme* plasmin.

Amniocentesis: A test performed during pregnancy in which amniotic fluid (the fluid that surrounds the baby in the womb) is withdrawn through a long needle and examined to check the fetus for certain defects. Although *hemophilia* cannot be detected this way, the sex of the baby can be accurately determined.

Anaphylactic reaction: An intense and potentially life-threatening allergic reaction to a foreign substance in the bloodstream, which can be fatal. A small number of *hemophilia* patients experience this reaction after infusion with *factor concentrates*.

Anemia: A lower than normal *red blood cell* count, the main symptom of which is fatigue.

Antibody: A blood protein produced by the immune system that normally seeks, attacks, and destroys bacteria, viruses, and foreign proteins in the blood system. Antibodies develop in response to stimulation by an invader and are specific to that invader; that is, they attack a certain virus or protein, and no other.

Antigen: A foreign protein, carbohydrate, or nucleic acid in the bloodstream that is introduced by bacteria, *viruses,* or other foreign proteins and that causes the immune system to produce specific *antibodies* to attack it.

Antihemophilic factor (AHF or *Factor VIII*):   A coagulation *factor* in *plasma,* the congenital lack of which results in the bleeding disorder known as *hemophilia A.*

Anti-inhibitor complex: An "activated" form of *PCC* that is used in the treatment of *hemophilia* patients with *inhibitors* to a *Factor.*

Apheresis: The collecting of individual components of blood instead of whole blood from the donor (e.g., *plasmapheresis,* plateletapheresis). The desired component is extracted from the whole blood as it is collected and the remaining blood is reinfused into the donor.

APCC: See *Activated prothrombin complex concentrate.*

ARC: See *AIDS-related complex.*

ARV: See *AIDS-related retrovirus.*

Assay: A laboratory test.

Asymptomatic: Without signs of illness. Many patients with *hepatitis C* do not show signs of illness and are considered asymptomatic.

ATF: AIDS Task Force, *National Hemophilia Foundation.*

Autologous: Derived from the same organism or one of its parts.

Autologous donation: A blood donation that is stored and reserved for return to the donor as needed, usually in elective surgery.

Azidothymidine (AZT; also known as Retrovir®, zidovudine [ZDV], or Compound S):   An antiretroviral nucleoside analog used to treat *HIV* infection and *AIDS.* This drug prevents HIV from multiplying in the body, thus prolonging life by reducing the number of infections contracted, and was the first anti-HIV agent approved in the United States.

AZT: See *Azidothymidine.*

B cell: See *B lymphocyte.*

Biochemical: Relating to the chemical processes and compounds occurring in living organisms.

Bioengineering: Use of engineering principles to solve biomedical problems, such as creating chemicals or drugs that do not naturally occur.

Biologic: A biological product that can be used as a vaccine, therapeutic serum, toxoid, or antitoxin against the agents of infectious diseases or their harmful byproducts.

Blood: The body's complex liquid mixture of *plasma,* specialized cells (*white blood cells, red blood cells,* and *platelets*), proteins, and other molecules, among whose functions are the transport of oxygen and nutrients to body tissues, removal of carbon dioxide and other wastes, transfer of hormonal messages between organs, prevention of bleeding, and transport of *antibodies* and infection-fighting cells to sites of infection.

Blood bank: General name for a facility or part of a facility (e.g., a hospital) that stores blood and blood components and that also may collect and process blood.

Blood-borne substances: Those substances that are present in the blood and are carried by it throughout the body. Blood-borne substances, such as *viruses,* can be passed on to others through blood *transfusions,* needle sharing, and even sharing a toothbrush if both people have bleeding gums.

Blood cells: *Red blood cells* (erythrocytes), *white blood cells* (leukocytes), or *platelets* (thrombocytes).

Blood center: A facility that provides a full range of blood services, including the collection, testing, processing, and distribution of blood and blood products, for a particular geographic area (e.g., community or region).

Blood components: Products separated from whole blood (i.e., *red blood cells, white blood cells, platelets,* and *plasma*). Compare with *Plasma derivatives.*

B lymphocyte (also called B cell):   A type of *white blood cell* associated with the *humoral immune response,* that produces *antibodies.* Each B lymphocyte produces a specific antibody for a specific *antigen,* much as a specific key is made for a specific lock. B lymphocytes proliferate under stimulation from factors released by *T lymphocytes.*

Carrier (of infection):   A person who appears healthy but has been infected with an organism and is capable of infecting and causing diseases in others.

CAT scan: See *Computed tomography.*

CD4 cell: A subtype of *T lymphocyte,* also referred to as a helper T cell, that plays a critical regulatory role in the *immune system,* including turning *antibody* production on and off, and whose deficiency is responsible for the immunodeficiency characteristic of *AIDS.* These *lymphocytes* have the marker protein CD4 (previously known as T4) on their surface, which makes the cells a target for destruction by *HIV.*

CD8 cell: A subtype of *T lymphocyte* that plays an essential role in the host's *immune response* to intracellular *pathogens* such as *viruses* or parasites. *Cyto-*

toxic T lymphocytes express the CD8 (previously known as T8) molecule on their surfaces, which facilitates their ability to recognize and kill host cells that display evidence of infection by foreign pathogens.

CDC: See *Centers for Disease Control.*

Centers for Disease Control and Prevention (CDC):   U.S. Public Health Services agency, based in Atlanta, Georgia. Established as the Communicable Disease Center in 1946 and later known as the Centers for Disease Control. The agency has led efforts to prevent the spread of such illnesses as malaria, polio, smallpox, toxic shock syndrome, Legionnaire's disease, AIDS, and tuberculosis. CDC's responsibilities as the nation's prevention agency have expanded over the years and will continue to evolve as the agency addresses contemporary threats to health such as injury, environmental and occupational hazards, behavioral risks, and chronic diseases, including *hemophilia.*

Chorionic villi sampling (CVS):   A test performed during the first trimester of pregnancy that samples tissue from the placenta and shows, among other things, the presence or absence of genetic markers for *hemophilia.*

Christmas disease: *Hemophilia B* or *Factor IX* deficiency; named for the first family diagnosed with this form of hemophilia.

Chromatography: A process that uses a column or tube containing a selective medium to separate a complex mixture into its constituent parts; such processes include *gel-permeation chromatography, ion exchange chromatography,* and *monoclonal antibody purification.* Chromatography is used to separate blood-clotting proteins from other proteins.

Chromosome: A thread-like structure in the nucleus of an animal or plant cell that carries the genetic information which determines the characteristics of the particular organism.

Chronic infection: An infection that lasts for a long time or that returns after it had seemed to be cured.

CIRC: Chapter Internal Relations Committee, *National Hemophilia Foundation.*

Clinical trial: A carefully controlled test conducted in humans to evaluate the effectiveness and safety of new medical products (such as all new drugs) and techniques.

CMV: See *Cytomegalovirus.*

Coagulation: The process of blood clotting, resulting in an insoluble fibrin clot.

Coagulation concentrates or complexes: Products obtained through selective purification of the proteins in *plasma,* resulting in concentrated forms that are needed for blood to coagulate (clot). *Immunoglobulins* and *albumin* are also obtained in this manner. See also *Cold ethanol precipitation technique.*

Coagulation factors or proteins: Naturally occurring proteins in *plasma* (e.g., *Factor VIII, Factor IX*) that aid in the coagulation of blood.

Coagulation system: The cascading effect of all the coagulation (clotting) factors whose final product is fibrin, which helps to form a clot.

CODP: Chapter Outreach Development Project, *National Hemophilia Foundation.*

Cofactor: Factors or agents that increase the probability of the development of disease in the presence of the basic etiologic agent of that disease.

Cohn Fraction I: A blood component produced by the fractionation process developed by Edwin Cohn and his group at Harvard in 1946. Cohn Fraction I yields antihemophilic activity in a more concentrated form than does *plasma* itself.

Cold ethanol precipitation technique: The principal method used to separate *plasma* into its major protein groups. A three-variable system (of temperature, ionic strength, and ethanol concentration) is used to precipitate different proteins in the following order: Fraction I (chiefly *Factor VIII* and *fibrinogen*); Fraction II (the *immunoglobulins*); Fractions III and IV (other coagulation proteins and trace components); Fraction V (the *albumins*); and Fraction VI (the remaining residue).

Complications: New medical problems that arise while treating existing ones.

Components: See *Blood components.*

Comprehensive care: A health care delivery model in which a multidisciplinary team of professionals works with the patient to cover all aspects of the patient's physical, emotional, financial, and mental well-being. Comprehensive care team members for *hemophilia* include those from hematology, psychology, social services, dentistry, physical therapy, and counseling; care is usually given in one place, a hemophilia treatment center (HTC). Most federally funded HTCs are located in teaching hospitals, often in academic medical centers.

Computed tomography (CT scan) or computerized axial tomography (CAT scan):   A cross-sectional image of the body used to detect abnormalities and bleeds (in *hemophilia,* especially useful in detecting cranial bleeds).

Concentrate: A product consisting of blood cells or proteins that have been separated from the rest of blood or *plasma* in concentrated form—for example, *platelet* concentrates. In particular, a freeze-dried, powdered product containing *Factor VIII* or *Factor IX,* derived from screened and pooled human blood and subjected to *inactivation* methods and perhaps *purification* methods to kill *viruses* and remove foreign substances. See also *Coagulation concentrates.*

Core protein: Any of the proteins that make up the internal structure or "core" of a *virus.* For example, the core proteins of *HIV* are p24, p15, and p18.

Crossmatching: Testing to determine compatibility of blood types between donor and recipient. See also *histocompatibility*.

Cryoprecipitate: The solid material (precipitate) remaining when fresh-frozen *plasma* is thawed at 2–4°C. This product is rich in clotting factors needed to treat *hemophilia A, von Willebrand's disease*, and *factor XIII* deficiencies.

CT scan: See *Computed tomography*.

CVS: See *Chorionic villi sampling*.

Cytomegalovirus (CMV):   One of a group of highly host-specific herpes *viruses* that infect humans, monkeys, or rodents. Infections may occur without causing any symptoms or may result in mild flu-like symptoms of aching, fever, mild sore throat, or enlarged lymph nodes. Severe CMV infections can result in retinitis, *hepatitis,* mononucleosis, or pneumonia, especially in immune-suppressed persons. CMV is shed in body fluids such as urine, semen, saliva, feces, and sweat.

Cytotoxic: Having a toxic effect on cells.

DDAVP: See *Desmopressin acetate*.

Desmopressin acetate (DDAVP, also known in intranasal form as Stimate®):   A synthetic drug used to stop bleeding in people with *von Willebrand's disease* or moderate or mild *hemophilia A*. Although not a clotting *factor,* it does stimulate the release of *Factor VIII* and *von Willebrand factor* from their storage, which temporarily increases activity levels in the body.

Directed donations: Donations from identified individuals, such as family and friends, intended to be used as the sole source of blood for the patient for whom the donations were made.

EIA: See *Enzyme-linked immunosorbent assay*.

ELISA: See *Enzyme-linked immunosorbent assay*.

Envelope: Proteins present on the surface of a *virus* that play an essential role in the initiation of virus infection of host target cells. The envelope proteins of *HIV* are composed of two subunits: gp120, which specifically binds to *CD4*, and gp41, which is embedded in the membrane of HIV and facilitates fusion with the cell surface membrane of the target cell during the earliest stages of the virus infection cycle.

Enzyme: Any of a group of catalytic proteins that are produced by living cells and that mediate and promote the chemical processes of life without themselves being altered or destroyed.

Enzyme-linked immunosorbent assay (ELISA; also referred to as EIA):   A lab test that detects *antibodies* in the bloodstream (such as *HIV* antibodies).

Erythrocytes: See *Red blood cells*.

Etiologic agent: A causative agent.

Factor: Blood components that help clot blood. Listed are twelve Factors, identified by Roman numerals. (A previously identified Factor VI has been removed from the list.) *Hemophilia A* is a result of a deficiency in Factor VIII, while *hemophilia B* is a deficiency in Factor IX. "Factor" is also popularly used for *Factor concentrate.*

Factor I *fibrinogen*

Factor II *prothrombin*

Factor III tissue factor (thromboplastin)

Factor IV calcium

Factor V proaccelerin (thrombogen)

Factor VII proconvertin (autoprothrombin I)

Factor VIII antihemophilic factor (AHF)

Factor IX plasma thromboplastin component (PTC, Christmas factor, factor B)

Factor X Stuart factor

Factor XI plasma thromboplastin antecedent

Factor XII Hageman factor

Factor XIII fibrin-stabilizing factor

Factor VIII assay: A laboratory test that determines the amount of active *Factor VIII* in a patient's bloodstream. The patient's *plasma* is added to a control plasma deficient in factor VIII; normal plasma corrects the coagulation deficiency of the control.

Factor VIII concentrate: A commercial product to treat bleeding resulting from *Factor VIII* deficiency. The product is derived from screened, donated, and pooled human blood that is heat-treated, pasteurized, or washed with *solvent-detergent* to destroy *viruses.* It can be further purified from extraneous proteins and freeze-dried and is stored in sterile bottles. Often popularly referred to just as "Factor."

FDA: See *Food and Drug Administration.*

Fetoscopy: A test performed during the first trimester of pregnancy, sampling blood in utero from the umbilical cord to check for the presence of *hemophilia.*

FFP: See *Fresh-frozen plasma.*

Fibrinogen: Factor I; a plasma protein, synthesized in the liver, which is involved in *coagulation* as the precursor of fibrin.

Filter needle: The needle used to transfer reconstituted Factor (Factor concentrate mixed with sterile water) into an empty sterile syringe. Its function is to trap any clumps of factor left in the bottle before they are inadvertently drawn into the syringe.

Food and Drug Administration (FDA):   A U.S. government agency charged with protecting the public health, which establishes safety and effectiveness guidelines and rules for healthcare products, including new drugs.

Fractionation: See *Plasma fractionation.*

Frenulum: The piece of skin that bridges the inside of the upper lip to the gum. Tearing of this in hemophilic children, common in the teething and toddler years, can cause bleeds.

Fresh-frozen plasma (FFP):   *Plasma* that has been frozen soon after collection to preserve the activity of the coagulation proteins. FFP was at one time a major treatment for *hemophilia,* and is now used for those *Factor* deficiencies for which concentrates are not available, such as Factor V. It can also be used when a family member wishes to store plasma to reduce the risk of viral transmission.

Gamma globulin: A separated fraction of proteins present in blood-derived *serum* that contains many types of *antibodies.*

Gel-permeation chromatography: A protein *purification* process for *Factor VIII* production using thousands of microscopic filters in a column through which Factor VIII solution is passed. The filters allow passage of the heavier Factor VIII molecules while the lighter foreign proteins and detergents are held back. Factor VIII is thus separated from extraneous material and left in a more pure and concentrated form.

Gene: The basic unit of heredity; an ordered sequence of nucleotide bases, comprising a segment of DNA. Located along *chromosomes,* genes contain chemical instructions for how the body cells will develop in the fetus and carry genetic traits such as hair color, eye color, and *hemophilia.*

Gene insertion therapy: A procedure in which normally functioning *genes* can be inserted into a patient's own cells so that those cells will in turn produce the specific protein controlled by the particular inserted genes. This is the major research priority in searching for a cure for *hemophilia.* For hemophilia the genes must be put into a cell that will deliver the *Factor VIII* or *Factor IX* protein into the bloodstream. Successful gene therapy also involves the "expression" of functioning clotting factor, long-term stability, simple and consistent procedures, and steady "normal" levels of clotting factor. There are two types of gene therapy: when the transfer occurs inside the patient, it is called "in vivo"; when it occurs outside the patient it is "ex vivo" transfer.

Genetically Handicapped Program: *Hemophilia* program for the state of California, which provides care and assistance to persons with hemophilia.

Genetic mutation: A change in a *gene* that scrambles the genetic instructions for bodily growth and processes. *Hemophilia* is a genetic mutation that scrambles the instructions for blood clotting.

Globulins: Simple proteins in the blood *serum* that contain molecules central to *immune system* functioning.

Half-life: For *hemophilia*, the time it takes for half the clotting activity of the infused product to disappear. New *Factor VIII* products have a half-life of 8–14 hours; that is, they are only half as effective 8–14 hours after being infused.

HANDI: See *Hemophilia and AIDS/HIV Network for the Dissemination of Information*.

HAV: See *Hepatitis A*.

HBV: See *Hepatitis B*.

HCV: See *Hepatitis C*.

Heat treatment: A viral *inactivation* method that heats *Factor* in a dry state to a high temperature for a certain amount of time without damaging the effectiveness of the Factor molecule.

Helper T cells: See *CD4 cell*.

Hemarthrosis: Swelling due to bleeding into the joints.

Hematocrit: The volume occupied by the *red blood cells* in relation to the total volume of blood.

Hematology: The science of blood, its nature, function, and diseases.

Hematoma: A large bump accompanied by a bruise, from bleeding under the skin.

Hematuria: Presence of blood in the urine.

Hemoglobin: The protein in *red blood cells* that carries oxygen to cells and carbon dioxide away from them.

Hemolytic transfusion reaction: An *antigen-antibody* reaction in the recipient of a blood *transfusion* that results in the destruction of *red blood cells*.

Hemophilia: A rare, hereditary sex-linked bleeding disorder caused by a deficiency in the ability to synthesize one or more of the *coagulation* proteins; e.g., *Factor VIII* (*hemophilia A*) or *Factor IX* (*hemophilia B*). Hemophilia is classified as severe, moderate, or mild.

Hemophilia A: A blood clotting disorder also known as *Factor VIII* deficiency or classical *hemophilia*.

Hemophilia and AIDS/HIV Network for the Dissemination of Information (HANDI):   A clearinghouse at the *National Hemophilia Foundation* whose mission is to provide information, resources, and referrals on *hemophilia* and *AIDS/HIV* to people with hemophilia, their families and the families who care for them, National Hemophilia Foundation chapters, other hemophilia organizations, and the general public.

Hemophilia B: A blood clotting disorder also known as *Factor IX* deficiency or *Christmas disease*.

Hemorrhage: The escape of blood from the vascular system; excessive bleeding.

Hemorrhaging: Heavy or uncontrolled bleeding.

Hemostasis: The maintenance of normal *coagulation* activity. For patients with *hemophilia,* this usually means treating an injury by infusing *Factor* to produce normal clot formation. Before the discovery of modern treatment methods, treatment of an injury consisted of immobilizing and applying ice. Current treatment involves infusion of either *heat-treated* or *solvent-detergent-*treated pooled *plasma* products or genetically engineered (*recombinant*) products.

Hepatic: Related to the liver.

Hepatitis: A disease that causes inflammation and potential deterioration of the liver. Like *HIV* it can be spread through certain bodily fluids, by blood *transfusions,* contaminated needles, and unprotected sexual contact. There are three main types of the disease: *hepatitis A, hepatitis B,* and *hepatitis C.*

Hepatitis A (HAV):   Formerly called infectious hepatitis, an *acute* infection of the liver that does not progress to *chronic* hepatitis or cirrhosis and is generally not considered very harmful. Most patients recover completely within 6–10 weeks. HAV is spread mainly via feces and contaminated food and water.

Hepatitis B (HBV):   Formerly called serum hepatitis, a very harmful *acute* or *chronic* infection of the liver; about 10 percent of cases progress to chronic hepatitis. Like *HIV,* HBV can be transmitted by sexual contact, contaminated needles, or blood products. Unlike HIV, it can also be transmitted through close casual contact. A *vaccine* is available.

Hepatitis C (HCV):   A very harmful form of hepatitis previously known as non-A, non-B hepatitis. The *CDC* estimates 28,000 new cases each year, 6–10 percent of which are *transfusion* related; the virus is resistant to *heat treatment* and has been eliminated in current, virus inactivated factor *concentrates.* Of patients diagnosed with hepatitis C, 40 percent have no identified risk factors. More than 85 percent with recent infection develop *chronic* hepatitis C and 20 percent develop cirrhosis.

Hepatitis D (HDV):   Also called delta hepatitis, a form of the disease that infects only patients who already carry *hepatitis B.* Rare in the United State, hepatitis D occurs primarily in recipients of multiple blood *transfusions,* including patients with *hemophilia* or those undergoing renal dialysis, and among those who share contaminated needles.

Hepatitis E (HEV):   Also referred to as enterically transmitted hepatitis C, an *acute* infection spread by fecal contamination in water that is much like *hepatitis A* and that occurs primarily in developing countries, rarely in the United States.

HEW: U.S. Department of Health, Education, and Welfare.

HHS: U.S. Department of Health and Human Services, successor to *HEW.*

Hill-Burton Act: A 1946 law providing federal support for hospital construction, with the requirement that any hospital receiving this support must provide medical care to the poor. This requirement was not enforced until the 1960s.

Histocompatibility: The extent to which individuals or their tissues are immunologically similar, which is relevant for *crossmatching* in blood transfusion, organ transplants, and the like, in order to prevent shock and rejection.

HIV: See *Human inmmunodeficiency virus.*

HIV-1:   The *retrovirus, human immunodeficiency virus* type 1, that is responsible for most cases of *AIDS* worldwide. HIV-1 was first discovered in 1983 by investigators at the Pasteur Institute and was demonstrated to be the *etiologic agent* of AIDS by investigators at the *National Institutes of Health* in 1984.

HIV-2:   A *retrovirus, human immunodeficiency virus* type 2, that is distantly related to *HIV*-1 and that is most common in West Africa but is seen with increasing frequency in regions of India, Asia, and the West Indies. HIV-2 infections result in a clinical syndrome of immunodeficiency that can be indistinguishable from HIV-1– induced AIDS.

HNN: *Hemophilia Newsnotes,* publication of the *National Hemophilia Foundation.*

HTC: Hemophilia Treatment Center; see *Comprehensive care.*

HTIE: *Hemophilia/HIV Treatment Information Exchange,* a *National Hemophilia Foundation* publication sent to persons with hemophilia, chapters, and *HTCs.*

HTLV-III: Former name for *human immunodeficiency virus* (HIV).

Human immunodeficiency virus (HIV):   The *virus* that causes *AIDS.* After infection (by exchange of bodily fluids, such as through unprotected sexual contact, intravenous needle sharing, breast-feeding, prenatally through the placenta, or through shared blood and blood products) it takes 3–6 months, on average, before *antibodies* to the virus appear in the bloodstream. At present, tests that detect these antibodies determine if a person has HIV, but during the period before antibodies appear, HIV can still be transmitted to others. This time period is popularly known as "the window."

Human T cell lymphotropic virus, type III (HTLV-III):   A name used to describe certain isolates of *HIV-1* shortly after the identification of the etiologic agents of *AIDS;* this terminology has been abandoned in favor of the term HIV-1 to refer to all related virus isolates.

Humoral: Relating to the *immune response* that involves *antibodies* secreted by *B lymphocytes* and circulating in bodily fluids.

Hyperimmune globulins: Immune *globulin* products derived from the *plasma* of donors with high titers (concentration) of *antibodies* specific for a given *antigen*, such as anti-Rh globulin used to prevent destruction of red blood cells in an Rh-positive newborn with an Rh-negative mother.

Iliopsoas (psoas):   Large group of muscles in the hip area that help flex the thigh. Bleeding into this area, which can happen spontaneously with hemophilia, is serious because pooled blood can put pressure on the nerves, causing numbness, loss of circulation, and death of the nerves, which can lead to paralysis.

Immune complexes: Combinations of *antibodies* and *antigens* that may either circulate in the blood or be deposited in the tissues. Immune complexes are found in certain infectious and autoimmune diseases.

Immune deficiency: Breakdown or inability of certain parts of the *immune system* to function. The inability of the body to attack and destroy invading bacteria, *viruses,* and foreign proteins leaves a person susceptible to diseases normally not contracted.

Immune globulin: See *Immunoglobulin.*

Immune response: See *immune system.*

Immune system: The complicated and highly integrated system of cells and cellular products that protect a host from infectious diseases or toxic substances. The immune response consists of both so-called cellular and *humoral* components. Cellular immune responses are initiated by direct interaction of host immune system cells such as *helper T cells* with foreign *antigens.* Humoral immune responses refer to those mediated by *antibodies* that are produced by *B lymphocytes,* but that can travel to and act at distant sites in the body.

Immunity: A natural or acquired resistance to a specific disease. Immunity may be partial or complete, long-lasting or temporary.

Immunoaffinity: The attraction of an *antibody* to an *antigen.* See *Monoclonal antibody purification.*

Immunogen: A preparation such as a *vaccine* (typically composed of protein or carbohydrate) that is administered to generate a specific *immune response.*

Immunoglobulin (also called immune globulin):   *Serum* proteins manufactured by *B lymphocytes* in response to *antigens.* Elevated levels of immunoglobulins have been seen in HIV-positive persons. Why this occurs is not fully understood but is believed to be caused by faulty regulation of the B cells.

Immunology: The branch of medicine that focuses on the immune system, immunity, and allergy.

Immunotherapy: Therapy that attempts either to reconstruct or enhance a damaged *immune system* or to kill cancer cells.

Inactivation: The destroying of blood-borne *viruses* such as *HIV* and *hepatitis,* through heat, pasteurization, or *solvent-detergent* treatment.

Infection: The result of the presence of harmful microorganisms in the body. Infections can be *acute* or *chronic.*

Infiltration: Leaking of *Factor concentrate* into the surrounding tissue, rather than into a vein, causing swelling at the *infusion* site.

Infusion: Inserting reconstituted (liquid) *concentrates* into the bloodstream via a vein, using a syringe with a special needle, to help stop bleeding by raising the amount of clotting factor in the body.

Inhibitor: An *antibody* to *Factor VIII* or *Factor IX.* Inhibitors are formed by approximately 10 percent of patients with severe *hemophilia* receiving Factor VIII infusions, and 2 percent of those receiving Factor IX infusions. As part of the *immune system,* this antibody does not recognize infused Factor VIII or IX as a normal part of the bloodstream and attempts to destroy it before the body can use it in blood clotting.

Interferon: A protein important in immune function and thought to inhibit viral infections. Many different cells, including liver cells, produce natural interferon; it can also be produced artificially.

Investigational drug: A new drug that is undergoing *clinical trials* to prove its effectiveness and safety.

IOM: Institute of Medicine, National Academy of Sciences, chartered in 1976 to enlist distinguished members of appropriate professions to help government in examining policy maters.

Ion exchange chromatography: A procedure used to purify proteins like *Factor VIII* that uses electrical (electrostatic) binding to attract Factor VIII molecules, rather like a magnet. When the Factor VIII molecules are bound to the sides of a column, the rest of the solution passes through, leaving a more pure and concentrated form.

Kaposi's sarcoma (KS):   A type of malignancy (cancer) commonly seen in persons with *AIDS,* resulting from the abnormal proliferation of the endothelial cells that line blood vessel walls. Although the disease is also seen in individuals not infected with HIV, it is much more severe in the setting of HIV infection. Recent studies suggest that Kaposi's sarcoma may be caused by a member of the herpes virus family.

LAS: See *Lymphadenopathy syndrome.*

LAV: See *Lymphadenopathy-associated virus.*

Leukocytes: See *White blood cells.*

Liver: The largest glandular organ in the body, whose many functions include, but are not limited to: the production of protein and cholesterol, the production of bile, the storage of sugar in the form of glycogen, and the breakdown of carbohydrates, fats, and proteins. The liver also breaks down and excretes many medications.

Liver cell transplants: Treatment of liver cell malfunction by the replacement or addition of a new liver. Historically whole livers from recently deceased donors have been used, but recently partial livers have been obtained from living donors. Although liver transplants can correct *Factor VIII* deficiencies and offer a cure for *hemophilia*, it is not considered at present a practical treatment because of the complications associated with the transplants.

Lymphadenopathy-associated virus (LAV):   The name used by investigators at the Pasteur Institute to describe a *retrovirus* they isolated in 1983 from an individual with *lymphadenopathy syndrome*. It is now known to be a member of the *HIV*-1 group.

Lymphadenopathy syndrome (LAS):   A condition that follows *HIV* infection and is characterized by lymphadenopathy (swollen lymph nodes) at multiple locations in the body. This syndrome was identified as one of the components of the *AIDS-related complex* (ARC) and was used as a marker for persons at risk of developing *AIDS* before HIV was identified. Like the term ARC, the term "lymphadenopathy syndrome" is now considered antiquated and is no longer used.

Lymphocytes: Specialized *white blood cells* involved in the *immune response*.

Lymphosarcoma: A subset of malignant diseases of *lymphocytes* known as lymphoma.

Lyophilized: Freeze-dried.

MANN: See *Men's Advocacy Network of the National Hemophilia Foundation*.

MASAC: Medical and Scientific Advisory Council of the *National Hemophilia Foundation*. This council was founded in the early years of NHF to advise the board. Kenneth M. Brinkhous was its first chair. Originally composed of physicians, it has expanded to include the chairs of various NHF committees such as Nursing and Mental Health.

MCH: Maternal and Child Health Bureau; originally known as the Office of Maternal and Child Health and from the late 1970s to 1991 as the Division of Maternal and Child Health. The key health agency at the federal level responsible for matters regarding systems of health care affecting families and children. MCH provides funding and administers programs, including the Hemophila Treatment Center Network Program since this program began in 1976.

Men's Advocacy Network of the *National Hemophilia Foundation* (MANN):   An organization that focuses on education, support, and advocacy. It strives to give men an avenue through which positive change can be made both personally and within the whole hemophilia community and beyond.

Monoclonal antibodies: Homogeneous *antibodies* derived from clones of a single cell. Monoclonal antibodies recognize and bind to only one chemical structure (*antigen*) and thus have remarkable specificity. They are easily produced in large quantities and have a variety of industrial and medical uses.

Monoclonal antibody purification: An *immunoaffinity* chromatography process used both in *Factor VIII* and *Factor IX concentrate* preparation, separating the Factor from extraneous proteins which might cause allergic reactions or a weakened *immune system*. For Factor VIII production, *cryoprecipitate* is poured through an immunoaffinity column that is coated with antibodies specific to Factor VIII or von Willebrand factor/Factor VIII complexes. These antibodies attract the Factor VIII molecules and cause them to stick to the sides of the column, while the rest of the solution, plasma, and proteins are washed away. Factor VIII can then be collected virtually free of extraneous proteins. Although this results in the purest plasma-derived *Factor concentrates* now available, there is still risk of viral transmission, because no *purification* method has been shown to be 100 percent effective.

MSSC: Medical and Scientific Steering Committee of the *National Hemophilia Foundation*.

National Hemophilia Foundation (NHF):   Nonprofit agency dedicated to the treatment and care of *hemophilia*, related bleeding disorders, and complications of those disorders or their treatment, including *HIV* infection, as well as improving the quality of life through research, education, and other services.

National Institutes of Health (NIH):   An agency of the U.S. Public Health Service whose mission is to uncover new knowledge that will lead to better health for everyone and which includes several specific institutes such as *NHLBI* or *NIAID*. NIH conducts research in its own laboratories and supports research conducted by scientists in universities, medical schools, hospitals, and research institutions throughout the country and abroad. NIH is one of eight health agencies of the Public Health Service, which in turn is part of *HHS*.

NEC: Nursing Executive Committee of the *National Hemophilia Foundation*.

NHF: See *National Hemophilia Foundation*.

NHLBI: National Heart, Lung, and Blood Institute, successor to *NHLI;* part of the *National Institutes of Health*.

NHLI: National Heart and Lung Institute, former name of an institute of the *National Institutes of Health*.

NIAID: National Institute of Allergy and Infectious Diseases, part of the *National Institutes of Health*.

NIH: See *National Institutes of Health*.

NNN: Nursing Network News, publication of the *National Hemophilia Foundation.*

Nonreplacement fee: An additional fee that may be charged to users of whole blood or red cells if no replacement donations are made.

Normal serum albumin: Concentrates of *albumin* obtained through *plasma fractionation* and used to maintain or restore plasma volume. The appropriateness of using albumin preparations instead of other fluids is under examination. See also *Plasma protein fraction.*

Nosocomial infection: A new infection acquired during a patient's treatment in a hospital. An example could be a person who enters a hospital for a blood *transfusion* or organ transplant and inadvertently acquires an infection.

NRCC: National Resource and Consultation Center of the *National Hemophilia Foundation;* established in 1986 as a national clearing house for *AIDS* information.

Opportunistic infection: A disease or infection caused by a microorganism that does not ordinarily cause disease but which, under certain conditions (e.g., impaired immune responses), becomes pathologic.

Organic solvent-detergents: See *Solvent-detergent treatment.*

p24 antibody: An *antibody* produced following *HIV* infection that recognizes a protein component of the *virus* core known as p24. The presence of such antibodies is used to make a diagnosis of active HIV infection.

p24 antigen: A protein component of the core of the *HIV* virus particle. The p24 antigen test detects the presence of this protein in the *serum* of infected persons, an indicator of active HIV replication. Because of the insensitivity of the test, however, it is being supplanted by more sensitive tests based on the detection of HIV RNA.

Partial thromboplastin time (PTT):   A laboratory test that assesses the function of the intrinsic *coagulation* pathway. A clotting agent is added to a sample of the patient's blood, thereby activating the intrinsic pathway, and the results are timed.

Passive immunity: Disease resistance in a person or animal due to the injection of *antibodies* from another person or animal. Passive immunity is usually short-lived. Compare with *Active immunity.*

Pasteurization: The process of heating in solution to just under boiling and maintaining this temperature for a certain time to kill bacteria and *viruses* present in the product. Some *Factor* products are pasteurized to inactivate viruses.

Paternalism: Controlling of another person's actions by such means as coercion or deception for what is believed to be that person's own good.

Pathogen: Any microorganism capable of causing disease.

PCC: See *Prothrombin-complex concentrates.*

Plasma: The liquid portion of blood, which contains nutrients, electrolytes (dissolved salts), gases, *albumin,* clotting *factors,* wastes, and hormones.

Plasma cells: Cells that derive from *B lymphocytes* and that produce *antibodies.*

Plasma derivatives: Products derived from the fractionation of *plasma* to concentrate selected proteins. Compare with *Blood components.*

Plasma fractionation: The separation of *plasma* into its major proteins. See also *Cold ethanol precipitation technique.*

Plasmapheresis: Collection of *plasma* by *apheresis.*

Plasma protein fraction (PPF):   A product of *plasma fractionation* that is at least 85 percent *albumin* and is used interchangeably with albumin preparations. See also *Normal serum albumin.*

Platelets (also called thrombocytes):   Sticky protoplasmic discs in the bloodstream that create a plug over an injury site in the blood vessel wall. These are essential for blood clotting.

Porcine: Related to pigs. Porcine *Factor VIII* concentrate is sometimes used as a treatment for hemophilic patients with *antibodies* to human Factor VIII.

PPF: See *Plasma protein fraction.*

Prophylaxis: In hemophilia treatment preventive treatment, such as regular *Factor infusions,* intended to maintain health and avoid spontaneous bleeds. Primarily because of cost, this has not been a widely used procedure in the United States.

Prothrombin: Factor II; an inactive plasma protein precursor of *thrombin.*

Prothrombin complex (PTC):   A product of *plasma fractionation* consisting of *Factors II, VII, IX,* and *X,* but mostly Factor IX; also known as Factor IX complex (concentrate). Used in the treatment of *hemophilia B.* An "activated" form of this concentrate is used in the treatment of *hemophilia A* patients with *inhibitor* to *Factor VIII.* See also *Anti-inhibitor complex.*

Prothrombin-complex concentrates (PCC):   *Factor IX concentrates* used to treat patients with Factor IX deficiency (*hemophilia B*). In some cases, PCC can also be used to treat patients with *Factor VIII* deficiency and inhibitors. See also *Activated prothrombin-complex concentrate.*

Prothrombin time (PT):   A laboratory test that assesses the function of the extrinsic *coagulation* pathway. Tissue thromboplastin and calcium are added to a sample of the patient's blood, thereby activating the extrinsic pathway, and the results are timed.

PTT: See *Partial thromboplastin time.*

Purification (of proteins):   The reduction in the amount of foreign protein substances in *Factor concentrates*. These foreign proteins can cause allergic reactions and can overly stimulate and later weaken the *immune system*. *Purification* processes include *gel-permeation chromatography, ion exchange chromatography,* and *monoclonal antibody purification.*

PWA: Person with AIDS.

Recombinant DNA techniques: Techniques that allow specific segments of DNA to be isolated and inserted into a bacterium or other host (e.g., yeast, mammalian cells) in a form that will allow the DNA segment to be replicated and expressed as the cellular host multiplies. The DNA segment is said to be "cloned" because it exists free of the rest of the DNA of the organism from which it was derived.

Recombinant Factor VIII: *Factor VIII* that has been synthetically produced in the laboratory by combining genetic material from two different sources. The human Factor VIII *gene* is spliced into a nonhuman cell that can be readily grown in a laboratory. Once in the cell, the gene instructs the cell to produce Factor VIII on its own. Because this is not Factor VIII derived from human blood sources it therefore does not carry the risk of *HIV* or *hepatitis.* These nonhuman cells also secrete traces of nonhuman proteins, which may contaminate these products. As of this date, however, these contaminants have caused no health problems in those who have received recombinant Factor VIII in experimental trials.

Reconstitution: Returning freeze-dried, powdered *Factor concentrates* to a liquid state by mixing with sterile water.

Recovered plasma: *Plasma* that is removed from outdated blood or that remains after the cells have been removed but has not been frozen in time to preserve the coagulation proteins; it is fractionated for the remaining proteins.

Red blood cells (also called erythrocytes):   The oxygen–carbon dioxide transporting cells of blood.

Retrovirus: A diverse family of *viruses* that share a common strategy for replicating, which depends on an enzyme known as reverse transcriptase. Retroviruses contain RNA which must be copied by reverse transcriptase into DNA during the early stages of the viral life cycle. The DNA copy of the retrovirus then integrates into the chromosomes of the host cell and produces the requisite RNA and protein constituents of additional virus particles.

Rh blood group: A major blood group defined by the presence or absence of genetically determined substances on the red blood cells of humans as well as other higher animals. Most humans are "Rh positive"; those without the factor are "Rh negative." The Rh factor is capable of inducing intense antigenic reactions. See also *ABO blood group.*

SAC: Special Assistance Council, a *National Hemophilia Foundation* initiative to seek compensation for persons with *hemophilia* who were infected with *HIV* through contaminated blood products.

Seroconversion: The point at which HIV antibodies become detectable, indicating infection; the change from HIV-negative to HIV-positive status.

Serology: A branch of medical testing that focuses on *serum,* particularly immune factors in serum.

Seropositive: Commonly used to refer to HIV-positive individuals.

Serum: The clear portion of any animal liquid separated from its more solid elements, especially the clear liquid (blood serum) that separates in the clotting of blood.

Solvent-detergent treatment: An *inactivation* method that destroys *blood-borne viruses* such as *hepatitis B, hepatitis C,* and *HIV.* An organic solvent-detergent is used to dissolve the fatty cover of the viruses, rendering them incapable of infecting cells, while leaving the clotting factor protein intact and functioning.

Source plasma: *Plasma* collected directly by *plasmapheresis* for fractionation into *plasma derivatives.*

Special Projects of Regional and National Significance (SPRANS):   A program of discretionary grants administered by *MCH,* which includes research, training, *hemophilia* diagnosis and treatment, genetic disease screening, and maternal and child health projects to demonstrate and test a variety of approaches intended to improve the health and services delivered to mothers, children, adolescents, and children with special health needs.

Surrogate markers: Laboratory tests that may predict clinical outcomes or indicate whether a drug is effective without having to wait for clinical endpoints. Surrogate markers under study in *HIV* disease include *CD4* counts, *p24 antigen,* beta-2 microglobulin, and plasma viremia. Surrogate markers may be used instead of clinical changes as the endpoints for a *clinical trial.*

Symptom: A noticeable change in the body or its functions that suggests the presence of a disease.

Syndrome: A group of symptoms and signs that together are indicative of a specific disease or medical condition.

T4 cell: See *CD4* cell.

T8 cell: See *CD8* cell.

T cells: See *T lymphocytes.*

Thrombin: An enzyme that induces clotting by converting *fibrinogen* to fibrin; precursor form in blood is *prothrombin.*

Titer: A laboratory measurement of the amount of a substance in solution. In *hemophilia* treatment, used in reference to *inhibitor antibody* level.

T lymphocytes (also called T cells):   *White blood cells* that are the primary effector cells for the host cellular *immune response*. They are derived from progenitor (precursor) cells produced in the bone marrow that then migrate to the thymus, where they mature into functional effector cells. Mature T lymphocytes leave the thymus and migrate to many areas of the body to provide protection from infectious pathogens or other foreign substances.

Tourniquet: A strip of rubber or cloth tied around the arm or leg to restrict blood flow, which allows veins to become more prominent so that *venipuncture* is easier.

Transfer needle: The double-ended needle used to allow sterile water from one bottle to flow into the *Factor concentrate* bottle, thus allowing it to reconstitute or mix.

Transfusion: The introduction of whole blood or components of blood (such as *plasma, platelets*) from one person—or from pooled material or sources—into the bloodstream of another.

Typing and screening (TS):   Determining *ABO* and *Rh blood groups* and screening of blood for unexpected *antibodies* prior to *transfusion*.

Vaccine: A preparation of killed organisms, living attenuated organisms, living fully virulent organisms, or parts of microorganisms, which is administered to produce or artificially increase immunity to a particular disease.

Venipuncture: Insertion of a needle into a vein.

Viral proteins: The main components of a *virus*. The core of *HIV* includes the proteins p24 and p18. Its envelope includes the proteins gp141 and gp120.

Virus: Any of a large and varied group of subcellular organisms composed of genetic material surrounded by at least one protein shell. Able to reproduce only within a living cell, a virus may subvert the host cell's normal functions, causing it to behave in a manner determined by the virus and resulting in disease and often ultimately the death of the host cell. Viruses can also play a positive role in *gene insertion therapy*. They have become the most common vector for gene insertion in in vivo transfers. DNA carrying the *Factor VIII* gene is combined with a deactivated virus capable of finding and infecting certain cells, thus delivering normal DNA to the cells.

von Willebrand factor (vWF):   A blood protein, important for normal *platelet* function, that circulates bound to *Factor VIII* and that is believed to help stabilize Factor VIII and carry it to bleeding sites.

von Willebrand's disease (vWD):   A combined disorder of *platelet* function and a mild to severe deficiency of *Factor VIII*. Von Willebrand's disease is transmitted genetically and can be expressed in males and females.

WFH: See *World Federation of Hemophilia*.

White blood cells (also called leukocytes; WBCs):   Specialized cells involved in defending the body against invasion by organisms and chemical substances and including the circulating white blood cells and the cells of the reticu-loendothelial system. *Granulocytes* and *lymphocytes* are particular types of white blood cells.

WONN: Women's Outreach Network of the *National Hemophilia Founda-tion,* a peer-led *hemophilia* and *HIV* education and support program initi-ated by women of the hemophilia community and the National Hemophilia Foundation.

World Federation of Hemophilia (WFH):   An international organization, founded by Frank Schnabel, whose overall mission is to advance and stimu-late services worldwide for people with *hemophilia* and related disorders. Its headquarters are in Montreal, Canada.

X chromosome: The chromosome, shaped like an "X," that carries the gene for instructions for the development of the female. Any gene on the X chro-mosome, which includes that for *hemophilia*, is said to be sex-linked.

Y chromosome: The chromosome, shaped like a "Y," that carries the gene for the development of the male.

APPENDIX B

Research Methods

*Thus while method and meaning can be treated as independent
themes, they are at the bottom inseparable. The choice of evidence
must reflect the role of history in the community.*

*Historical information need not be taken away from the
community for interpretation and presentation by the
professional historian. Through oral history the community can
and should be given the confidence to write its own history.*
Paul Thompson, *The Voice of the Past: Oral History*

My goal, from the very beginning of this project, was to produce a participatory social history of the U.S. hemophilia community, reflecting the varied perspectives, "the voices," of the wide range of members of that community, traversing the local, regional, and national levels. Three important factors have shaped my undertaking and should be discussed before I describe the linear research process.

First, my research was conducted within the context of a school of public health, based in a medical school, and I received a doctoral dissertation grant from a federal government agency. As a result, my research design and approach were subject not only to the scrutiny of a multidisciplinary doctoral committee whose members were from the Columbia University of Public Health and Teachers College, but also to the rigors of the medical school's Institutional Review Board (IRB), which is charged by government regulation with protecting the rights of human research subjects. This did not pose any problems so far as I was concerned, since it reinforced anthropology's ethical standards, by granting "informants"—i.e., research subjects or patients—the right to anonymity and confidentiality. Accordingly, I identified the persons with hemophilia who were my original informants in 1990–91 by code names, assigning a first name alphabetically in order of the date of the initial interview or contact and giving them all a last initial of "H.," representing hemophilia, thus, "Adam H.," "Brett H.," "Cliff H.," etc.

By 1994, in the months just prior to my defense of my dissertation, several other informants indicated discomfort with revealing their identities because of the political and legal climate then surrounding hemophilia, HIV, and the blood supply. After consultation with Columbia University's legal counsel, I chose to use coded names for everyone mentioned in the chapters covering the AIDS Era in my dissertation. In 1997, when I undertook to update the story for publication as this book, I was outside of the academic setting, and I presented the option of revealing true identities in the AIDS Era and the updated portion to all informants, whether they were persons with hemophilia or not. The result is that only three of the informants with hemophilia who are still living and two other informants have elected to retain their coded identities. I have respected their sensitivity and hope that readers will appreciate my decision. (However, I use the coded names for all informants with hemophilia through Chapter 10.) Also, since the time of the initial interviews seven informants have passed away; six were men with hemophilia, and one was the wife of a man with hemophilia. The widow of one man has asked that his name be used. Out of respect for the desire expressed by the others to maintain privacy, I have retained their coded names throughout. I use the term "informants" throughout the book, because all these research participants were selected within an ethnographic study framework.

Second is the question of my role as researcher and writer. When one does research outside of the walls of a laboratory, in the "real world," no matter how rigorous the design of the research, the influence or bias of the researcher inevitably enters into or "contaminates" the data gathered to some extent. It is important from the outset to acknowledge this as possible under these circumstances.

Third, my research was shaped by the traditions of public health, anthropology, and oral history. A number of books and articles that enriched my understanding of these approaches can be found in the bibliography.

The Researcher's Role

My introduction to the hemophilia community began in 1979 when I was hired by the National Hemophilia Foundation as the education director of the Educational Resources Project. As a public health educator who has worked in a variety of community and health care delivery settings, I consider myself a culture broker between providers and consumers of health care. Previous jobs included sensitizing providers to the lifestyle and culture of the consumers while concurrently empowering the consumers, enabling them to become, through educational means, full partners in planning and carrying out their health care.

In the first two years at the National Hemophilia Foundation I worked with the NHF Nursing Committee to develop an interactive teaching tool, known as the Patient/Family Model, for providers to use with patients and their families. The process of assessing educational needs and developing and field-testing the tool entailed traveling throughout the United States. In the course of these activities, I worked with many members of the multidisciplinary teams at the hemophilia treatment centers and met many hemophilia families.

As time went on and that project was completed, I became the overall education director for the National Hemophilia Foundation. I began to work both nationally and internationally, in conjunction with the World Federation of Hemophilia, to acquaint hemophilia treatment center teams throughout the world with the use of the teaching guide.

After matriculating at Columbia University as a doctoral student in the School of Public Health in 1983, I began to play a dual role, continuing to work at NHF on a part-time basis while pursuing my studies. My expressed interest in studying anthropology led to immersion in the Applied Anthropology Colloquium at Teachers College as part of my course work. For my summer fieldwork experience in 1983, I studied leadership and interaction on a hemophilia treatment center multidisciplinary team. Assuming the role of participant observer, I took field notes and administered a structured questionnaire. I was able to gain access to the setting because of my previous work with the medical directors and other team members. I experienced some strain in keeping my roles separate, which I described in the paper produced at the end of the experience:

Maintaining the dual role of NHF Education Director / anthropology student had both advantages and disadvantages. Initial access was facilitated by my role at NHF. During the summer experience, however, it became clear that Alice (known as "Ann" in the study), the nurse clinician, and several other team members felt more comfortable introducing me as the education director from NHF than as a student, particularly with outside visitors such as a representative from a pharmaceutical company. I found it difficult at times to maintain the student/observer role. This was the case when I identified a "teachable moment," a time when there was an opportunity to integrate education into a particular activity. I had to restrain myself on several occasions from bringing patients together who were seated at opposite ends of the conference room who were asking about AIDS. Facilitating a group discussion, and perhaps enabling them to develop a support group, would have been appropriate for the health educator but not for the student observer. At that particular moment I chose to restrain myself and instead to raise these points at a later time with selected team members.

My paper also included a discussion of my bias: "As a health educator who believes that patient education should be integrated into the delivery of health care, I bring a bias which I must acknowledge. I feel that the patient and his family should be fully participatory as active learners, not passive recipients of information."

In the summer of 1989, while working as a part-time Consultant for Education and Evaluation at NHF, I returned to this HTC to replicate the fieldwork project and found my sense of tension was eased. All team members were fully involved in educating patients about HIV and AIDS, and my comfort with the researcher role had grown over the passage of time. After defending my doctoral dissertation proposal in 1989 and securing funding from the U.S. Agency for Health Policy Research in the form of a doctoral dissertation research grant in the summer of 1990, I gave my notice at NHF in order to focus on my dissertation research on a full-time basis.

From the time when I decided to study the social history of hemophilia, I had become a participant observer during all hemophilia activities. While serving as the liaison between the National Hemophilia Foundation and the consulting firm of J. William Flynt, M.D., evaluating the impact of funding for HIV–risk reduction, and participating on various committees, I carried a small green notebook in which I jotted down notes related to expressions used, repetition of particular beliefs, changes in provider-patient relationships, and other behaviors with cultural significance. Attaining access to institutional and personal files and gaining the cooperation of informants was definitely made easier by my being an insider, a member of the community. Having worked in the past with both providers and consumers, I felt at ease with the wide range of interviewees.

The most difficult aspect of the interviewing process was to try to sit impassively when hemophilia informants, some of whom had become good friends, showed evidence of being in pain, coughed incessantly, and perspired profusely. One informant, "Eugene H.," placed a bottle of his medication in front of me during the interview, stating visually what he would not verbalize: he had AIDS. It was difficult (both personally and professionally) to sit in smoke-filled rooms, watching persons with hemophilia chain-smoke, a very common behavior at the time. Reminding myself that the interview was a time-limited situation helped. Taking notes about the context of the interview became a useful coping mechanism, though admittedly it was particularly difficult when a three-year-old was bouncing up and down on the stomach of his bedridden father who was having "a bleed"—or when a physician's office windows were shaking from the mild earthquake that had just occurred (only 3.5 on the Richter scale). As time went on, I learned to carry tissues for informants shedding tears, whether doctors, nurses, persons with hemophilia, or their family members.

Each interview brought fresh insights and revelations. Some interviews brought joy rather than sadness. It was exciting to share one scientist's step-by-step search for a cure for hemophilia and another's optimism about AIDS vaccine trials. An article entitled "Pearls, Pith, and Provocation: Research Alert! Qualitative Research May Be Dangerous to your Health!" describes one researcher's emotional reactions while conducting a qualitative research study. The author, Linda Dunn, considers it essential that qualitative researchers describe not only their observations but also their experiences. She describes awakening in the middle of the night and experiencing severe headaches while conducting a study of battered women—physical and emotional experiences that were parallel to those of the subjects of her study. She expresses feelings of powerlessness during the interviews when her informants cried. Although she wished to make things better for them, she had to confine herself to listening actively instead. For me, this article struck a chord. Not only while interviewing informants in person, but often while listening to the tapes of those interviews, I had to evoke coping mechanisms so as not to experience a physical expression of shared pain. It became evident that researchers as well as health providers are not impervious to anguish.

Analysis of Data: Common Themes and Terms

Doing research with an ethnographic orientation includes the concurrent collection and analysis of data. One type of analysis is to look for recurrent themes and terms of reference. Using an application called ZY Index, I was able to do this by searching the transcripts of the interview audiotapes for previously identified themes and repeated descriptive terms. When a term appeared in several interviews, I would then use it with future informants to determine whether it was, in fact, widely used as part of the hemophilia community's "culture." Such terms were useful as probes and have been compiled as Appendix E, "Linguistic Markers along Historical Pathways."

Research Methods and Strategies

BACKGROUND: VIEWING LIFE
THROUGH A BLOOD-STAINED LENS

In 1989, there was no written chronicle or historical account of the U.S. hemophilia community. At the time, the community seemed all too close to fulfilling the role described as being "the canary in the mine shaft," warning others about the danger in the U.S. blood supply and perishing in the process. Before this community and its culture vanished, I wanted to capture its essence, to understand how it began, expanded, flourished, and then fell victim to technology gone awry. When I began my research, I underestimated the community's resiliency and did not realize the extent of the lessons to be learned, by subgroups and society as a whole. Since anthropologists often combine complementary skills, tools, and strategies to study communities in depth while examining social and cultural change, I decided to employ ethnographic strategies—observation and description of a culture—and what anthropologists call an "emic" approach to capture this social history. The "emic" orientation involves using semistructured interviews and the compilation of life stories to elucidate community insiders' perspectives and sense of meaning. As stories are told, patterns emerge. As data is gathered, it is "triangulated," or verified by finding it repeated in other sources—in the words of other informants or in documents and other writing, as identified by "content analysis"—and then used to explore other issues.

Before I started my own research with informants, in order to enrich the contextual information I would bring to the process, I began to familiarize myself with the available scientific and medical literature and with a variety of writings about the social, economic, and political climate from 1948 to the present. Two articles offering the medical view of the disease—"A Short History of Hemophilia, with Some Comments on the Word 'Hemophilia'" by Dr. Kenneth Brinkhous and "The History of Haemophilia" by Dr. G. I. C. Ingram—were useful in constructing the scientific and technological context for what I came to see as distinct time frames in this period. There was substantial agreement of science between the two authors, the former American and the latter British.

Original documents, such as minutes of meetings and personal correspondence, furnished at a later date by informants from their files, further augmented my understanding of each of these time periods. Two medical directors of hemophilia treatment centers, Dr. Frederick Rickles and Dr. Charles Abildgaard, guided me in defining scientific milestones and in identifying potential informants who had been involved in shaping scientific and medical progress. In the summer of 1983, before I began formal research for my dissertation, I had, as described above, used an ethnographic strategy called "participant observation" to study the informal structure of a multidisciplinary team at a hemophilia treatment center based in an urban academic medical center. I was particularly interested in studying the structure of the team, the leadership patterns, and the nature of the physician-patient relationship. I had spent every day in the treatment center observing and writing "field notes." The use of a structured interview instrument enhanced the reliability of my observations. In the summer of 1989, I repeated the study at the same HTC, using the same interview instrument and was able to observe what things had changed and what things had stayed the same. These field data, across five years of the AIDS Era, were used to corroborate data later furnished by informants, thus further establishing reliability. The 1989 findings indicated an erosion of trust in the physician-patient relationship and shifting leadership of the team in the HTC. There was a sense that the medical director was no longer in charge and not available. His presence in the clinic had decreased. By 1989, the nurse coordinator was perceived by both the team members and patients as "a hero" and "a leader." The data also confirmed perceptions voiced later on that there was "an old team" and "a new team," those who had a hemophilia background and those with AIDS and hospice training.

SELECTION OF INFORMANTS

Since ethnographic research is not statistical, but descriptive, the meaning and richness of the data are enhanced, not by the numbers of informants, but by selecting persons acknowledged by their peers to have played a role in shaping events or making discoveries. The cultural context is enriched by extrapolating repetitive themes that emerged from life stories of persons with hemophilia who were willing to share their personal experience of the illness and of community membership.

In the summer of 1990, the first step I took was to select a "key informant," who would serve as my guide during the entire research process. "Adam H.," an older person with hemophilia, was recognized at that time by all segments of the community as a key shaper and leader. He would direct me to other leaders, representing the entire range of treatment center providers, leaders at the involved government and nongovernment agencies, plasma manufacturers, and eleven other men with hemophilia representing different age cohorts, men then in their twenties, thirties, forties, and fifties. Two other community leaders, a younger person with hemophilia and a physician, also suggested informants. The total selection was then approved by another physician and another person with hemophilia. All indicated their understanding of the importance of selecting informants who could contribute their knowledge of events and issues or share the process of making an important discovery and worked with me to accommodate limitations in both travel budget and time that made it necessary to select people in geographical clusters.

Ultimately my informants, who are listed in Appendix D, included people who staff hemophilia treatment centers—hematologists, an orthopedist, pediatricians, a psychiatrist, nurses, social workers, and administrators—federal government agency bureau, division, and program directors, a plasma manufacturing company representative and an executive, epidemiologists, an NHF Executive, a WFH executive, chapter volunteers, a consultant, two parents, and two wives of men with hemophilia. All thirty-six of these selected leaders and shapers of events agreed to be interviewed. Although some are not quoted directly as individuals in this book, the opinions and expressions of feeling of all of them truly "inform" the overall story. The group of twelve persons with hemophilia includes three cohorts: four men who were children in the 1940s and 1950s, who were in their forties or fifties at the time of the interview; six men who were children in the late 1950s and the 1960s, who were in their thirties; and the youngest, two men who were in their twenties when interviewed. One man was gay, another African American. Both urban and rural dwellers from all sections of the United States were included. All have attended college, and many have received graduate degrees. At the time of the interviews two were ministers (one teaching at the graduate level and the other counseling HIV-positive persons with hemophilia), one was a physician/researcher, two were attorneys, four worked in the plasma manufacturing or home care industry, one was a professor, one directed a community outreach project, and the other, a scientist, was an executive of a major corporation. One hundred percent of the selected hemophilia informants agreed to be interviewed, and in fact, rather than the struggle I had feared to locate willing informants, I had to tell ten people that I hoped to establish a project in the future in which they could be included. The richness in depth of this sample reflects the universe being studied. During the course of the interviews, informants from both groups mentioned additional individuals who they thought should be interviewed.

Seventeen trips were planned during the year and a half (August 1990–December 1991) of informant interviewing. A list of core themes, defining events, and issues was sent to each informant prior to the interview. The basic outline of the interview is contained in Appendix C. Questions included defining "the hemophilia community" and explaining whether it is a community and who is in it; changes in health care delivery; what the historical milestones are; identification of problems and barriers; the greatest strengths in the community; and the future of the community. In addition to these issues, I prepared special questions for persons with hemophilia. Since informants were from the macro (federal government and national agency) level and the micro (chapter, local treatment center) level, gathering information about both context and role also became important.

Terms that had appeared recurrently in the literature and the media provided useful probes; among them were denial, isolation, complaints, independence, and support systems. Two examples of recurring themes raised by informants during interviews included discussing events surrounding their circumcision and the exact number of days absent from school each year. Another repeated theme was the cost of blood products, which is a key ongoing issue. In addition to inserting these themes in subsequent interviews, I also developed special questions for people telling their life stories.

Using oral history techniques, I produced archival quality audiotapes and transcripts for interviews with the forty-eight informants. The tapes ranged from one and a half hours to nine hours in length. Informants were given the opportunity to review and edit their transcripts prior to my using the material. These tapes will eventually be deposited in the Columbia University Oral History Collection; they will be known as "reminiscence."

THE UPDATED PORTION—THE SECOND ROUND

When I undertook to update this history for publication, the relatively brief time frame for doing research and writing about the years from 1989–98 set limits on the extent and depth of my exploration. However, guidance from the academic and hemophilia community mentors enabled me to proceed rapidly. In order for me to maintain congruency with the original research conducted, I set about to interview informants who are acknowledged leaders and shapers at the current time. (These are also listed in Appendix D.) The two key informants, Glenn Pierce and Bea Pierce, identified other potential informants, who in turn selected others. Again, using a snowball sample, I asked Fred Rickles, who had guided me originally regarding the scientific domain, to do so again. Charles Abildgaard had retired, so I asked Dr. Shelby Dietrich to serve as my other physician guide, because of her long-term presence in the leadership role in the hemophilia community. The eleven informants selected represent the diversity of the community as it is today. Just as before, they all had the opportunity to edit the transcripts. In addition I had brief telephone conversations with seven other informants.

The ethnographic approach enabled me to see the hemophilia community through the eyes of these informants. Taping their voices helped me to hear what this diverse group had to say, not limiting this social history to the official literature. I am grateful to everyone who shared their feelings and thoughts and feel honored to bring them to the readers.

Informant Interview Discussion, 1990–92

As discussed in Appendix B, I used the following discussion guide in the interviews conducted in 1990–91. Depending on the informant's preference, I either asked these questions directly or, if the informant began by telling his or her story, I would interject the topics as appropriate. I tried to cover all the core issues with all of the informants.

Themes and Issues to Be Raised with Informants:

The concept of "the hemophilia community." Why is it or isn't it a community? If it's not a community, what is it?

Who is in this community?

Changes in: the role of the patient, the role of the providers, the patient-provider relationship

Changes in team structure, changes in health care delivery

Changes in treatment such as use of freeze-dried product, monoclonal, Amicar®, DDAVP?

What were the historical milestones? What about cryoprecipitate?

Who were the leaders in the hemophilia community then and now?

What has happened in the hemophilia research that is important, 20 years ago, 10 years ago?

What are treatment issues? The changing role of the National Hemophilia Foundation? The changing role of the pharmaceutical companies? The changing role and different participants since the advent of AIDS? Changes in the kinds of research? Changing technology?

What were the main problems and barriers 20 years ago? 10 years ago? Today?

What are the greatest strengths of the hemophilia community?

What can we offer those with other chronic illnesses? With AIDS?

What is the future of the hemophilia community?

The following recurring terms appear in the literature and in the media. Useful to mention as probes:

Denial: Is this helpful or counterproductive in the AIDS Era?

Isolation: A tendency to be a community turned inward?

Compliance: Is this a medical-model concept (that is, physician framed and controlled)?

Independence: Is this a goal of hemophilia care today?

Support system: What does this consist of for you? For others?

Special Questions for Life Stories, Persons with Hemophilia:

What were your first perceptions of having hemophilia?

Role of parents: Were they involved in an NHF chapter?

Personal recollections of childhood

Isolation

Acting out

Blood Brothers

Costs to family

Pain

Control

Being different

Developing intellectually

Being HIV-positive

Decision making

Being normal: What's normal?

Themes and Issues That Emerged During Interviews, Raised with Informants and Persons with Hemophilia as Interviews Progressed

The medical model

A consumer model

A family-centered model

Tri-agency model

Managed care

Strengths and weaknesses of the hemophilia model, the community

Should there be a generic chronic illness model?

Is NHF a "sick organization" because it has "sick people" on its board?

Should physicians be in the forefront today?

What are the technologies fostering a sense of community?

Should the HTC provider teams become HIV experts? Should others be brought in to care for AIDS patients?

Did "the ascendancy of the shrinks and social workers" begin at the beginning of the AIDS Era?

Gene insertion therapy

APPENDIX D

Informants

All interviews (in the form of audiotapes and transcripts) for this book have been conducted by Susan Resnik and will eventually be deposited in the Columbia University Oral History Collection. There they will be known as "reminiscences." In the following lists, "+" indicates a "key informant"; "(d.)" indicates that the person is now deceased.

Persons with Hemophilia, Interviewed 1990–91

As explained in Appendix B, the initial understanding for these interviews was that the hemophilia informants would be referred to by code names. When I sought to update material for this book, three of the original twelve informants still living were willing to have their real names used. In addition, the widow of another has granted permission to use her husband's real name. In conformity with the original research code of ethics, however, code names are used for all these informants through Chapter 10. Age cohort abbreviations are "O," oldest; "M," middle; Y, "youngest."

Informant	Age Cohort	Date of Interview
+"Adam H."	O	August 21, 1990; October 3, 1991
"Brett H." (d.)	M	September 10, 1990
"Cliff H." (Charles Carman, d.)	O	September 12, 1990
"Daniel H." (Glenn Pierce)	M	October 24, 1990
"Eugene H." (d.)	M	October 26, 1990

Informant	Age Cohort	Date of Interview
"Frank H."	O	December 4, 1990
"Gregory H."	M	July 24, 1991
"Harold H." (d.)	Y	August 7, 1991
"Irwin H." (Richard Johnson)	O	September 5, 1991
"James H." (Dana Kuhn)	M	September 9, 1991
"Kent H." (d.)	Y	October 4, 1991 (initial conversation, September 10, 1991)
"Lloyd H." (d.)	M	September 16, 1991

Other Informants, Interviewed 1990–92

Informant	Date of Interview	
Charles Abildgaard, M.D.	October 24, 1990	former HTC director; researcher
David Agle, M.D.	September 12, 1990	psychiatrist; former chair NHF Mental Health Committee
Sharon Barrett	January 15, 1991	former director, MCH Hemophilia Program
G. William Bissell	August 6, 1990	attorney; former NHF board member
Sheila Brading	November 21, 1990	former executive, WFH
Kenneth M. Brinkhous, M.D.	November 29, 1991	pioneer coagulation researcher; first chair MASAC
Regina Butler, R.N.	December 19, 1990	HTC nursing coordinator; former chair NHF Nursing Committee
Barbara Chang	October 26, 1990	former marketing director, plasma manufacturing company
Maribel Clements, R.N., M.A.	December 16, 1990	HTC nursing coordinator, former chair NHF Nursing Committee
Shelby Dietrich, M.D.	October 26, 1990	former HTC director; pioneer in comprehensive care model

Informant	*Date of Interview*	
Bruce Evatt, M.D.	June 7, 1991	former director, Host Factors Division, CDC; director, Hematologic Diseases Branch, CDC
Lisa Flam, M.P.H.	December 19, 1990	former assistant executive director, NHF
J. William Flynt, M.D.	January 16, 1991	consultant, MCH; former director, Diabetes Program, CDC
Marvin S. Gilbert, M.D.	January 4, 1991	orthopedist; former medical co-director, NHF
Ed Gomperts, M.D.	October 26, 1990	former HTC director; plasma manufacturing company executive
Mary Gooley	December 10, 1990; May 5, 1991	former HTC director; former director, NHF Chapter Program
Tony Gorenc	August 8, 1990	HTC administrator
Mrs. J. Green	June 2, 1992	pioneer parent
Paul Haas	September 10, 1990	former president, NHF
Peggy Heine, M.S.W.	September 13, 1990	social worker; former director, NRCC
Margaret Hilgartner, M.D.	December 13, 1990	pediatric hematologist; former HTC director; former medical co-director, NHF
Vince Hutchins, M.D.	February 2, 1990	former deputy director, MCH
Craig Kessler, M.D.	October 14, 1991	former co-medical director, NHF; HTC director
Dale Lawrence, M.D.	October 11, 1991	chief, Clinical Development Section, Vaccine Bureau, Division of AIDS, NIAID; former CDC epidemiologist
Peter H. Levine, M.D.	December 6, 1990	former NHF co-medical director; former HTC director; medical center CEO
Richard Lipton, M.D.	April 25, 1991	HTC medical director

Informant	*Date of Interview*	
Merle MacPherson, M.D., M.P.H.	April 25, 1990	acting director, MCH; former director, Habilitative Services, MCH
Karen Meredith, R.N., M.P.H.	January 15, 1991	former chief, Hemophilia Program; CDC; former NHF Nursing Committee consultant
"Mindy H." (d.)	November 29, 1990	wife of hemophilia patient
"Paul Phillips," M.P.H., M.S.W.	October 29, 1990	former executive director, NHF
Bea Pierce ("Diane H."), M.S.N.	October 24, 1990	wife of Glenn Pierce ("Daniel H."); vice-president, NHF
Oscar Ratnoff, M.D.	November 5, 1991	pioneer coagulation researcher; former HTC medical director
Frederick Rickles, M.D.	December 5, 1990	researcher; HTC director; assistant director, Hematologic Diseases Branch, CDC
Frank Schnabel (d.)	taped statement obtained November 11, 1990	founder and former president, WFH
Billie Sullivan	October 24, 1990	former HTC counselor
"Marcus Victor," M.D.	January 9, 1991; February 12, 1991	former medical co-director, NHF

Informants for Update, Interviewed 1997

Val Bias	July 15, 1997	MANN; NHF liaison, Marc Associates
Sally Crudder, R.N.	May 26, 1997	director, Hemophilia Program, CDC
+Shelby Dietrich, M.D.	June 16, 1997	former HTC director; pioneer in comprehensive care model
Bruce Evatt, M.D.	August 26, 1997	former director, Host Factors Division, CDC; director, Hematologic Diseases Branch, CDC

Informant	*Date of Interview*	
Kathy Gerus	August 27, 1997	WONN; former vice-president, NHF; member, Presidential HIV Advisory Council
Keith Hoots, M.D.	September 2, 1997	HTC director
Richard Johnson ("Irwin H.")	August 28, 1997	CUDP leader
Laureen Kelley	July 17, 1997	parent; publisher, *Parent Exchange Newsletter*
+Bea Pierce, M.S.N. ("Diane H.")	April 14, 1997	wife of Glenn Pierce ("Daniel H."); vice-president, NHF
+Glenn Pierce, Ph.D., M.D. ("Daniel H.")	May 1, 1997	former president, NHF
+Frederick Rickles, M.D.	May 26, 1997	researcher; HTC director; assistant director, Hematologic Diseases Branch, CDC

Telephone Conversations for Update, Conducted 1997

Informant	*Date of Conversation*	
Dana Kuhn, Ph.D. ("James H.")	September 10, 1997	MANN leader, legislative advocate
Dale Lawrence, M.D.	September 1, 1997	chief, Clinical Development Section, Vaccine Bureau, Division of AIDS, NIAID; former CDC epidemiologist
Richard Lipton, M.D.	September 25, 1997	HTC medical director
Kathy McAdam	August 27, 1997	social worker; WONN; wife of Bill McAdam (d.)
"Paul Phillips"	September 30, 1997	former executive director, NHF
Fred Rosner, M.D.	August 27, 1997	physician and Talmudic scholar
Linda Smith	August 28, 1997	WONN; wife of Nathan Smith (d.)

Linguistic Markers
along Historical Pathways

Whilst I never forget the medical status of the deaf, I now have to see them in a new "ethnic" light, as a people, with a distinctive language, sensibility, and culture of their own.
Oliver Sacks, *Seeing Voices: A Journey into the World of the Deaf*

As I researched the history of hemophilia and the people who either have the condition or treat it, I discovered a shared belief that there is a hemophilia community. During interviews and conversations certain terms came up over and over again to describe aspects of living with hemophilia. Often these are markers for specific time frames. I have chosen to call these terms "linguistic markers," and I perceive them as part of the shared hemophilia culture.

The Dismal Era	The Golden Era	The AIDS Era	Looking into the Future
The Bad Old Days	Golden Years	The Black Cloud	The Green Years
The Royal Disease	Miracle time	The Hemophilia Holocaust	Years of Hope
Clotters	Treaters, "Hemophilia Flying Circus"	"I.D.s" (infectious disease doctors)	Gene cloners (vectorologists)
Victims, sufferers	Patients	Fallen soldiers	Virgins, pups
Bleeders	Blood brothers	Young bloods, PWHs (persons with hemophilia), PWAs (persons with AIDS)	
Viper venom	Blood shots, infusions, cryo, Factor, the Blood Business	Heat-treated and solvent-detergent-treated products, recombinants	Gene therapy
Parents' horror stories	Patients' war stories	Testimony, articles, books	
"Pioneer parents"	Parents	Wives, mothers, partners	
The Red Bed* (Ohio)	Money getters* (New York), Chapterland* (Rochester, N.Y.)		

*Terms used in certain geographical areas.

Federal Hemophilia Program Regions

The federal hemophilia program has divided the country into ten regions, listed here. Readers can refer to the NHF or MCH for the Directory of Hemophilia Treatment Centers and Facilities for the names and addresses of MCH Regional Directors and Coordinators.

Region I:	Connecticut, Maine, Massachusetts, New Hampshire, Rhode Island, Vermont
Region II:	New Jersey, New York, Puerto Rico, Virgin Islands
Region III:	Delaware, District of Columbia, Maryland, Pennsylvania, Virginia, West Virginia
Region IV:	Alabama, Florida, Georgia, Kentucky, Louisiana, Mississippi, North Carolina, South Carolina, Tennessee
Region V:	Illinois, Indiana, Michigan, Minnesota, North Dakota, Ohio, South Dakota, Wisconsin
Region VI:	Arkansas, Oklahoma, Texas
Region VII:	Iowa, Kansas, Missouri, Nebraska
Region VIII:	Arizona, Colorado, Montana, New Mexico, Utah, Wyoming
Region IX:	California, Guam, Hawaii, Nevada
Region X:	Alaska, Idaho, Oregon, Washington

Changes in Death Rates and Causes of Death in Persons with Hemophilia A, 1979–89

	Years						1987-1989/ 1979-1981	
	1979-1981		1983-1985		1987-1989			
	Rate	(No.)	Rate	(No.)	Rate	(No.)	Risk Ratio	95% CL
Total	0.4	250	0.6	403	1.2	853	3.2	2.9 - 3.7
Gender								
Male	0.7	228	1.1	368	2.3	815	3.3	2.9 - 3.8
Female	0.1	22	0.1	35	0.1	38	1.6	1.0 - 2.7
Race								
White	0.4	219	0.6	356	1.2	769	3.3	2.9 - 3.9
Black	0.4	29	0.5	42	0.9	79	2.4	1.6 - 3.7
Other Races	0.1	2	0.2	5	0.2	5	1.5	0.3 - 7.8
Age Group								
0-9	0.2	17	0.2	18	0.2	26	1.4	0.8 - 2.6
10-19	0.1	14	0.2	21	0.8	38	7.1	4.0 -12.4
20-29	0.2	22	0.3	33	1.1	133	6.0	3.8 - 9.4
30-39	0.2	22	0.5	52	1.4	173	6.2	4.0 -10.0
40-49	0.4	26	0.7	50	1.5	128	3.9	2.5 - 5.9
50-59	0.5	37	0.8	53	1.2	78	2.3	1.5 - 3.3
60-69	0.9	52	1.1	66	1.6	97	1.7	1.2 - 2.4
70+	1.2	60	2.0	110	2.1	130	1.8	1.3 - 2.4
Region								
Northeast	0.5	66	0.6	95	1.3	190	2.8	2.1 - 3.7
North Central	0.4	61	0.5	93	1.2	204	3.3	2.5 - 4.4
South	0.4	84	0.6	142	1.2	291	3.1	2.5 - 4.0
West	0.3	39	0.5	73	1.1	168	3.7	2.6 - 5.2

Hemophilia A Annual Death Rates (per 1,000,000 Persons), United States, 1979-1981, 1983-1985, and 1987-1989. Data provided by CDC.

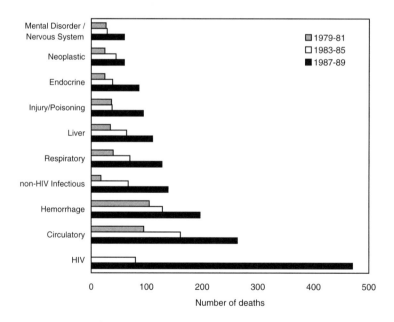

Number and percentage of hemophilia A deaths by cause of death listed on death certificates for leading causes of death, by period, United States, 1979-1981, 1983-1985, and 1987-1989. Data provided by CDC.

Hemophilia Treatment Center Data Collection and Presentation: A Historical Overview

The earliest hemophilia treatment center data collection activities began on the two coasts of the United States in the 1960s and early 1970s. The hemophilia program at Los Angeles Orthopaedic Hospital, under the direction of Shelby Dietrich, M.D., collected data and issued a report entitled *Hemophilia : A Total Approach to Treatment and Rehabilitation*, in 1968. Tables documented the decline in the number and duration of hospital admissions and stays that resulted from Dietrich's "total approach," making the case for supporting rehabilitation and keeping patients out of the hospital rather than on welfare support. Concurrently, HTCs in Rochester, N.Y., under the direction of Mary Gooley, and in Worcester, Mass., supervised by Peter Levine, M.D., collected data showing the cost effectiveness of home care. These data were presented to insurance companies to make the case for coverage for home care for hemophilia.

Levine took the next step by publishing his data in *The Annals of Internal Medicine* in 1973 and also presenting it to Congress in support of the effort to pass legislation that would create a federally funded hemophilia treatment center program. The federal Hemophilia Program that resulted was placed under the administration of the Office of Maternal and Child Health. Levine then assumed a leadership role in expanding data collection efforts throughout the national network of HTCs on an annual basis, continuing to illustrate the cost effectiveness of comprehensive care and home therapy. These data were useful to MCH, with its focus on systems of health care and health services. Data were collected by either nurses or social workers as part of their job. Renewal of funding for the federal program was bolstered by presentation of these annual reports.

Beginning in the early 1980s, when it became known that the hemophilia population was "at risk" for HIV and AIDS, risk reduction efforts were initiated. Collaboration between the Centers for Disease Control and the National Hemophilia Foundation began with research protocols to examine whether family members of persons with HIV were at risk from "casual contact." (It was found that they were not.) In 1988 MCH hired J. William Flynt, M.D., as a consultant to evaluate efforts at risk reduction efforts then being made. Flynt's report suggested that the CDC take the leadership role in data collection for risk reduction, since it was the agency with the relevant expertise. During this time the "minimal data set" was developed. Data were collected, as before, on an annual basis by various kinds of hemophilia treatment center personnel who often allowed inconsistencies in definitions and methods of collection. A sample of data collected in 1993 (with some of these shortcomings) is given below.

During the 1990s the CDC initiated more sophisticated procedures, such as surveillance studies. (See Chapter 12.) Currently, data collectors at health departments on the local level receive training and supervision from CDC personnel. More reliable data are becoming available through the Hemophilia Surveillance System, currently in place in six states. Sample data from this survey are given below.

Minimal Data Set for Risk Reduction, National Totals, 1993

I. Characteristics of Active Patients

1. Estimated number of persons with
   hemophilia A or hemophilia B: 17,435
2. Number of active patients with hemophilia
   A, hemophilia B, and other bleeding
   disorders, including von Willebrand's
   disease: 19,845
3. Number of active patients that died in 1993:   419
4. Number of active patients with:
   A. Hemophilia A   10,382 (52%)
   B. Hemophilia B   2,835 (14%)   (67%)
   C. von Willebrand's and other   6,628   (33%)
                     (A + B + C should = #2) = 19,845
5. Number of active female patients with
   bleeding disorder: 2,959
6. Number of active patients in the following
   age groups:
   A. <13 years   6,997 (35%)
   B. 13–19 years   3,022 (15%)
   C. >19 years   9,420 (47%)
   D. Age unknown   406 (2%)
                     (A + B + C + D should = #2) = 19,845

7. Number of active patients in the following racial/ethnic groups:

A. White, non-Hispanic	14,556	(73%)
B. Black, non-Hispanic	1,862	(9%)
C. Hispanic	1,729	(9%)
D. Other	1,133	(6%)
E. Unknown	565	(3%)

$(A + B + C + D + E \text{ should} = \#2) = 19,845$

II. Risk Reduction Information—Patients

8. Number of active patients who are known to have received potentially contaminated products between 1978 and the end of 1985:   9,741   (49%)

9. Of the above, the number:

A. Known to be HIV-positive	3,897
B. Known to be HIV-negative	5,326
C. Not tested	356
D. Whose test result is not known	162

$(A + B + C + D \text{ should} = \#8) = 9,741$

Of the number not tested ("C" above), the number:

E. Refusing testing	297
F. Not offered testing	56

10. Number of active patients that are HIV-positive, not tested, or whose test status is unknown: $9A + 9C + 9D = 4,415$

11. Number of active patients for whom it is unknown if they received potentially contaminated products: 553

12. Number of active patients that received potentially contaminated products (total for #8) and have been provided pre–HIV test counseling:

A. Ever	9,451	(97%)
B. This last year (Jan. 1, 1993– Dec. 31, 1993)	1,012	

13. Number of active patients that received potentially contaminated products (total for #8) receiving their *first* HIV test this last year (Jan. 1, 1993–Dec. 31, 1993):   206

14. Number of active known HIV-positive patients who are:

A. White, non-Hispanic	2,968	(76%)
B. Black, non-Hispanic	481	(12%)
C. Hispanic	317	(8%)
D. Other	116	(3%)
E. Unknown	15	(<1%)

$(A + B + C + D + E \text{ should} = \#9.A) = 3,897$

15. Number of active HIV-positive, not
tested, or test status unknown patients
(#10) who have been:
A. Sexually active in 1993   2,084 (47%)
B. Not sexually active in 1993   1,599 (36%)
C. Sexually active status unknown for
1993   732 (17%)
(A + B + C *must* = #10) = 4,415

III. Risk Reduction Information—Partners

	Current ('93) partner	Past partner	Total	
16. A. Number of sexual partners of active HIV-infected, exposed and not tested, or exposed and test status unknown patients (#10):	2,010	2,070	4,080	
16. B. Of the total above, the number of sexual partners that were reported to the HTC for the first time in 1993:			411	(10%)
17. Of the total for #16.A, the number that ever received: (information optional— please refer to Instructions for Completion. Please supply "current partner" numbers, even if "past partner" data is not available. All must include Totals)				
A. Pretest counseling	581	322	2,378	(58%)
B. An HIV test	529	299	2,407	(59%)
18. Number of current and past sexual partners tested between Jan. 1, 1993, and Dec. 31, 1993:			850	(21% of all partners)
19. Of the above number, the number of partners receiving:				
A. Initial HIV tests	166	(20%)		
B. Repeat HIV tests	685	(80%)		

(A + B should = #18) = 851

20. Number of current and past sexual partners of active patients tested by:
    A. Treatment center (ever)   1,748
    B. Other providers (ever)   841

21. Number of HIV tested current and past partners of active patients who are:

                                                Seroprevalence (proportion at any one time):

    A. HIV-positive   241 (10.7%)
    B. HIV-negative   2,018
    C. HIV serostatus unknown   149   (6%)

(A + B + C should = #17.B) = 2,408

IV. Pregnancy Information

22. Number of pregnancies among HIV-positive and at-risk couples:
    A. Between Jan. 1993 and Dec. 1993   81
    B. Cumulative (between Jan. 1980 and Dec. 1993)   1,194

23. Number of cumulative still births or spontaneous or elective abortions to HIV-positive mothers: 40

24. Number of *cumulative* live births to HIV positive mothers: 152

25. Of the above, the
    A. Number of living infants who are HIV-symptomatic or >17 months and persistently HIV-positive   18
    B. Number of infants who are HIV-positive, <19 months of age and not symptomatic   4
    C. Number of infants who are HIV-negative   92

D. Number of de-
ceased infants from
known or presump-
tive HIV disease   12
E. Number of infants
whose status is
unknown (e.g. lost
to follow-up)   26

$$(A + B + C + D + E \text{ must} = \#24) = 152$$
$$\text{Perinatal transmission: } 30/122 = 25\%$$

V. Counseling Information

26. Estimate the number
of individual counsel-
ing sessions by staff
during Jan. 1–Dec. 31,
1993, for the following
HIV-infected or at-risk
persons (#10):   Total = 41,555
A. Adult patients
(>19 years)   20,425
B. Sexual partners   5,285
C. Child patients
and/or parents   4,441
D. Adolescent patients
(13–19 years)
and/or parents of
adolescent patients   7,669
E. Other family
members   3,735

27. Estimate the number
of individual counsel-
ing sessions by staff
during Jan. 1–Dec. 31,
1993, for the following
persons who are neither
HIV-infected nor at-risk: Total = 23,309
A. Adult patients
(>19 years)   7,217
B. Sexual partners   1,409
C. Child patients
and/or parents   9,388
D. Adolescent patients
(13–19 years)
and/or parents of
adolescent patients   3,874
E. Other family
members   1,421

28. Estimate the number of group counseling sessions by staff during Jan. 1–Dec. 31, 1993, for the following groups of HIV-infected or at-risk persons: Total = 2,828

    A. Adult patients (>19 years)   934

    B. Sexual partners   634

    C. Child patients and/or parents   456

    D. Adolescent patients (13–19 years) and/or parents of adolescent patients   476

    E. Other family members   328

29. Estimate the number of group counseling sessions by staff during Jan. 1–Dec. 31, 1993, for the following groups of persons who are neither HIV-infected nor at-risk: Total = 1,604

    A. Adult patients (>19 years)   375

    B. Sexual partners   164

    C. Child patients and/or parents   482

    D. Adolescent patients (13–19 years) and/or parents of adolescent patients   360

    E. Other family members   223

VI. Deceased Patient Information

30. Number of patient deaths:

    A. Between Jan. 1, 1992, and Dec. 31, 1992   382   (15% of cumulative)

    B. Cumulative death (1980–92)   2,504

31. Number of cumulative deaths between 1980 and 1992 that were primarily (choose only one):

A. HIV-related			1,654	(66%)
B. Hemophilia-related			364	(15%)
C. Other			393	(16%)
D. Unknown cause			96	(4%)

32. Number of patients that died between 1980 and 1992 and:

			Cumulative	Seroprevalenc
A. Were known to be HIV-positive	1,928	(77%)	5,825	(51%)
B. Were known to be HIV-negative	209	(8%)	5,535	
C. Were not tested	330	(13%)		
D. Tested, but test status is unknown	40	(2%)		

$(A + B + C + D \text{ should} = \#30.B) = 2,507$

33. Number of sexual partners of patients who died between 1980 and 1992 that

A. Have been HIV-counseled	831
B. Have been HIV-tested	767

Of the above in #33.B, the number who were:

C. HIV- positive	121
D. HIV- negative	622
E. HIV serostatus unknown	25

$(C + D + E \text{ should} = B) = 768$

F. Are currently being followed at your center (i.e., had contact with the partner this last year)   207

VII. Inactive Patient Information

34. Number of inactive patients   6,954

Selected Data from the Hemophilia Surveillance System, 1993–95

Table 1. *Number of Prevalent Male Cases of Hemophilia A (HemA) and Hemophilia B (HemB) Identified in Six U.S. States during 1993–95*

	1993		1994		1995	
State of residence	HemA No.	HemB No.	HemA No.	HemB No.	HemA No.	HemB No.
Colorado	177	50	181	51	185	49
Georgia	358	70	389	82	413	89
Louisiana	194	75	196	80	197	82
Massachusetts	305	61	309	61	315	62
New York*	905	253	902	263	902	267
Oklahoma	158	45	158	49	157	52
TOTAL	2,097	554	2,135	586	2,169	601

*Two persons had both hemophilia A and B and are included as cases in both columns for all 3 years.

Table 2. *Number of Incident Male Cases of Hemophilia A (HemA) and Hemophilia B (HemB) Identified in Six U.S. States during 1993–95*

	1993		1994		1995	
State of residence	HemA No.	HemB No.	HemA No.	HemB No.	HemA No.	HemB No.
All States	36	12	35	12	42	9

NOTE: The number of cases with birthdates in the year of the surveillance. This number will be an undercount of new cases of hemophilia because a diagnosis of hemophilia is often not made until the child is more than 5 years old, especially for children with mild cases of disease. Since these data were collected during 1994–97, cases among persons born in 1993–95 may not yet have been diagnosed.

Table 3. *Age Distribution of Males with Hemophilia Residing in Six U.S. States in 1993*

Hemophilia type		Age group (years)																TOTAL
		0–4	5–	10–	15–	20–	25–	30–	35–	40–	45–	50–	55–	60–	65–	70–	75+	
A	N	228	242	259	195	182	202	185	150	135	93	68	43	42	29	22	22	2,097
	%	10.9	11.5	12.4	9.3	8.7	9.6	8.8	7.2	6.4	4.4	3.2	2.0	2.0	1.4	1.0	1.0	
B	N	67	63	52	56	48	55	51	41	29	31	14	14	12	5	9	7	554
	%	12.1	11.4	9.4	10.1	8.7	9.9	9.2	7.4	5.2	5.6	2.5	2.5	2.2	0.9	1.6	1.3	

Table 4. *Age Distribution of Males with Hemophilia Residing in Six U.S. States in 1994*

Hemophilia type		0–4	5–	10–	15–	20–	25–	30–	35–	40–	45–	50–	55–	60–	65–	70–	75+	TOTAL
									Age group (years)									
A	N	225	253	264	217	168	192	189	162	135	102	63	40	50	31	21	23	2,135
	%	10.5	11.8	12.4	10.2	7.9	9.0	8.8	7.6	6.3	4.8	3.0	1.9	2.3	1.4	1.0	1.1	
B	N	66	74	58	51	57	49	55	40	35	37	17	12	12	6	8	9	586
	%	11.3	12.6	9.9	8.7	9.7	8.4	9.4	6.8	6.0	6.3	2.9	2.0	2.0	1.0	1.4	1.5	

Table 5. *Age Distribution of Males with Hemophilia Residing in Six U.S. States in 1995*

Hemophilia type		0–4	5–	10–	15–	20–	25–	30–	35–	40–	45–	50–	55–	60–	65–	70–	75+	TOTAL
								Age group (years)										
A	N	239	265	253	237	168	185	179	159	136	119	59	39	50	30	24	27	2,169
	%	11.0	12.2	11.7	10.9	7.8	8.5	8.2	7.3	6.3	5.5	2.7	1.8	2.3	1.4	1.1	1.2	
B	N	63	82	61	56	52	51	50	50	35	32	21	13	14	6	8	7	601
	%	10.5	13.6	10.2	9.3	8.6	8.5	8.3	8.3	5.8	5.3	3.5	2.2	2.3	1.0	1.3	1.2	

Notes

Chapter 1

1. National Hemophilia Foundation, *What You Should Know About Hemophilia*, 1. Twenty thousand is the figure currently used by the NHF and cited in the literature and in the press. Before 1972, newspapers in Rochester, N.Y., and Los Angeles, Calif., stated that there were 100,000 Americans with hemophilia. The origin of this figure is unclear. In 1972 the National Institutes of Health *Pilot Study of Hemophilia Treatment in the U.S.* stated that there were 25,000 hemophiliacs being treated in the United States. Ensuing studies undertaken by the NHF and the CDC have revised the figure downward.

2. See C. E. Rosenberg, "Disease in History," 1.

3. See Turner, *The Ritual Process*. "Communitas" pertains to cult membership that transects village and lineage membership. Here I use the term to describe a "community of suffering" that defines itself by its shared affliction.

4. On purposive sampling and snowball strategies, see Babbie, *The Practice of Social Research*, 178.

5. Information on hemophilia is from the following: interview with Shelby Dietrich, M.D. (June 16, 1997), conducted by Susan Resnik, 34, 35; NHF, *What You Should Know About Hemophilia*, esp. 1; and Miller, *The Inheritance of Hemophilia*, esp. 3, 4, 9.

Chapter 2

1. The epigraph quotation appears in Rosner, *Medicine in the Bible and the Talmud*, 43. (Dr. Rosner generously provided clarification of the difference between the Babylonian and Jerusalem mishnahs and elucidation of all references

in a telephone conversation, Aug. 27, 1997.) See also Ingram, "The History of Haemophilia," 3.

2. Rosner, *Medicine in the Bible and the Talmud,* 43 (Albucasis), 44 (Maimonides), 46 (Shulhan Arukh).

3. Ibid., 43.

4. K. M. Brinkhous, "A Short History of Hemophilia," 3–12.

5. Ingram, *History of Haemophilia,* 4.

6. Ibid. Ingram comments that "Many people know about the Romanov hemophilia from reading Dorothy Sayers's (1932) novel *Have His Carcase,* and, more importantly, R. K. Massie's (1968) book *Nicholas and Alexandra,* and the film version made for Columbia Pictures by Sam Spiegel."

7. Ibid., 6. Ingram notes that historians have debated this point but that "the strain on the Royal household is clear enough."

8. Brinkhous, "Short History of Hemophilia," 3. See also Ingram, "The History of Haemophilia," 4; Ingram writes that Fildes (who was later knighted) made his contribution to "haemophilia" while still a medical student and that Bulloch "meticulously traced out the spread of Victoria's mutant gene through the Royal houses of Europe."

9. Ingram, "The History of Haemophilia," 6.

10. Ibid., 4.

11. Brinkhous, "Short History of Hemophilia," 11.

12. Ingram, "The History of Haemophilia," 9, 11.

13. Brinkhous, "Short History of Hemophilia," 13. Brinkhous notes that plasma was used by "force of circumstances": a paternal donor had red cells that were incompatible with his hemophilic son's, so Feissly harvested his plasma and discovered that it was as effective as whole blood. The history of fractionation of plasma to give a preparation with antihemophilic factor (AHF) activity probably began in 1911, according to Brinkhous; Drs. Patek and Taylor then produced "a crude fraction which lowered the whole blood clotting time in hemophiliacs" (13).

14. Interview with Oscar Ratnoff, M.D. (Nov. 5, 1991), conducted by Susan Resnik, 2.

15. Interview with Kenneth M. Brinkhous, M.D. (Nov. 29, 1991), conducted by Susan Resnik, 3.

16. P. Starr, *The Social Transformation of American Medicine,* 338–40. Although, as Starr notes, critics have suggested that congressmen were more willing to spend money to save hogs than people, he also points out that agricultural research did yield medical advances. Discoveries in veterinary medicine led to better comprehension of transmission of disease, and other agricultural research led to the discovery of antibiotics.

17. Brinkhous interview, 11.

18. Interview with Peter H. Levine, M.D. (Dec. 6, 1990), conducted by Susan Resnik, 4.

19. Lederman, "Yesterday, Today, and Tomorrow" (Summer 1984), 4.

20. Lederman, "Yesterday, Today, and Tomorrow" (Fall 1982–Winter 1983), 5.

21. Ingram, "The History of Haemophilia," 9. In discussing the treatments attempted in the 1930s, Ingram states that "most of these treatments must have been based on little more than guess-work, and their general ineffectiveness is testified to by the extensive mortality and morbidity recorded by Carol Birch in her 1937 monograph."

22. De Neffe, "Sharing the Pulse," 13.

23. C. Levine, "How Wartime Needs Changed Medicine."

24. De Neffe, "Sharing the Pulse," 13.

25. D. Starr, "Again and Again in World War II," 130.

26. Ibid., 134–35.

27. De Neffe, "Sharing the Pulse," 13.

28. Brinkhous, "A Short History of Hemophilia," 11.

29. Littell, "Bearer Is a Hemophiliac," 215–17.

30. Interview with "Adam H." (Session #1, Aug. 21, 1990), conducted by Susan Resnik, 11, 16, 17.

31. P. Starr, *The Social Transformation of American Medicine*, 332.

Chapter 3

1. Interview with Kenneth M. Brinkhous, M.D. (Nov. 29, 1991), conducted by Susan Resnik, 20.

2. Smith, *A History of the National Hemophilia Foundation*, 2.

3. Ibid., 12.

4. Pemberton, "Bleeder Dogs," 1, 64. Despite Brinkhous's recollection in his interview, Pemberton has discovered that it was actually in 1947 that Brinkhous, then chairman of the Pathology Department at the University of North Carolina at Chapel Hill, began breeding dogs with an inherited bleeding disorder for the explicit purpose of conducting research on hemophilia. Brinkhous received a grant from the NIH for $14,000 to cover his expenses, beginning June 1, 1947. Pemberton also discusses Brinkhous's prior exposure to the use of dogs as laboratory technology as part of the Iowa Group, which was doing coagulation research at the University of Iowa (36).

5. Ibid., 36, 77, 2.

6. Brinkhous interview, 2.

7. Ibid., 18, 20.

8. Interview with Frederick Rickles, M.D. (Dec. 5, 1990), conducted by Susan Resnik, 8.

9. Interview with Oscar Ratnoff, M.D. (Nov. 5, 1991), conducted by Susan Resnik, 8.

10. Ibid., 21.

11. P. Starr, *The Social Transformation of American Medicine*, 338, 342, 343.

12. Ibid., 336.

13. Ibid.

14. Ibid., 347.

15. Ibid., 336.

16. Ibid.

17. Stevens, *American Medicine and the Public Interest,* 274.

18. P. Starr, *The Social Transformation of American Medicine,* 359.

19. Stevens, *American Medicine and the Public Interest,* 269.

20. P. Starr, *The Social Transformation of American Medicine,* 359.

21. Ibid., 348.

22. Ibid., 357.

23. Ibid.

24. Ibid., 358.

25. Interview with Marvin Gilbert, M.D. (Jan. 4. 1991), conducted by Susan Resnik, 12, 13.

26. Interview with Mary Gooley (Session #1, Dec. 10, 1990), conducted by Susan Resnik, 2, 6.

27. Interview with "Cliff H." (Charles Carman; Sept. 12, 1990), conducted by Susan Resnik, 4, 32.

28. Interview with "Irwin H." (Richard Johnson; Sept. 5, 1991), conducted by Susan Resnik, 1, 2, 4.

29. Ibid., 6, 8, 9, 22.

30. Interview with "Adam H." (Session #1, Aug. 21, 1990), conducted by Susan Resnik, 3, 8, 9.

31. Ibid., 12, 15.

32. Titmuss, *The Gift Relationship,* 47.

33. Ibid., 53, 56, 59.

34. Ibid., 160, 163.

35. P. Starr, *The Social Transformation of American Medicine,* 238, 244.

36. Ibid., 331.

37. Smith, *History of the National Hemophilia Foundation,* 1, 2.

38. "Interview with Robert Lee Henry," 9.

39. Smith, *History of the National Hemophilia Foundation,* Appendix B.

40. "Interview with Robert Lee Henry," 9. Despite the article's title, it also includes an interview with Betty Jane Henry.

41. American Diabetes Association, *The Journey and the Dream,* 1.

42. Gooley interview (Session #1), 10, 20.

43. Smith, *History of The National Hemophilia Foundation,* 2–5.

44. Massie and Massie, *Journey,* 39, 40.

45. Gooley interview (Session #1), 11.

46. Interview with Mrs. J. Green (June 2, 1992), conducted by Susan Resnik, 4, 10.

47. Brinkhous interview, 26.

Chapter 4

1. Interview with Frederick Rickles, M.D. (Dec. 5, 1990), conducted by Susan Resnik, 2, 9.

2. Ibid., 2.

3. Interview with Charles Abildgaard, M.D. (Oct. 24, 1990), conducted by Susan Resnik, 2, 3.

4. Interview with Margaret Hilgartner, M.D. (Dec. 13, 1990), conducted by Susan Resnik, 5.

5. Interview with Kenneth M. Brinkhous, M.D. (Nov. 29, 1991), conducted by Susan Resnik, 28, 29, 34.

6. Interview with Barbara Chang (Oct. 26, 1990), conducted by Susan Resnik, 46.

7. Brinkhous interview, 28.

8. Abildgaard interview, 16.

9. Brinkhous interview, 30; interview with Oscar Ratnoff, M.D. (Nov. 5, 1991), conducted by Susan Resnik, 14.

10. Rickles interview, 4.

11. Ratnoff interview, 14.

12. Smith, *History of the National Hemophilia Foundation,* 15.

13. Abildgaard interview, 16.

14. Smith, *History of the National Hemophilia Foundation,* 15.

15. Ibid.

16. Interview with "Adam H." (Session #1, Aug. 21, 1990), conducted by Susan Resnik, 48, 56.

17. Interview with "Daniel H.,"(Glenn Pierce, Ph.D., M.D.; Oct. 24, 1990), conducted by Susan Resnik, 1–2. Later in the interview, "Daniel H." indicated that his third period was that of Factor treatment.

18. Ibid., 39, 4.

19. Interview with "Lloyd H." (Sept. 16, 1991), conducted by Susan Resnik, 3.

20. Ibid., 9.

21. P. Starr, *The Social Transformation of American Medicine,* 9, 363.

22. C. E. Rosenberg, *The Care of Strangers,* 3.

23. P. Starr, *The Social Transformation of American Medicine,* 334.

24. Interview with "Gregory H."(July 24, 1991), conducted by Susan Resnik, 7.

25. Edward Carey, "President's Report," minutes of meeting of Board of Trustees of the National Hemophilia Foundation, Mayflower Hotel, Washington, D.C., Dec. 4, 1964. I thank Mary Gooley for directing me to this report.

26. Ibid.

27. Ibid.

28. American Blood Resources Association, *Coagulation Concentrates,* 6.

29. Brinkhous interview, 32–34. In a 1998 telephone conversation, Steven Pemberton emphasized that this technique resulted in no significant side effects.

30. Deutsch and Deutsch, "Dr. Thelin's Fight Against Hemophilia," 93.

31. Ibid., 93, 94; Brinkhous interview, 34.

32. Interview with Marvin Gilbert, M.D. (Jan. 4, 1991), conducted by Susan Resnik, 5.

33. Ibid., 2, 3.

34. Interview with Shelby Dietrich, M.D. (Oct. 26, 1990), conducted by Susan Resnik, 1, 2.

35. Ibid., 2, 3,

36. Ibid., 4.

37. Ibid., 4, 6.

38. Ibid., 7, 8.

39. Ibid., 8.

40. Dietrich, *Hemophilia: A Total Approach,* 4.

41. Dietrich interview, 9.

42. Ibid.

43. Vils, "Transfusion of Interest."

44. Dietrich interview, 10, 11.

45. "Normal Lives Possible: New Shots Will Help Hemophilia Victims," *Los Angeles Times,* May 12, 1966, 1.

46. James, "Hope for Bleeders." The article went on to say, "Ever more effective preparations are on the way, giving doctors the hope that hemophiliacs may eventually be able to control their ailment entirely through periodic injections, much as diabetics use insulin." Other papers ran headlines, "Shots to Cure Hemophilia."

47. Dietrich, *Hemophilia: A Total Approach,* 1, 11.

48. "Lloyd H." interview, 10, 11, 14.

49. Ibid., 11, 12, 15, 14.

50. Interview with "Dr. Marcus Victor" (Session #1, Jan. 9, 1991), conducted by Susan Resnik, 4, 5.

Chapter 5

1. Smith, *History of the National Hemophilia Foundation,* 7.

2. Interview with David Agle, M.D. (Sept. 12, 1990), conducted by Susan Resnik, 4, 5. As a result of this work, Agle and "Victor" established the NHF Mental Health Committee in 1975 to coordinate hemophilia mental health activities throughout the country. The most important recognition of the psychosocial component of hemophilia care came in the requirement of the law establishing the HTC program, which stipulated that centers must address psychoscocial, vocational, and financial needs of families. In 1980 a committee chaired by Agle used the hemophilia mental health program as a model for services to all children with chronic illnesses. The psychosocial features that were listed as common to all such diseases include interference with achievement of normal social and vocational goals, social isolation, a sense of being different and defective, impact on nonaffected siblings and parents, anger, and guilt. The HIV/AIDS epidemic has further illustrated the need for psychosocial services.

3. Martin C. Rosenthal, M.D., "Memorandum on meeting with the American Red Cross," May 10, 1967; I thank Mary Gooley for providing a copy of this memorandum from her files.

4. Smith, *History of the National Hemophilia Foundation,* 10.

5. Ibid.

6. Interview with "Dr. Marcus Victor" (Session #1, Jan. 9, 1991), conducted by Susan Resnik, 4.

7. The poem, given here in its entirety, is contained in Herbert Russalem, "Memorandum on the Greystone Conference," The National Hemophilia Foundation, Aug. 26, 1969, 7, 8. I thank Mary Gooley for providing a copy of this memorandum from her files. The meeting was held at Greystone, an old mansion owned by Columbia University, and according to Mary Gooley "may be the most important ever held by the National Hemophilia Foundation" (interview, Session #1, Dec. 10, 1990, conducted by Susan Resnik, 35).

Medical Summary

Dr. Brinkhous reviewed the Medical Scene,
Predicts progress and, friends, that's not drinkmanship.
He thinks advances will come but very slowly
Please take his word, 'cause that's not Ken's Brinkmanship.

Chapters and Staff all tend to agree.
For once all factions mesh their gears.
If they do, hallelujah! Well on our way,
Offering a program of Blood, Sweat, & Tears.

A stronger supply of human blood,
Plus medical research with national dough.
Educate M.D.'s and the chapter members,
And take steps to make costs reasonably low.

To implement these and others too
And to make it produce all it ought,
This is the charge that our chapters make
To our own Doctors Gilbert and "Victor."

A concern of the chapters, so they say,
In working with doctors, even those with honors,
Is to find ways and means of coping with
The vagaries of medical prima donnas.

A solution suggested to deal with this case
Is have one or two become chapter leaders.
The problem is that we depend upon them
While, alas, these men practically never need us.

Should our medical people construct for us
Medical standards for local groups?
Our participants say yes to this, indeed,
And to bring up standards, help them out with national troops.

When we send to the locals these national teams
To help the chapters at the local roots,

Add to the team some good physicians
And we'll all get substantial fruits.

Without engineers, let's all build bridges
Between national and local medical boards.
Through meeting together they'll have integration
And become tied together with umbilical cords.

Let national set up minimum programs,
Have chapters self-study where they are,
And if chapter boards find they're falling short,
They can ask national teams to bring them to par.

Centers or not, that is the question,
They're needed for rurals, but less in a city
If a center you have, be careful that
Community interest doesn't flag an itty-bitty.

Diagnostic centers are badly needed,
With behavioral sciences taking part,
But to the national staff, we have a message:
Doctors and Behaviorals be nice to each other and have a heart.

With concentrates still in short supply
Who should receive the best we have got?
The national staff should study this problem,
Even though the issue is definitely hot.

So this is our charge to our medical advisors.
We know our physicians are the best, nothing else.
Please do not mind us, "Victor" and Gilbert,
When from time to time we take your pulse

8. Goodwin, *Remembering America*, 9.

9. Interview with Mary Gooley (Session #2, May 10, 1991), conducted by Susan Resnik, 85.

10. Russalem, "Memorandum on the Greystone Conference," 5. The memo summarized the various committee reports, including the report from the Legislation Committee.

11. P. Starr, *The Social Transformation of American Medicine*, 381.

12. Jonas, *Health Care Delivery in the United States*, 106.

13. Nixon's "Health Message to the Congress on February 15, 1971" is quoted in Department of Health, Education, and Welfare (HEW), *Report of the President's Committee on Health Education*, 2.

14. HEW, *Report of the President's Committee on Health Education*, 13, 28, 31, 24, 11.

15. Ibid., 19.

16. National Institutes of Health (NIH), *Pilot Study* (citations to roman numbered pages refer to the general introduction of the *NHLI's Blood Resource Studies*, of which the *Pilot Study* is volume 3), ix.

17. Ibid., iii, 88, 44, 50, 56, 106. See note 2 to Chapter 1.

18. Ibid., 193–98, quote on 195.

19. Ibid., 83–92.

20. Ibid., 121, 114, 181.

21. Friedson, *Professional Dominance*, 108. This pattern conforms to Talcott Parson's "theory of technical competence," on which Friedson draws in his discussion of the sources of power and authority among the medical profession. Friedson suggests that professional dominance occurs when professionals do not view the client as a responsible adult person.

22. NIH, *Pilot Study*, 68.

23. Ibid., 141, 150.

24. Ibid., 24.

25. Interview with Oscar Ratnoff, M.D. (Nov. 5, 1991), conducted by Susan Resnik, 13, 12, 5, 36.

26. Ibid., 35, 18, 10.

27. NIH, *Pilot Study*, 160, 161, 156, 235.

28. Smith, *History of the National Hemophilia Foundation*, 16, 25.

29. Ibid., 26.

30. Ibid., 25, 14.

31. American Diabetes Association, *The Journey and the Dream*, 164, 166, 148.

32. Ibid., 148.

33. Interview with Peter H. Levine, M.D. (Dec. 6, 1990), conducted by Susan Resnik, 9.

34. Ibid., 7, 8, 10.

35. Ibid., 7.

36. Ibid.

37. *Fact Sheet* (National Hemophilia Foundation, December 1981), 1. The Omnibus Reconciliation Act of 1981 cites the report of the House Committee on the Budget to accompany H.R. 3982 (Washington, D.C.: U.S. Government Printing Office, 1981, 69): "The Committee notes that hemophilia is one of the biomedical and medical success stories of the decade."

Chapter 6

1. Smith, *History of the National Hemophilia Foundation*, 21, 22.

2. Ibid., 29.

3. Ibid., 30, 31.

4. "Marcus Victor," M.D., telephone conversation with Susan Resnik, July 24, 1994. In this conversation "Dr. Victor" provided commentary and clarification regarding his perception of what he did and why he did it, to augment the statement in Nathan Smith's *A History of the National Hemophilia Foundation* about balancing manufacturers.

5. Smith, *History of the National Hemophilia Foundation*, 31.

6. Ibid.

7. Interview with Mary Gooley (Session #1, Dec. 10, 1990); conducted by Susan Resnik, 62, 63.

8. Interview with "Cliff H." (Charles Carman; Sept. 12, 1990), conducted by Susan Resnik, 40.

9. American Diabetes Association (ADA), *The Journey and the Dream,* 164.

10. Interview with Mary Gooley (Session # 2, May 10, 1991), conducted by Susan Resnik, 72.

11. Interview with "Adam H." (Session #1, Aug. 21, 1990), conducted by Susan Resnik, 60.

12. ADA, *The Journey and the Dream,* 51.

13. Interview with Marvin Gilbert, M.D. (Jan. 4, 1991), conducted by Susan Resnik, 15.

14. Interview with "Marcus Victor," M.D. (Session #1, Jan. 9, 1991), conducted by Susan Resnik, 8.

15. "Adam H." interview (Session #1), 8.

16. Interview with "Lloyd H." (Sept. 16, 1991), conducted by Susan Resnik,

17. Interview with "Daniel H." (Glenn Pierce, Ph.D., M.D.; Oct. 24, 1990), off-tape conducted by Susan Resnik, 21. The importance of being in control was expressed by most informants.

18. John Grupenhoff, "Memorandum to Bettijane Eisenpreiss, with respect to attached draft article concerning 'Passage of the Hemophilia Centers Legislation,'" 1. The "attached article" is one of eight included in Eisenpreiss, "Draft Report: Hemophilia Treatment Center History Project," 1987, prepared for the Maternal and Child Health Bureau, describing ten years of experience with the Hemophilia Program.

19. Ibid., 3, 1.

20. Gilbert interview, 18.

21. Grupenhoff, "Passage of the Hemophilia Centers Legislation," in Eisenpreiss, "Draft Report," 9.

22. ADA, *The Journey and the Dream,* 164.

23. Grupenhoff, "Passage of the Hemophilia Centers Legislation," in Eisenpreiss, "Draft Report," 41.

24. Ibid., 9.

25. Ibid., 8.

26. Ibid., 9.

27. Both Peter H. Levine, M.D. (interview conducted by Susan Resnik, Dec. 6, 1990) and Craig Kessler, M.D. (interview conducted by Susan Resnik, Oct. 14, 1991) emphasized the importance of MCH and its directors and staff. Levine said in an off-tape conversation that the Golden Era had really begun in the Maternal and Child Years.

28. Henry T. Ireys and Merle McPherson, "Perspectives on the Hemophilia Treatment Center Program: Looking Toward Future Care for Chronically Ill Children," in Eisenpreiss, "Draft Report," 4–6.

29. "Victor" interview (Session #1), 11.

30. Gooley interview (Session #2), 62.

31. Levine interview, 19.

32. P. Starr, *The Social Transformation of American Medicine*, 405.

33. Levine interview, 19–20.

34. Ibid.

35. "Brett H.," in an early conversation (field notes, Jan 3. 1988), introduced Dr. Ratnoff's name and described him as both "a voice in the wilderness" and a "Cassandra."

36. Friedson, *Professional Dominance*, 19.

37. P. Starr, *The Social Transformation of American Medicine*, 389.

38. "Brett H.," field notes, Jan 3, 1988.

39. Maternal and Child Health Bureau, "Report on the Conference on Hemophilia Care," 1.

40. Lewis and Sheps, *The Sick Citadel*, 12.

Chapter 7

1. Interview with "Kent H." (Oct. 4, 1991), conducted by Susan Resnik, 8, 15, 21.

2. Ibid., 42–45.

3. Interview with "Harold H." (Aug. 7, 1991), conducted by Susan Resnik, 10.

4. Ibid., 15–17, 22.

5. Ibid., 25, 62, 63.

6. Ibid., 65, 78, 95.

7. Interview with "James H." (Dana Kuhn; Sept. 19, 1991), conducted by Susan Resnik, 1–2, 10–11.

8. Interview with "Brett H." (Sept. 10, 1990), conducted by Susan Resnik, 3–5, 10.

9. Interview with "Eugene H." (Oct. 26, 1990), conducted by Susan Resnik, 1–5.

10. Ibid., 6.

11. "Brett H.," 1990 telephone conversation with Susan Resnik, field notes.

12. Interview with "Adam H." (Session #1, Aug. 21, 1990), conducted by Susan Resnik, 75, 78, 87. The doctor "Adam" challenged in the meeting, "Marcus Victor," offers a different retrospective recollection of his approach to solving these problems, claiming that he regularly presented issues to the board and gained their full support. Other physicians queried were noncommittal.

13. Interview with "Cliff H." (Charles Carman; Sept. 12, 1990), conducted by Susan Resnik, 13–14, 18.

14. Smith, *History of the National Hemophilia Foundation*, 39, 42.

15. Ibid., 43, 46.

16. Interview with Barbara Chang (Oct. 26, 1990), conducted by Susan Resnik, 2–3.

17. Interview with Peter H. Levine, M.D. (Dec. 6, 1990), conducted by Susan Resnik, 19.

18. "Adam H." interview (Session #1), 89, 91. "Adam" used the phrase "create a culture" in an untaped portion of the conversation.

19. Ibid., 96–98.

20. Interview with G. William Bissell (Aug. 6, 1990), conducted by Susan Resnik,, 2, 3, 13.

21. Ibid., 26–27.

22. Ibid., 42, 45, 41.

23. G. William Bissell to Mr. M., Apr. 24, 1979; this letter is now in my collection.

24. Bissell interview, 47, 23.

25. Ibid., 12, 49, 47.

26. "Cliff H." interview, 28, 29.

27. Ibid., 30–32.

28. Bissell interview, 29, 30.

29. "Cliff H." interview, 32, 36, 33.

30. Ibid., 33.

31. Interview with Maribel Clements, R.N. (Dec. 16, 1990), conducted by Susan Resnik, 2, 23, 24, 13, 3.

32. Interview with Regina Butler, R.N. (Dec. 19, 1990), conducted by Susan Resnik, 3, 5, 6.

33. Ibid., 10, 49.

34. Interview with Karen Meredith, R.N. (Jan. 15, 1991), conducted by Susan Resnik 3, 5, 18, 26, 35.

35. Peter S. Smith and Peter H. Levine, "Health and Economic Outcomes," in Eisenpreiss, "Draft Report."

36. "Paul Phillips" and Merle McPherson, "Regionalization," in Eisenpreiss, "Draft Report," 1.

37. Several physicians mentioned similar successes in their interviews. These statements come from Frederick Rickles (interview, Dec. 5, 1990, conducted by Susan Resnik, 19) and Richard Lipton (interview, Apr. 25. 1991, conducted by Susan Resnik, 50).

38. Lipton interview, 43.

39. In his interview "Cliff H." alluded to this in an untaped portion of the conversation.

40. Shilts, "HIV's Startling Spread among Hemophiliacs."

Chapter 8

1. Rehr and Rosenberg, *The Changing Context of Social Health Care*, 100.

2. Interview with Bruce Evatt (June 7, 1991), conducted by Susan Resnik, 11.

3. Interview with "Paul Phillips" (Oct. 29, 1990), conducted by Susan Resnik, 20.

4. "My center" and "my patients" are terms frequently used by many of the treaters in interviews.

5. "Paul Phillips" and Merle McPherson, "Regionalization," in Eisenpreiss, "Draft Report," 1, 2. Regionalization is a proven method of conserving scarce resources, controlling costs, and improving the accessibility and quality of services; from the beginning, the system of primary hemophilia treatment centers with affiliates recognized the importance of some kind of regional grouping. In 1980 medical directors who were on the MCH Ad Hoc Advisory Committee gave formal commitment to regionalization and appropriate linkages to state agencies as critical to the survival of the comprehensive care concept.

6. Interview with Oscar Ratnoff, M.D. (Nov. 5, 1991), conducted by Susan Resnik, 11.

7. Interview with "Adam H." (Session #1, Aug. 21, 1990), conducted by Susan Resnik, 92.

8. Shilts, *And the Band Played On,* 19. "Before" means before AIDS, in Shilts's terminology describing the effect of the AIDS epidemic on the gay community. Shilts speaks of the AIDS epidemic "cleaving lives in two; before and after," likening it to the way a great war or depression presents a commonly understood point of reference around which an entire society defines itself.

9. Bayer, *Private Acts, Social Consequences,* 5. Bayer discusses the complexity of the issues and the conflicts surrounding the gay community's sense of their "right to privacy" against the public's need for protection from a spreading epidemic, AIDS.

10. Newton, *Cherry Grove, Fire Island,* 186–87. Newton, an anthropologist, describes the history of Cherry Grove, "the oldest gay and lesbian town in America," as remembered by its inhabitants, her informants. They depict a unique community, away from the mainland where they could live the American dream. She describes an area frequented by gay men called "The Rack" as similar to the gay baths: "sexuality stripped of social condition which can foster communitas, the diffuse but powerful feeling of group solidarity transcending the usual social divides." In *AIDS in the Mind of America,* Dennis Altman states that "for many of us a certain sexual style was inextricably intertwined with being gay: 'for gay men, sex, that most powerful implement of attachment and arousal, is also an agent of communion, replacing an often hostile family and even shaping politics'" (7).

11. Shilts, *And the Band Played On,* 13, 19, 14, 15.

12. Ibid., xxii.

13. Ibid., 68; Relman, "AIDS: The Emerging Ethical Dilemmas," 1.

14. Relman, "AIDS," 1.

15. Altman, *AIDS in the Mind of America,* 16.

16. Ibid., 17.

17. Ibid., 21, 33, 13.

18. Ibid., 13.

19. Ibid., 33–35.

20. Krim, "AIDS: The Challenge to Science and Medicine," 3.

21. "Phillips" interview, 7–8.

22. Evatt interview, 9, 4.

23. Ibid., 5–6.

24. Ibid.

25. Interview with Dale Lawrence, M.D. (Oct. 11, 1991), conducted by Susan Resnik, 7. Lawrence noted that he "was very much interested in population genetics, because that's part of our human heredity, and ethnicities and the control of immune responses that may differ between populations and markers for that." He added that he had expected to continue doing research in this area when he received a call concerning "an outbreak of pneumocystis carinii pneumonia in a gay population in two cities." In the ensuing months, it appeared that this was a bigger epidemic than anticipated. Then he was called by Bruce Evatt and informed about a hemophilia case (10).

26. Ibid., 10, 18.

27. Ibid., 11, 12.

28. Ibid., 12, 15, 16.

29. Ibid., 23, 24.

30. Ibid., 38, 39, 36.

31. Evatt interview, 9.

32. Interview with "Marcus Victor, M.D." (Session #2, Feb 12, 1991), conducted by Susan Resnik, 4.

33. "Pneumocystis Carinii Pneumonia Among Persons with Hemophilia A," *Morbidity and Mortality Weekly Report* (*MMWR*), July 16, 1982, 13, 14.

34. Evatt interview, 8.

35. "Victor" interview (Session #2), 4.

36. Camus, *The Plague,* 34, 40, 36, 37.

37. Evatt interview, 11–13. In this section of the interview, Evatt noted that "There was a sense of arrogance on the part of some of the physicians towards the young hotshots from the CDC," and that "The trends were very vivid to us and we knew it was going to be a matter of time."

38. Dale Lawrence, telephone conversation with Susan Resnik, Sept. 9, 1997. Lawrence said that MASAC was the first audience of non-CDC staff to hear him present his idea that the incubation period for AIDS was several times longer than any case had yet demonstrated or any case they then "knew"; Evatt had told him that the hemophilia community must hear this.

39. Interview with Regina Butler, R.N. (Dec. 19, 1990), conducted by Susan Resnik, 26; the last remark was made in an untaped portion of the conversation.

40. Ibid., 18, 21, 25.

41. Ibid., 20, 27, 29, 32.

42. Interview with "Adam H." (Session #2, Oct. 3, 1991), conducted by Susan Resnik, 2, 7.

43. "Brett H." made this statement in an untaped portion of his interview (Sept. 10, 1990; conducted by Susan Resnik).

44. *NHF Narrative Chronology* (NHF, Dec. 1992).

45. "Update on Acquired Immune Deficiency Syndrome (AIDS) Among Patients with Hemophilia," *MMWR,* Dec. 10, 1982, 644–48.

Chapter 9

1. *Morbidity and Mortality Weekly Report*, Dec. 10, 1982, 652; quoted in a combined NHF Medical Bulletin #4, Chapter Advisory #5, Dec. 21, 1982.

2. Combined NHF Medical Bulletin #4, Chapter Advisory #5, Dec. 21, 1982; emphasis in original.

3. Interview with Bruce Evatt, M.D. (June 7, 1991), conducted by Susan Resnik, 10.

4. Shilts, *And the Band Played On*, 220.

5. Ibid., 221.

6. Evatts interview, 10.

7. Shilts, *And the Band Played On*, 221.

8. *Recommendations to Prevent AIDS in Patients with Hemophilia*, The National Hemophilia Foundation Medical and Scientific Advisory Council, Jan. 14, 1983.

9. "Medical Bulletin #5," "Chapter Advisory #6," *Hemophilia Newsnotes*, NHF, Jan. 17, 1983.

10. Interview with "Paul Phillips" (Oct. 29, 1990), conducted by Susan Resnik, 65. In a faxed memo to me dated June 1, 1998, "Phillips" noted that during the early 1980s he maintained a close working relation with Rodger Mac-Farlane, the founding director of The Gay Men's Health Crisis (GMHC): "MacFarlane counseled me and assisted NHF in addressing these difficult issues while maintaining the public health primacy of the blood donor screening issue. At the national level NHF also maintained an ongoing relationship with the gay physicians group American Association of Physicians for Human Rights (AAPHR) and was an active member of the AIDS Action Council" (2).

11. Interview with "Adam H." (Session #2, Oct. 3, 1991), conducted by Susan Resnik, 23.

12. Ibid.

13. Ibid.

14. As happens in many organizational situations, "Victor's" resignation was brought about as a result of pressure from the NHF Executive Committee. A special meeting of the Executive Committee was held via telephone conference call on April 16, 1983. Nathan Smith convened this meeting to discuss his desire to replace "Victor" as medical co-director. Smith visited "Victor" the next day to seek his resignation. Smith had requested and received the committee's informal approval, since he did not need formal approval to take this action. The minutes of the telephone meeting of the Executive Committee are available through the NHF HANDI clearinghouse.

15. "Adam H." interview (Session #2), 23.

16. Ibid.

17. "Eugene H." made this comment in an untaped portion of the conversation in the interview conducted by Susan Resnik, Oct. 26, 1990.

18. "Adam H." interview (Session #2), 52.

19. Interview with Oscar Ratnoff, M.D. (Nov. 5, 1991), conducted by Susan Resnik, 16, 32.

20. "Eugene H." interview, 27.

21. Interview with "Irwin H." (Richard Johnson; Sept. 5, 1991.), conducted by Susan Resnik, 43, 44.

22. Ibid., 45.

23. Interview with "Daniel H." (Glenn Pierce, Ph.D., M.D.; Oct. 24, 1990), conducted by Susan Resnik, 14, 15, 19.

24. Interview with "Gregory H." (July 24, 1991), conducted by Susan Resnik, 97.

25. Interview with Shelby Dietrich, M.D. (Oct. 26, 1990), conducted by Susan Resnik, 33

26. Interview with Frederick Rickles, M.D. (Dec. 5, 1990), conducted by Susan Resnik, 33.

27. Ibid., 19–26.

28. Dietrich interview, 24, 25.

29. Interview with Craig Kessler, M.D. (Oct. 14, 1991), conducted by Susan Resnik, 43.

30. Interview with David Agle, M.D. (Sept. 12, 1990), conducted by Susan Resnik, 13.

31. Evatt interview, 25.

Chapter 10

1. Interview with "Lloyd H." (Sept. 16, 1991), conducted by Susan Resnik, 22–23.

2. Interview with "Irwin H." (Richard Johnson; Sept. 5, 1991), conducted by Susan Resnik, 44. As quoted in Chapter 9, "Irwin" stated that he "was never . . . told that I had an option" (45).

3. Interview with Richard Lipton, M.D. (Apr. 25, 1991), conducted by Susan Resnik, 47, 52, 49.

4. Interview with "Mindy H." (Nov. 29, 1990), conducted by Susan Resnik, 4.

5. Interview with "Diane H." (Bea Pierce; Oct. 24, 1990), conducted by Susan Resnik, 15.

6. Interview with Sharon Barrett (Jan. 15, 1991), conducted by Susan Resnik, 18.

7. Ibid., 19. Barrett uses the term "medical model" here as it is commonly used in conversations among many members of the hemophilia community.

8. Koop, *Koop,* 227. See also White and Cunningham, *Ryan White.*

9. "Paul Philips," faxed memo to Susan Resnik, June 1, 1998, 3.

10. In a telephone conversation on Sept. 30, 1997, "Paul Phillips" remarked that there was a split within the NHF at the time. Leadership tried to penetrate the denial but was frustrated.

11. Resnik, "Field Notes." This statement was in response to a question asking for a description of "the team." The 1989 study replicated the ethnography undertaken in the same hemophilia treatment center during the summer of 1983 (see Appendix B) and sought to observe differences in team structure and team leadership between the two periods.

12. In a conversation on Sept. 25, 1997, "Paul Phillips" called the demand for materials a form of success, because in reaching out to the NRCC the community was beginning to break through its denial.

13. Interview with J. William Flynt, M.D. (Jan. 16, 1991), conducted by Susan Resnik, 2.

14. Ibid., 4.

15. Ibid., 8. Flynt also remarked that AIDS had changed the hemophilia community by "showing some of the weaknesses of the medical model . . . [where] physicians say: 'Okay, I want to be in control of everything. I want to make all decisions.'" This could not continue when "you have so many different people that need to be involved, including other interests in addition to hemophilia." He also noted that because dealing with AIDS necessitated "behavior change" and "the person you're changing has to be part of the process . . . it's not enough to be didactic" (13).

16. Koop, *Koop*, 207.

17. Ibid.

18. Ibid.

19. Resnik, "Field Notes."

Chapter 11

1. Quoted in Navarro, *The Politics of Health Care Policy*, 99.

2. Epstein, *Impure Science*, 1, 221.

3. Ibid., 288.

4. Ibid., 206.

5. Davidson, "Strange Blood," 1.

6. "Paul Phillips," faxed memo to Susan Resnik, June 1, 1998, 4.

7. Interview with Glenn Pierce, Ph.D., M.D. ("Daniel H."; May 1, 1997), conducted by Susan Resnik, 13.

8. "Phillips" memo, June 1, 1998, 5.

9. Epstein, *Impure Science*, 290. "Paul Phillips," Glenn Pierce, and "Adam H." assert that it was actually the NHF that launched a campaign, forming the NHF/NIAID/AIDS Clinical Trials Working Group that met with officials at NIAID "in face-to-face confrontation as they sought to exclude people with hemophilia because of their liver enzyme levels." "Phillips" recalls, "We also secured bill report language directing NIAID to include hemophilia patients. The concrete result was to open up the trials and to create a special hemophilia section of the AIDs clinical trial group within NIAID to insure that all people with hemophilia were included" ("Phillips" memo, June 1, 1998, 5). Pierce notes that Wadleigh's contributions took place following this groundwork (telephone conversation, June 2, 1998).

10. National Hemophilia Foundation, *Annual Report*, 1989, 2.

11. Ibid.

12. Interview with Bruce Evatt, M.D. (Aug. 26, 1997), conducted by Susan Resnik, 5.

13. Interview with Richard Johnson ("Irwin H."; Aug. 28, 1997), conducted by Susan Resnik, 8.

14. Interview with Bea Pierce ("Diane H."; Apr. 14, 1997), conducted by Susan Resnik, 7, 4.

15. Ibid.

16. Linda Smith, telephone conversation with Susan Resnik, Aug. 28, 1997.

17. Cathy McAdam, telephone conversation with Susan Resnik, Aug. 27, 1997.

18. B. Pierce interview, 4.

19. Dale Lawrence, M.D., telephone conversation with Susan Resnik, Sept. 1, 1997.

20. This list, gathered by Bea Pierce and Cathy McAdam, was included in a paper entitled "A Hemophilia Community Model for the Prevention of Heterosexual and Perinatal Transmission of HIV," which I presented in the Maternal and Child Health Session at the annual meeting of the American Public Health Association, Oct. 23, 1989.

21. Interview with Kathy Gerus (Aug. 27, 1997), conducted by Susan Resnik, 28, 30.

22. Interview with Val Bias (July 15, 1997), conducted by Susan Resnik, 55.

23. National Hemophilia Foundation, *Annual Report,* 1990, 4.

24. G. Pierce interview, 2.

25. Verma, "Gene Therapy," 68.

26. Interview with Frederick Rickles, M.D. (May 26, 1997), conducted by Susan Resnik, 35.

27. Schwartz et al., "Human Recombinant DNA-Derived Antihemophilic Factor," 1800.

28. Interview with Laureen Kelley (May 16, 1997), conducted by Susan Resnik, 9, 10.

29. Ibid., 14.

Chapter 12

1. Navarro, *The Politics of Health Care Policy,* 205.

2. Browning, "Proposals to Reform the U.S. Health Care System," 223.

3. Blumenthal, "Sounding Board," 465–66.

4. Richard Lipton, M.D., telephone conversation with Susan Resnik, Aug. 25, 1997.

5. *Echo Magazine* 15, 6 (Nov.–Dec. 1994): 7, 6. *Echo* is published by Cutter Biodivision of Cutter Laboratories, Inc., to provide education and communication "for hemophiliacs and others."

6. Interview with Shelby Dietrich, M.D. (June 16, 1997), conducted by Susan Resnik, 22, 23

7. "HIV Financial Assistance Schemes in WFH Member Countries," information sheet from World Federation of Hemophilia, Montreal, Canada, April 2, 1996.

8. "NHF Will Seek Special Assistance for People with Hemophilia and HIV/AIDS," *Hemophilia Newsnotes,* Feb. 1993, 1.

9. "Paul Phillips," telephone conversation with Susan Resnik, Sept. 30, 1997. "Phillips" reminded me that there was, in fact, a struggle by then between himself and some supporters and the chapters, as he sought to "raise the organization's profile" in dealing with HIV. Also, he recalled the "wartime mentality," where the NHF staff and many professional volunteers worked around the clock to ameliorate the AIDS situation by fighting for funding and providing information and support as best as they could.

10. M. Rosenberg, "The Time for Business as Usual Has Passed," 7.

11. Interview with Val Bias (July 15, 1997), conducted by Susan Resnik, 57.

12. "New NHF Leadership Elected at Annual Meeting," *Hemophilia Newsnotes*, Feb. 1995, 8.

13. Ibid., 6, 3.

14. Ibid., 7.

15. Dana Kuhn, in a telephone conversation, Sept. 10, 1997, noted that he had compiled "The Trail of AIDS," which contained chronologically arranged documents and notes that served to inform a wide variety of audiences, including the Institute of Medicine (IOM) Committee at a later date.

16. Wadleigh's comments are in *The Common Factor*, April 1992.

17. "Paul Phillips," faxed memo to Susan Resnik, June 1, 1998, 4.

18. Interview with Glenn Pierce, Ph.D., M.D. ("Daniel H.", May 1, 1997), conducted by Susan Resnik, 37, 11.

19. *The Common Factor*, April 1992.

20. M. Rosenberg, "The Time for Business as Usual Has Passed."

21. *The Common Factor*, April 1992.

22. G. Pierce interview, 41.

23. "Gene Therapy for Hemophilia," Workshop Agenda, Bethesda, Md., NHLBI, March 18–19, 1992; NHF press release, contact Alan Ampolsk.

24. G. Pierce interview, 51–53, 56.

25. Ibid., 66.

26. "Blood, Money, and AIDS: Hemophiliacs Are Split," *New York Times*, June 11, 1996, D1.

27. "Blood Money," *San Francisco Examiner*, June 8, 1997, 1.

28. Leveton, Sox, and Stoto, eds., *HIV and the Blood Supply*, v.

29. Ibid., v, 218–30.

30. Ibid., 231, 233.

31. "Paul Phillips," *Community Alert* 1, 1, March 1994.

32. According to Kevin C. Kelley, "The first clinical trials for a cure for hemophilia could actually start in 1998—pending approval by the FDA. Transkaryotic Therapies, Inc., a Cambridge, Massachusetts–based company, has filed for permission to begin gene therapy on humans" ("Which Gene Therapy Will Your Child Use?" *Parent Exchange Newsletter* 8, 1 [Feb. 1998]: 9).

33. Michael Soucie, "Memo: Information on Blood Safety," CDC Information, 2–4.

34. Dietrich interview, 47.

Chapter 13

1. Pellegrino, "The Metamorphoses of Medical Ethics," 1158–59.
2. Ibid., 1159–60.
3. Drucker, "The Global Economy and the Nation State," 167–68.
4. This concept is discussed in Huntington, "The Erosion of American National Interests," 37.

Bibliography

Altman, Dennis. *AIDS in the Mind of America: The Social, Political, and Economic Impact of a New Epidemic.* Garden City, N.Y.: Doubleday, 1986.

American Blood Resources Association. *Coagulation Concentrates: A 1988 Status Report.* Annapolis, Md.: American Blood Resources Association, 1988.

American Diabetes Association. *The Journey and the Dream: A History of the American Diabetes Association, 1940–1990.* n.p., American Diabetes Association, Inc., 1990.

Arensberg, Conrad, and Solon T. Kimball. *Culture and Community.* New York: Harcourt, Brace, and World, 1965.

Babbie, Earl. *The Practice of Social Research.* Belmont, Calif.: Wadsworth, 1983.

Bayer, Ronald. *Private Acts, Social Consequences: AIDS and the Politics of Public Health.* New York: Free Press, 1989.

Bloch, Marc. *The Historian's Craft.* New York: Knopf, 1953.

Blood Policy and Technology. Washington, D.C.: U.S. Congress, Office of Technology Assessment, OTA-H-260, January 1985.

Blumenthal, David. "Medicare: The Beginning." In *Renewing the Promise: Medicare and Its Reform,* ed. David Blumenthal, Mark Schlesinger, and Pamela Brown Drumheller. New York: Oxford University Press, 1988.

———. "Sounding Board: Health Care Reform—Past and Future." *New England Journal of Medicine* 332, 7 (Feb. 16, 1995): 465–67.

Brandt, Allan M. "AIDS in Historical Perspective: Four Lessons from the History of Sexually Transmitted Diseases." *American Journal of Public Health* 78, 4 (Apr. 1988): 367–71.

Brinkhous, K. M. "A Short History of Hemophilia, with Some Comments on the Word 'Hemophilia.'" In *Handbook of Hemophilia.* New York: American Elsevier, 1975, 3.

Browning, Susan. "Proposals to Reform the U.S. Health Care System: A Critical Review." In *North American Health Care Policy in the 1990s*, ed. Arthur King, Thomas Hyclak, and Robert Thornton. Chichester, Eng.: John Wiley and Sons, 1993.

Camus, Albert. *The Plague*. New York: Vintage Books, 1972.

"Counterpoint: The COTT Caveat." *The Parent Exchange Newsletter* 5, 1 (Apr. 1995).

Davidson, Michael. "Strange Blood: Hemophobia and the Unexplored Boundaries of Queer Nation." In *Beyond the Binary: American Identity and Multiculturalism*, ed. Timothy Powell. New Brunswick, N.J.: Rutgers University Press, 1998.

De Neffe, Larkey Sheldon. "Sharing the Pulse: A History of Blood Transfusion." Research paper, 1985.

Department of Health, Education, and Welfare, Health Services and Mental Health Administration. *The Report of the President's Committee on Health Education*. New York, 1972.

De Prince, Elaine. *Cry Bloody Murder: A Tale of Tainted Blood*. New York: Random House, 1997.

Deutsch, Patricia, and Ron Deutsch. "Dr. Thelin's Fight Against Hemophilia." *Readers Digest,* Aug. 1967, 90–94.

Dietrich, Shelby. *Hemophilia: A Total Approach to Treatment and Rehabilitation*. Los Angeles: Los Angeles Orthopaedic Hospital, 1968.

Dollard, John. *Criteria for Life History*. New Haven: Yale University Press, 1935.

Dolnick, Edward. "Deafness as a Culture." *Atlantic Monthly,* Sept. 1993, 37–53.

Drucker, Peter F. "The Global Economy and the Nation State." *Foreign Affairs: 75th Anniversary, the World Ahead* 76, 5 (Sept.–Oct. 1997): 167–69.

Dunaway, David K., and Willa K. Baum, eds. *Oral History: An Interdisciplinary Anthology*. Nashville, Tenn: American Association for State and Local History, in cooperation with the Oral History Association, 1987.

Dunn, Linda. "Pearls, Pith, and Provocation: Research Alert! Qualitative Research May Be Hazardous to Your Health!" *Qualitative Research* 1, 3 (Aug. 1991): 338–92.

Dutton, Diana B. *Worse Than the Disease: The Pitfalls of Medical Progress*. New York: Cambridge University Press, 1992.

Eisenpreiss, Bettijane, ed. "Draft Report: Hemophilia Treatment Center History Project." Manuscript. Rockville, Md.: Maternal and Child Health Bureau, 1987.

Epstein, Steven. *Impure Science: AIDS, Activism, and the Politics of Knowledge*. Berkeley: University of California Press, 1996.

Fox, Renee C., and Judith P. Swazey. *The Courage to Fail*. Chicago: University of Chicago Press, 1978.

Friedson, Elliot. *Professional Dominance: The Social Structure of Medical Care*. New York: Atherton Press, 1970.

Gaffney, John C., Susan Browning, and Edward B. Hirschfeld. "Forces for Reforming the U.S. Health Care System: A Review of the Cost and Access

Issues." In *North American Health Care Policy in the 1990s*, ed. Arthur King, Thomas Hyclak, and Robert Thornton. Chichester, Eng.: John Wiley and Sons, 1993.

Glaser, Barney G., and Anselm L. Strauss. *The Discovery of Grounded Theory: Strategies for Qualitative Research*. New York: Aldine, 1967.

"Glossary." In Leveton, Lauren B., Harold C. Sox, Jr., and Michael A. Stoto, eds. *HIV and the Blood Supply: An Analysis of Crisis Decision Making*.

Goodwin, Richard N. *Remembering America: A Voice from the Sixties*. Boston: Little, Brown, 1988.

The Hemophilia Patient/Family Model. New York: National Hemophilia Foundation, 1981.

Hoffman, Alice M., and Howard S. Hoffman. *Archives of Memory: A Soldier Recalls World War II*. Lexington: University Press of Kentucky, 1990.

Huntington, Samuel P. "The Erosion of American National Interests." *Foreign Affairs: 75th Anniversary, the World Ahead* 76, 5 (Sept.–Oct. 1997): 28–49.

Ingram, G. I. C. "The History of Haemophilia." *Journal of Clinical Pathology* 29, 6 (June 1976): 3.

"Interview with Robert Lee Henry." *Hemophila Newsnotes*, Winter 1986–87.

Ives, Edward D. *The Tape-Recorded Interview*. Knoxville: University of Tennessee Press, 1974.

James, Richard D. "Hope for Bleeders: End to Hemophilia Peril May Become Possible with New Preparations." *Wall Street Journal*, Mar. 26, 1968.

Jensen, Donald, M.D. *Understanding Hepatitis: A Glossary of Terms*. Thousand Oaks, Calif.: Amgen Pharmaceutical Co., 1996.

Jonas, Steven, M.D., with contributors. *Health Care Delivery in the United States*. New York: Springer, 1981.

Kaufman, Sharon R. *The Ageless Self: Sources of Meaning in Late Life*. Madison: University of Wisconsin Press, 1986.

Kelley, Laureen. *Raising a Child with Hemophilia*. © Laureen A. Kelley, Georgetown, Mass., 1993.

Kirk, Jerome, and Marc L. Miller. *Reliability and Validity in Qualitative Research*. Beverly Hills, Calif: Sage Publications, Inc., 1986

Koop, C. Everett. *Koop: The Memoirs of America's Family Doctor*. New York: Random House, 1991.

Krim, Mathilde. "AIDS: The Challenge to Science and Medicine." In Carol Levine and Joyce Bermel, eds., *Hastings Center Report Special Supplement*.

Lane, Harlan. *When the Mind Hears: A History of the Deaf*. New York: Random House, 1984.

Langness, L. L., and Frank Gelya. *Lives: An Anthropological Approach to Biography*. Novato, Calif.: Chandler and Sharp, 1981.

Lederman, Ben. "Yesterday, Today, and Tomorrow." *Hemophilia Newsnotes* (National Hemophilia Foundation). Fall 1982–Winter 1983, 5.

———. "Yesterday, Today, and Tomorrow." *Hemophilia Newsnotes* (National Hemophilia Foundation). Summer 1984, 4.

Leveton, Lauren B., Harold C. Sox, Jr., and Michael A. Stoto, eds. *HIV and the Blood Supply: An Analysis of Crisis Decision Making*. Report of the IOM Committee to Study HIV Transmission through Blood and Blood Products, Division of Health Promotion and Disease Prevention, Institute of Medicine. Washington, D.C.: National Academy Press, 1995.

Levine, Carol. "How Wartime Needs Changed Medicine." *The Hastings Center Report*. Dec. 1984, 3.

Levine, Carol, and Joyce Bermel, eds. *A Hastings Center Report Special Supplement*. Hastings on Hudson, N.Y.: Institute of Society, Ethics, and Life Sciences, 1985.

Levine, Peter H., and Anthony F. Britten. "Supervised Patient Management of Hemophilia: A Study of 45 Patients with Hemophilia A and B." *Annals of Internal Medicine* 78, 2 (Feb. 1973): 195–201.

Lewis, Irving J., and Cecil G. Sheps. *The Sick Citadel: The American Academic Medical Center and the Public Interest*. Cambridge, Mass.: Oehlschlager, Gunn, and Hain, 1983.

Lindenbaum, Shirley. *Kuru Sorcery: Disease and Danger in the New Guinea Highlands*. Palo Alto, Calif.: Mayfield, 1979.

Littell, Robert. "Bearer Is a Hemophiliac." *Readers Digest* 74 (Apr. 1959): 214–18.

Lusher, J. M., and C. M. Kessler. "Gene Therapy for Hemophilia." In *Hemophilia and von Willebrand's Disease in the 1990s: A New Decade of Hopes and Challenges*, ed. Lusher and Kessler. Proceedings of the Nineteenth Congress of the World Federation of Hemophilia. Elsevier Science Publishers, 1991.

Massie, Robert, and Suzanne Massie. *Journey*. New York: Warner Books, 1976.

Maternal and Child Health Bureau. "Report on the Conference on Hemophilia Care." La Jolla, Calif., Jan. 8–10, 1976.

Miller, Connie. *The Inheritance of Hemophilia*. New York: National Hemophilia Foundation, 1992.

Morse, Janice M. Editorial. *Qualitative Health Research* 1, 4 (Nov. 1991): 403–6.

National Hemophilia Foundation. *Glossary*. New York: National Hemophilia Foundation, n.d.

———. *The National Hemophilia Foundation Annual Report, 1989*. New York: National Hemophilia Foundation, 1989.

———. *The National Hemophilia Foundation Annual Report, 1990*. New York: National Hemophilia Foundation, 1990.

———. *What You Should Know About Hemophilia*. New York: National Hemophilia Foundation, 1991.

National Institutes of Health, Department of Health Education and Welfare. *Pilot Study of Hemophilia Treatment in the United States*. Vol. 3 of *NHLI's Blood Resources Studies*. Bethesda, Md.: NIH, June 30, 1972.

Navarro, Vincente. *The Politics of Health Care Policy: The U.S. Reforms, 1980–1994*. Cambridge, Mass: Blackwell, 1994.

Neustadt, Richard E., and Harvey V. Fineberg. *The Swine Flu Affair*. Washington, D.C.: U.S. Department of Health, Education, and Welfare, 1978.

Newton, Esther. *Cherry Grove, Fire Island: Sixty Years in America's First Gay and Lesbian Town*. Boston: Beacon Press, 1993.

"NHF Will Seek Special Assistance for People with Hemophilia and HIV/AIDS," *Hemophilia Newsnotes*, Feb. 1993, 1.

Orthopaedic Hospital. *Hemophilia and the Regional Center Concept: Final Report of RD-2522-M*. Los Angeles: Orthopaedic Hospital, 1971.

Patton, Michael Quinn. *Qualitative Evaluation Methods*. Beverly Hills, Calif: Sage, 1980.

Pearson, Maggie. "Book Review: Leprosy, Racism, and Public Health; Social Policy and Chronic Illness Control." *Medical Anthropology Quarterly* 4 (Dec. 1991): 404.

Pellegrino, Edmund. "The Metamorphosis of Medical Ethics: A 30-Year Retrospective." *Journal of the American Medical Association* 269, 9 (Mar. 3, 1993): 1158–62.

Pelto, Pertti J., and Gretel H. Pelto. *Anthropological Research: The Structure of Inquiry*. Cambridge, Eng.: Cambridge University Press, 1970.

Pemberton, Stephen Gregory. "Bleeder Dogs and the Framing of Hemophilia Management: From Dismal Prospects to Potent Medicine in the Laboratory of Kenneth Brinkhous, M.D., 1930–1960." Master's thesis. University of North Carolina at Chapel Hill, 1987.

"Pneumocystis Carinii Pneumonia among Persons with Hemophilia A." *Morbidity and Mortality Weekly Report* (Centers for Disease Control). July 16, 1982, 14.

Poirier, Richard. "AIDS and Homophobia." *Social Research*. Special issue: *In Time of Plague: The History and Social Consequences of Lethal Disease* 55, 3 (Autumn 1988): 461.

Potts, D. M., and W. T. W. Potts. *Queen Victoria's Gene: Hemophilia and the Royal Family*. Phoenix Mill, U.K.: Alan Sutton Publishing, 1995.

Preuss, Julius. *Biblical and Talmudic Medicine*. Trans. F. Rosner. New York: Sanhedrin Press, 1978.

Rabiner, S., and Jack Lazerson. "Home Management and Prophylaxis of Hemophilia." In vol. 3 of Elmer B. B. Brown, ed. *Progress in Hematology*. Grupe and Stratton.

Ragucci, Antoinette. "The Ethnographic Approach and Nursing Research." In *Health and Human Condition: Perspectives in Medical Anthropology*, ed. Michael H. Logan and Edward E. Hunt, Jr. North Scituate, Mass: Doubleday, 1978.

Redman, Eric. *The Dance of Legislation*. New York: Simon and Schuster, 1973.

Rehr, Helen, and Gary Rosenberg, eds. *The Changing Context of Social Health Care: Its Implications for Providers and Consumers*. New York: Haworth Press, 1991.

Relman, Arnold S. "AIDS: The Emerging Ethical Dilemmas." *Hastings Center Report, Special Supplement,* ed. Carol Levine and Joyce Bermel. Hastings on Hudson, N.Y.: Institute of Society, Ethics, and Life Sciences, 1985.

Resnik, Susan. "Field Notes: Fieldwork Experience Replicating Summer 1983 Experience in a Hemophilia Treatment Center." Unpublished manuscript, 1989.

————. "The Social History of Hemophilia in the United States (1948–1988): The Emergence and Empowerment of a Community." Dr.P.H. diss. Columbia University, Division of Health Policy and Management, School of Public Health, 1994.

Resnik, Susan, Ashaki Taha, and Peggy Heine. "A Hemophilia Community Model for the Prevention of Heterosexual and Perinatal Transmission of HIV," American Public Health Association Annual Meeting, October 23, 1989, Maternal and Child Health Sector, Session 1017.

Review of the Public Health Service's Response to AIDS: A Technical Memorandum. Washington, D.C.; U.S. Congress Office of Technology Assessment, Feb. 1985.

Rosen, George. *A History of Public Health.* New York: M.D. Publications, 1958.

Rosenberg, Charles E. *The Care of Strangers: The Rise of America's Hospital System.* New York: Basic Books, 1987.

————. "Disease in History: Frames and Framers." *The Milbank Quarterly* 67, supp. 1 (1989).

Rosenberg, Michael P. "The Time for Business as Usual Has Passed." *The Common Factor,* Apr. 1992, 7.

Rosner, Fred. *Medicine in the Bible and the Talmud,* rev. ed. New York: Yeshiva University Press, Ktav Publishing House, 1995.

Rothman, David, and Stanton Wheeler. *Social History and Social Policy.* New York: Academic Press, 1981.

Sachs, Oliver. *Seeing Voices: A Journey into the World of the Deaf.* Berkeley: University of California Press, 1989.

Scheiderman, Lawrence J. "Ethics in Clinical Practice." In *The Doctor-Patient Relationship,* SBS course syllabus, University of California San Diego Medical School.

Schwartz, Richard S. et al. (the Recombinant Factor VIII Study Group). "Human Recombinant DNA–Derived Antihemophilic Factor (Factor VIII) in the Treatment of Hemophilia." *New England Journal of Medicine* (Dec. 27, 1990): 1800–1805.

Shilts, Randy. *And the Band Played On.* New York: St. Martin's Press, 1987.

————. "HIV's Startling Spread among Hemophiliacs." *San Francisco Chronicle,* Dec. 5, 1989, A11.

Smith, Nathan. *A History of the National Hemophilia Foundation.* New York: National Hemophilia Foundation, 1984.

Sontag, Susan. *AIDS and Its Metaphors.* New York: Farrar Strauss and Giroux, 1989.

Spradley, James. *Participant Observation.* New York: Holt, Rinehart, and Winston, 1980.

Starr, Douglas. "Again and Again in World War II, Blood Made the Difference." *Smithsonian* 25, 12 (Mar. 1995): 125–38.

Starr, Paul. *The Social Transformation of American Medicine.* New York: Basic Books, 1982.

Stevens, Rosemary. *American Medicine and the Public Interest.* New Haven, Conn.: Yale University Press, 1971.

Thompson, Paul. *The Voice of the Past: Oral History.* New York: Oxford University Press, 1988.

Titmuss, Richard. *The Gift Relationship: From Human Blood to Social Policy.* New York: Vintage, 1972.

Tomes, Nancy. "Oral History in the History of Medicine." *Journal of American History* (Sept. 1991): 607–17.

Turner, Victor. *The Ritual Process: Structure and Anti-Structure.* Hawthorne, N.Y.: Aldine, 1982.

"Update on Acquired Immune Deficiency Syndrome (AIDS) among Patients with Hemophilia A." *Morbidity and Mortality Weekly Report* (Centers for Disease Control), Nov. 1982, 365–67, 577–80.

Vansina, Jan. *Tradition in Historical Methodology.* Trans. H. M. Wright. London: Routledge and Kegan Paul, 1965.

Verma, Inder. "Gene Therapy." *Scientific American.* Nov. 1990, 68–84.

Vils, Ursula, "Transfusion of Interest Aids War on Hemophilia," *Los Angeles Times,* Aug. 12, 1965, VI.

Watson, Lynne, Jeanette Irwin, and Sharon Michalske. "Pearls, Pith, and Provocation: Researcher as Friend: Methods of the Interviewer in a Longitudinal Study." *Qualitative Health Research* 1, 4 (Nov. 1994): 497–514.

White, Ryan, and Anne Marie Cunningham. *Ryan White: My Own Story.* New York: Penguin Books, 1992.

Index

Abildgaard, Charles, 4, 38, 40, 41, 226, 228, 234
ABO blood group, 199, 219
academic medicine, 26, 38–39, 87–88, 131
acquired immune deficiency syndrome. *See* AIDS/HIV
activated prothrombin complex concentrate (APCC), 199
active immunity, 199–200
ACT UP (AIDS Coalition To Unleash Power), 150–51, 155, 174; Women's Caucus of, 152
"Adam H.," 4, 18, 19, 29–30, 42–43, 76–78, 95, 99–102, 112, 123–24, 128–30, 140, 157, 227, 233, 265n12, 271n9
African Americans, 29, 158, 172, 227
Agency for Health Policy Research, U.S., 224
Agle, David, 57, 135, 234, 260n2
Agriculture, U.S. Department of, 15
AIDS Action Council, 269n10
AIDS/HIV, 1, 2, 112–63, 187–90, 192, 202, 203, 208, 218, 222, 224, 226, 227, 271n15, 273n9; activist response to, 150–52, 174–75; and attitudes about disease, 120–24; compensation for blood product infection with, 174, 176–77, 179, 182, 185; defined, 199, 210; discrimination against people with, 153–54; education on, 152–53, 155, 223; emotional impact of, 138–40, 260n2; first cases in hemo-

philia patients of, 115–19, 193; in gay men, 113–15, 267nn8–10; incubation period for, 268n38; informants and, 231, 232; IOM report on, 183; Kaposi's sarcoma in, 113, 114, 119, 133, 212; lymphadenopathy in, 213; managed care and, 172, 173; peer outreach approach to, 158–63, 167–68; research projects related to, 147–49, 156–57; and resistance to safeguarding blood supply, 125–28, 194–96; risk reduction programs for, 143–46, 157, 159, 184, 244; surrogate markers in, 218; testing technologies for, 136, 137, 215; treatments for, 178, 179, 201; and Tri-Agency Leadership model, 141–47, 157; viral inactivation techniques for, 129–32, 135–37, 156
AIDS-related complex (ARC), 200, 213
AIDS-related retrovirus (ARV), 200
Albucasis, 8
albumin, 17–18, 32, 39, 200, 203, 204, 216; normal serum, 215
Al Tasrif (Albucasis), 8
Altman, Dennis, 267n10
American Association for Labor Legislation (AALL), 33
American Association of Blood Banks (AABB), 126–28
American Association of Physicians for Human Rights, 269n10
American Blood Commission, 95

American Cancer Society, 24
American Diabetes Association (ADA), 34, 69–70, 76, 77, 82
American H/HIV/PEER Association, 174, 181
American Medical Association (AMA), 64, 79; Council on Medical Education and Hospitals, 26
American Nurses Association, 83
American Public Health Association, 272n20
American Red Cross, 17, 46, 47, 50, 57, 119, 126
American Society of Hematology, 119
Amicar (aminocaproic acid), 166, 200
amniocentesis, 200
anaphylactic reaction, 200
And the Band Played On (Shilts), 112, 131
animal research, 21–22, 38; on gene insertion therapy, 185
Annals of Internal Medicine, 243
antibodies, 201, 208, 211, 216; to Factor VIII or Factor IX, 212; in gamma globulin, 207; to HIV, 210, 215; monoclonal, 214; test for detection of, 205
antigens, 201, 202, 208, 211, 214, 215
anti-hemophilic factor (AHF). *See* Factor VIII
anti-inhibitor complex, 201
apheresis, 201
arthritis, 49
AZT (azidothymidine), 154, 156, 201

Babylonian Talmud, 8
Barrett, Sharon, 141–42, 145, 161, 162, 234, 270n7
Bayer, Ronald, 267n9
Bentsen, Lloyd, 150
Bias, Katie, 162
Bias, Val, 162–63, 172, 175, 177–80, 185, 236
Biggs, Rosemary, 23
Birch, Carol, 257n21
Bissell, G. William (Bill), 99–102, 234
blood banks, 17, 31–32, 41–42, 46, 74, 202; AIDS and, 119, 126–28, 195; gay community donations to, 113
blood-borne diseases, 66, 74, 131, 184, 202, 218. *See also* AIDS/HIV; hepatitis
blood centers, 202
blood components, 17, 202. *See also specific components*

Blue Cross–Blue Shield, 33, 70–71, 75
Blumenthal, David, 170
B lymphocytes, 202, 210, 211, 216
Boeing Corporation, 101
Booz, Allen, and Hamilton, 63
Brading, Sheila, 234
"Brett H.," 4, 93–94, 96, 124, 233
Brinkhous, Kenneth, 14, 15, 18, 20–22, 36, 37, 39, 40, 47–48, 226, 234, 256n13, 257n4
Britten, Anthony, 15
Browning, Susan, 169
Bulloch, W., 13, 256n8
Bush, George, 150
Butler, Regina, 104, 105, 122–23, 234

California, University of, San Francisco, 200
California Hemophilia Foundation, 50–51, 69
Camus, Albert, 120–21
Canada, government subsidies in, 174, 179
Canadian Hemophilia Society, 18
Carman, Charles ("Cliff H."), 28–29, 76, 95, 96, 101–3, 112, 123–24, 128, 154, 159, 178, 233
Carman, Patsy, 159–60
carriers, 6, 202; testing of, 112
Carter, Richard, 24
Carter Blood Center (Fort Worth), 36
Case Western Reserve University, 37
CD4 cells, 202, 218
CD8 cells, 202–3
Centers for Disease Control (CDC), 109, 113–22, 124–28, 130, 132–34, 136, 143–47, 149, 152, 156–58, 160, 186–88, 195, 196–97, 199, 203, 209, 244, 255n1, 268n37; Hematologic Diseases Branch, 186, 187; Hemophilia Program, 187; Host Factors Division, 115, 116, 157; Human Leukocyte Antigen Lab, 116; Immunology Division, 116, 117; Sexually Transmitted Diseases (STD) group, 115, 116
Chang, Barbara, 98, 234
Children's Hospital (Los Angeles), 39
Children's Hospital (Philadelphia), 105, 194
Children's Memorial Hospital (Chicago), 38
chorionic villi sampling (CVS), 203
Christmas disease, 5–6, 203, 208

chromatography, 203
chromosomes, 203, 207
Clements, Maribel, 104–5, 234
"Cliff H." *See* Carman, Charles
clinical trials, 151, 177, 203, 212; exclusion
    of women of childbearing age from,
    152; inclusion criteria for, 156
Clinton, Bill, 169–71, 189, 191, 196, 198
Clinton, Hillary Rodham, 169, 170
cloning, 112, 163, 164
coagulation, 203, 206, 209, 215; research
    on, 13–25, 27, 37–41, 47, 67, 86
coagulation concentrates, 203. *See also*
    concentrates
coagulation factors. *See* Factor VIII; Fac-
    tor IX
Cohen, Wilbur, 170
Cohn, Edwin, 17–18, 21, 204
Cohn Fraction I, 18, 21, 204
cold ethanol precipitation technique, 204
Colorado, University of, 61
Columbia University, 221, 222; Medical
    School, 14, 221; Oral History Collec-
    tion, 228, 233; School of Public Health,
    221, 223; Teachers College, 223
Committee of Ten Thousand (COTT),
    155, 174–75, 177, 178, 181
Committee on Health Education, 61
Common Factor, The, 175, 177–79, 181
Community Alert, 177–78, 180
complementary medicines, 177
comprehensive care, 50–55, 59, 75, 78, 86,
    110, 120, 204; and access to concen-
    trates, 93, 94; cost-efficacy of, 71, 85,
    106; international movement for, 108.
    See also hemophilia treatment centers
computed tomography (CT scan), 204
concentrates, 47–49, 55, 66, 88, 110, 204;
    access to, 86, 93–95; AIDS and, 123–26,
    133–35; allergic reaction to, 200; com-
    mercial availability of, 52–53; genetically
    engineered, 112; heat-treated, 130–32,
    135–37; hepatitis risk from, 66–67; infu-
    sion of, 78, 91, 212; lyophilized, 74, 131,
    135; purification of, 217; reconstitution
    of, 217
Congress, U.S., 23, 25, 60–61, 63, 66, 71,
    75, 77, 106, 110, 142, 145, 170–72, 174.
    See also House of Representatives, U.S.;
    Senate, U.S.
Cook County Hospital (Chicago), 17

Cornell University, 21
Creutzfeldt-Jakob disease, 186
Crippled Children Services (CCS), 69, 83
Crudder, Sally, 187, 236
Cry Bloody Murder (De Prince), 188
cryoprecipitate (cryo), 40–44, 66, 67, 88,
    124, 125, 205, 214, 230; AIDS and,
    130–33, 135; concentrates of, 47–49; des-
    ignated-donor program for, 122–23;
    Red Cross as supplier of, 57
Curran, Jim, 115
Cutter Laboratories, Inc., 40, 47; Cutter
    Biodivision, 272n5
Cystic Fibrosis Foundation, 69
cytomegalovirus (CMV), 205
cytotoxic T lymphocytes, 199, 202–3

"Daniel H." *See* Pierce, Glenn
Davidson, Michael, 153–54
Democratic Party, 150, 170
Denver Hemophilia Treatment Center
    Program, 117, 139
Depression, 19, 33
De Prince, Elaine, 188
desmopressin acetate (DDAVP), 205
de Wine, Mike, 184
Diabetes Detection and Education
    Act, 76
Diagnostic-Related Groups (DRGs), 156
"Diane H." *See* Pierce, Bea
Dictionary of Medical Specialists, 26
Dietrich, Shelby, 50–53, 55, 134–35, 172–73,
    190, 228, 234, 236, 243
directed donations, 205
Disraeli, Benjamin, 12
Drew, Charles, 17
Drucker, Peter F., 197–98
Dubin, Corey, 181, 182
Dukakis, Michael, 150
Duke University, 22, 38
Dunn, Linda, 224

Earnshaw, Kathryn, 68–69
Echo Magazine, 272n5
Education of All Handicapped Children
    Act, 93
ELISA (enzyme-linked immunosorbent
    assay) test, 136, 205
Emerson, Ralph Waldo, 179
England: blood donation program in, 31;
    orthopedic surgery in, 49

Enthoven, Alain, 170
Enthoven-Kronick plan, 170–71
envelope proteins, 205
Epstein, Steven, 151, 155
"Eugene H.," 94–95, 130, 132, 224, 233
Evatt, Bruce, 115–19, 121–22, 126, 127, 136, 145, 157–58, 186, 235, 236, 268nn25,37,38
excessive Lyonization, 6

Factor VIII (antihemophilic factor; AHF), 5, 21, 22, 52, 53, 63, 66, 92, 178, 199, 205, 206, 256n13; and AIDS, 116, 124; antibodies to, 212, 216; cloning of, 112, 163; components of, 67; cost of, 68, 78; defined, 201; discovery of, 15; half-life of, 208; liver transplants and, 213; purification of, 111, 203, 207, 212, 214; recombinant, 112, 156, 158, 163–65, 217; research on, 38, 40–42, 47, 48; in von Willebrand's disease, 219. See also concentrates; cryoprecipitate
Factor IX, 6, 22, 38, 63, 68, 78, 154, 163, 164, 201, 204, 206–8, 212, 214
Factor XII, 22, 206
Factor XIII, 205, 206
factor concentrates. See concentrates
Fahey, Tom, 178
family systems therapy, 57
Fantus, Bernard, 17
Federal Trade Commission, 32
Federation of American Societies of Experimental Biology, 15
Feissly, D. R., 14, 256n13
fibrinogen, 14, 203, 206; AHF-rich, 38
Fildes, P., 13, 256n8
Flam, Lisa, 235
Flynt, J. William, 144–45, 157, 224, 235, 244, 271n15
Food and Drug Administration (FDA), 116, 121, 126, 130, 136, 151, 156, 183–84, 186, 197, 207, 273n33; Blood Products Advisory Committee, 127, 183, 186, 196–97; Center for Biologics Evaluation Research, Division of Hematology, 186
Ford, Gerald R., 82, 83
Foreign Affairs, 197
France, HIV from blood transfusions in, 174
"Frank H.," 234
fresh-frozen plasma (FFP), 35, 42, 43, 50, 207

Friedland, Louis, 73, 79–81
Friedson, Elliot, 87, 263n21

gamma globulin, 32, 207
"Gay Cancer," 113–14
gay community, 112–15, 122, 134, 140; AIDS activism in, 151, 152; donor screening opposed by, 126–28; interaction of hemophilia community with, 153–55, 157, 179; safer sex in, 152–53
Gay Men's Health Crisis (GMHC), 152, 269n10
gel-permeation chromatography, 203, 207, 217
gene insertion therapy, 1, 163–64, 180, 185, 190, 207, 219
Genentech, 112
genes, 207; defective, 5
Genetically Handicapped Persons Program, 69, 207
genetic engineering, 111–12, 124, 149
genetic mutation, 207
Gerus, Kathy, 189, 237
Gift Relationship, The (Titmus), 31–32
Gilbert, Marvin S., 27, 48–50, 58, 69, 71, 73, 77, 81, 88, 97, 235
Gilliard, Pierre, 12–13
Goldwater Hospital, 14
Gomperts, Ed, 235
Gooley, Mary, 27–28, 34, 35, 59, 75, 84–85, 235, 243, 261n7
Gore, Al, 169
Gore, Tipper, 169
Gorenc, Tony, 235
Goss, Porter J., 182, 184
"Great Society," 45
Green, Mrs. J., 36, 235
"Gregory H.," 46, 133, 234
Greystone Conference (1969), 58–60, 261n7
GRID (gay-related immune deficiency), 113–14
Grupenhoff, John T., 80–82, 172
Grupenhoff and Endicott Associates, 80, 172
Gulf Oil, 101
Gulf States Hemophilia Program, 190
Gulf States Hemophilia Treatment Center, 108

Haas, Paul, 235
Hageman Factor, 22

Halden, Richard, 36
"Harold H.," 91–93, 124, 234
Harvard University, 17, 18, 114, 204;
    Medical School, 21, 150–51; Thorndike
    Laboratories, 14
Hatch, Orrin, 143
Hay, John, 9
health education, 61–62
Health, Education, and Welfare (HEW),
    U.S. Department of, 62, 80
health insurance, 19, 31–33, 45–46, 51, 61, 94;
    and cost-efficacy of comprehensive care,
    71, 75; group, 64; and inequality of treat-
    ment, 92; national, 25, 60, 85, 90, 150
Health Insurance Association of
    America, 171
health maintenance organizations
    (HMOs), 172
Health Manpower Act (1968), 61
Health Reform Task Force, 169, 170
Health Resources and Services Adminis-
    tration (HRSA), 157–58
Health Security Act, 170
heat treatment, 129–32, 135–37, 147, 148,
    208, 209, 212
Heine, Peggy, 139, 235
helper T cells, 211
hematology, 27, 37, 54, 64–65, 208; pedi-
    atric, 39, 106
hemophilia A, 5, 91, 115, 124, 201, 205, 208
Hemophilia Act (1973), 80
Hemophilia and AIDS/HIV Network for
    the Dissemination of Information
    (HANDI), 147, 180, 208
hemophilia B, 5, 203, 208
Hemophilia Foundation, 5, 20, 33–35,
    56. See also National Hemophilia
    Foundation
Hemophilia Newsnotes, 118, 175, 177
Hemophilia Surveillance System, 187, 244
hemophilia treatment centers (HTCs), 27,
    38, 70, 107, 108, 187–88, 204, 260n2;
    AIDS and, 112, 117, 122, 123, 131, 135,
    144, 158, 175, 223, 226, 232; data collec-
    tion and presentation, 243–54; federal
    funding of, 60, 78, 83; managed care
    and, 171–73; MCH and, 84–88, 98, 143;
    national network of, 60, 71, 75, 86, 110;
    nurse practitioners in, 61; plasma indus-
    try and, 110; risk reduction programs in,
    157. See also specific centers

Hemophilic Arthropathy (Jordan), 49
hemostasis, 209
Henry, Betty Jane, 34–35, 56
Henry, Lee, 34
Henry, Robert Lee, 20, 33–36, 56
hepatitis, 66, 86, 123, 124, 196, 205, 209;
    antibody to, 74; commercial blood
    banks and, 32; heat treatment and, 130,
    135; inactivation of virus causing, 212
hepatitis B (HBV), 209, 218; as surrogate
    marker, 126–28
hepatitis C (HCV), 200, 201, 209, 218
heterosexual transmission of HIV, 140
Hilgartner, Margaret, 38–39, 59, 71, 79,
    101, 235
Hill-Burton Act (1946), 25, 210
Hippocratic Oath, 193
hip replacement, 49
Hispanics, 158
histocompatibility, 210
HIV (human immunodeficiency virus).
    See AIDS/HIV
HIV Advisory Council, 189
HIV and the Blood Supply (IOM report),
    183, 195
HIV Treatment Information Exchange,
    180, 210
home therapy, 68–69, 74, 75, 78, 86, 104,
    110, 166–67; AIDS and, 135; cryo in, 123
Hoots, Keith, 108, 190, 237
Hopff, Frederick, 9
House of Representatives, U.S., 82,
    184–85; Committee on the Budget,
    263n37
human T cell lymphotropic virus
    (HTLV), 210
humoral immune response, 202, 210, 211
Hutchings, Jack, 84–85
Hutchins, Vince, 84, 235
Hyland, Clarence, 39
Hyland Laboratories, 38–40, 47, 48, 50,
    52, 53, 98
hyperimmune globulins, 211

iliopsoas, 211
Illinois, University of, Medical School, 38
immune deficiency, 211. See also
    AIDS/HIV
immune system, 199, 202, 207, 211, 212,
    214, 217, 219; genetics of, 116
immunoglobulin, 203, 204, 211

Impure Science (Epstein), 151
inactivation methods, 204, 208, 212, 214
infection, 212; acute, 200, 209, 212;
    chronic, 203, 209, 212; nosocomial, 215;
    opportunistic, 114, 154, 215
infusion, 36, 65, 91, 212; home, 74,
    78–79, 86, 92, 94, 110, 166–67; prophy-
    lactic, 189
Ingram, G. I. C., 13, 226, 256nn6–8,
    257n21
inhibitors, 199, 212
Institute of Medicine (IOM), 182–84, 186,
    195–97, 212, 273n15
insurance industry. *See* health insurance
interferon, 212
Internet, 186
ion exchange chromatography, 203,
    212, 217
Iowa, University of, 14, 257n4
"Irwin H." *See* Johnson, Richard

Jackson, Jesse, 150
James, Richard D., 260n46
"James H." *See* Kuhn, Dana
Javits, Jacob, 80, 81
Johns Hopkins University, 67
Johnson, Lyndon, 45, 61, 170
Johnson, Richard ("Irwin H."), 29, 30,
    132–33, 158–59, 234, 237
Jordan, Henry, 35, 49, 54
Journal of Biological Chemistry, 15
Journal of Clinical Investigation, 13
*Journal of the American Medical Associa-
    tion,* 193
Journey (Massie), 79
Judah, R., 8
Judaism, 8–9
Juvenile Diabetes Foundation, 69–70

Kansas City Hospital Association, 32
Kaposi's sarcoma (KS), 113, 114, 119,
    133, 212
Kelley, Kevin C., 167, 273–74n33
Kelley, Laureen, 165–68, 189, 237
Kelley, Tommy, 166
Kennedy, Edward M., 182
Kennedy, John F., 45
"Kent H.," 91, 234
Kessler, Craig, 135, 235, 264n27
kidney dialysis, 77–78
Koop, C. Everett, 142, 147, 148, 157

Krim, Mathilde, 114
Kronick, Richard, 170
Kuhn, Dana ("James H."), 93, 162, 163,
    185, 234, 237, 273n15

Lancet, 114, 118
Langmuir, Alexander, 117
Lasker, Mary, 24
Laun, Dick, 112
Lawrence, Dale, 116–18, 121, 122, 160, 235,
    237, 268nn25,38
Lazerson, Jack, 106
Lederman, Ben, 16
legionella, 116
Lenfant, Claude, 180
Lenox Hill Hospital (New York), 35,
    49, 54
Leopold, Duke of Albany, 12
leukocytes. *See* white blood cells
Levine, Peter, 15–16, 70–71, 75, 80, 83–86,
    97, 106, 167, 176, 235, 243, 264n27
Levy, Jay, 200
Lipton, Richard, 107–8, 139–40, 235, 237
liver, 212–13
liver cell transplants, 213
"Lloyd H.," 44, 54, 137–38, 234
Long Island Jewish Medical Center, 107
Los Angeles Orthopaedic Hospital, 50–55,
    59, 243; Department of Physical Ther-
    apy, 51; Division of Vocational Rehabili-
    tation, 51; Hemophilia Rehabilitation
    Project, 53; Hemophilia Treatment
    Center, 51; Model Program, 75
Lusher, Jeanne, 188–89
lymphadenopathy-associated virus
    (LAV), 213
lymphadenopathy syndrome (LAS),
    200, 213

McAdam, Kathy, 159–61, 237, 272n20
MacArthur, Gen. Douglas, 21
MacFarlane, R. G., 13, 23
MacFarlane, Rodger, 269n10
MacPherson, Merle, 84, 86, 236
Maimonides, 8
Maldonado, Daniel, 172
managed care, 171–73, 190
Marc Associates, 172, 176, 185
Massie, Bobby, 79
Massie, Robert, 79, 256n6
Massie, Suzanne, 79

Maternal and Child Health (MCH), Office of, 83–88, 90, 97–98, 104, 109, 138, 141, 143–47, 157–58, 172, 175, 186, 213, 240, 264n27; Ad Hoc Advisory Committee, 267n5; Habilitative Services, 84, 111; Hemophilia Program, 106, 161, 243

MCA-TV, 73

Medicaid, 60

medical education, 25–26, 38, 194

Medicare, 60, 77, 156, 170, 171

Memphis Theological Seminary, 93

Mendelian laws of heredity, 5

Merck, 47

Meredith, Karen, 104, 106, 236

Michael Reese Hospital (Chicago), 38

"Mindy H.," 140, 236

Minot, George, 14

Mintzer, Catherine, 97

Mishneh Torah, The (Maimonides), 8

monoclonal antibody purification, 111, 203, 214, 217

Morbidity and Mortality Weekly Report, 113, 118–19, 123, 125, 136, 188

Mt. Sinai Hospital (New York), 35; Department of Hematology, 49; Hemophilia Clinic, 48, 55, 58; Hemophilia Treatment Center, 149; Medical School, 88

Muir, Kathy, 189

multidisciplinary team approach, 50–55, 60–61, 70

"Nancy H.," 78

Nasse's Law, 9

National AIDS Commission, 157

National Association for Mental Health, 83

National Blood Resource Program (NBRP), 63

National Center for Health Education, 61–62

National Gay Task Force, 126, 127

National Health Council, 46

National Health Program (NHP), 150

National Health Services Corps, 82

National Heart and Lung Institute (NHLI), 214; Gene Therapy for Hemophilia workshop, 180; *Pilot Study* conducted by, 63–68, 88

National Heart Institute, 23

National Hemophilia Foundation (NHF), 34, 46, 73, 112, 167, 184, 187, 197, 214, 222–24, 227, 230–32, 240, 255n1, 261n7; Administrative Committee, 97; advocacy activities of, 71, 75–76, 79, 80, 82–83, 110; in AIDS era, 115–20, 122–32, 137–49, 156–63, 174–81, 244, 269n10, 270n10, 271n9, 273n9; AIDS Task Force, 128, 129, 154, 155, 177; Board of Directors, 154–55, 176; Bylaws Committee, 99, 100; Central Pennsylvania Chapter, 44; changes in leadership of, 56–60, 68–69, 99–103, 108, 185, 189; Chapter Outreach Demonstration Project (CODP), 158–59, 175, 186; and coagulation research, 25, 27, 36; Compassionate Care Program, 156; comprehensive care advocated by, 53, 55; cost issues in policies of, 66; creation of, 20; and cryoprecipitate, 41, 42; Educational Resources Project, 222; Executive Committee, 58, 102, 128–29, 269n14; and gene therapy research, 163–64; Health Education Advisory Committee, 103–4; informant's experiences with local chapters of, 91–96; Legislation Committee, 59; Maternal and Child Health Bureau and, 84–88; Medical and Scientific Advisory Council (MASAC), 36, 49, 58, 97, 99–100, 122–24, 126, 128, 129, 134, 136, 164, 176, 188, 190, 213, 268n38; Men's Advocacy Network of NHF (MANN), 162–63, 168, 174, 186, 213; Men's Executive Committee, 175; Mental Health Committee, 97, 105, 138–39, 260n2; Metropolitan New York Chapter, 42; National Resource and Consultation Center (NRCC), 138–39, 141, 143–44, 147, 153, 161, 271n12, 215; Nursing Committee, 97, 103–6, 122, 195, 223; plasma manufacturers and, 97–98, 195; Service Program Review, 59; Social Work Subcommittee, 97; Special Assistance Council (SAC), 176, 180–81, 218; spirit of "communitas" in, 76–77; staff turmoil in, 96–97; Strategic Plan, 185; Women's Outreach Network of NHF (WONN), 162, 175, 186–89, 220

National Institute of Allergy and Infectious Diseases (NIAID), 151, 156, 214, 271n9

National Institutes of Health (NIH), 20, 21, 23, 37, 47, 55, 126, 210, 214, 255n1, 257n4

National Science Foundation, 23

New England Hemophilia Association AIDS Task Force, 155

New England Hemophilia Treatment Center, 97

New England Journal of Medicine, 71, 80, 113, 131, 165

New England Medical Center Hospital, 15

"New Frontier," 45

Newton, Esther, 267n10

New York Blood Center, 42, 127

New York Department of State, 20

New York Hospital, 37, 79; Pediatric Hemophilia Clinic, 39

NHF Narrative Chronology, The, 124

NHF/NIAID/AIDS Clinical Trials Working Group, 271n9

Nixon, Richard M., 60–62, 65, 71, 77, 101, 196

North Carolina, University of, Medical School (Chapel Hill), 21, 23, 35, 36, 37, 39, 47–48, 91, 257n4

nurse practitioners, 61

Nurse Training Act (1964), 61

Nurse Training Program, 82

Office of Scientific Research and Development, 23

O'Hare, Donna, 85

Omnibus Reconciliation Act (1981), 263n37

opportunistic infections, 114, 154, 215

Oregon, University of, Medical School, 92

orthopedics, 27, 48–49, 51, 54, 81

Otto, John Conrad, 9

Paper, Renee, 189

Parent Exchange Newsletter, 167

Parsons, Talcott, 263n21

partial thromboplastin time (PTT), 215

passive immunity, 215

Pasteur Institute, 210, 213

pasteurization, 215

Patek, A. J., 14, 256n13

Patient/Family Model, 103–6, 144, 195, 223

Pearl Harbor, 17

Pellegrino, Edmund, 193

Pemberton, Stephen G., 21, 257n4, 259n29

Penn Central Railroad, 101

pentamidine, 116

People With AIDS (PWAs), 152, 179

Pharmaceutical Manufacturers Association, 126

"Phillips, Paul," 34, 103, 110, 112, 115, 118, 123, 142–43, 154–56, 177, 179, 185, 236, 237, 269n10, 270n10, 271nn9,12, 273n9

physical therapy, 51, 54

Pierce, Bea ("Diane H."), 140, 146, 159, 161, 186, 189, 197, 228, 236, 237, 272n20

Pierce, Glenn ("Daniel H."), 43, 133, 137, 154, 160, 163, 164, 175, 177–82, 190, 228, 233, 237, 259n17, 271n9

Plague, The (Camus), 120–21

Planned Parenthood, 83

plasma, 18, 30, 74, 91, 92, 202, 204, 205, 209, 216; AIDS virus in, 1; albumin in, 200; blood banks and, 31, 32; in clotting process, 13, 203; coagulation factors in, 204, 206; concentration of, 47 (*see also* concentrates); derivatives of, 216, 218; fractionation of, 17, 21, 215, 216; fresh-frozen (FFP), 35, 42, 43, 207; home infusion of, 36; isolation of proteins in, 22; manufacturers of, 97–98, 104, 110, 119, 120, 124, 129–30; marketing of components of, 39–40; recovered, 217; safety of, 197; transfusions of, 14, 27. *See also* cryoprecipitate

plasmapheresis, 57, 74, 201, 218

plasma protein fraction (PPF), 216

plasmathromboplastin. *See* Factor IX

plastic bags, technology for production of, 41–42

platelets, 18, 38, 67, 202, 216; concentrates of, 204

pneumocystis carinii pneumonia, 113, 115–16, 134

polio vaccine, 24

Pool, Judith Graham, 40–41, 47

porcine Factor VIII, 216

Presbyterian Hospital (New York), 17

prophylaxis, 189, 216; cost of, 68; joint health and, 91

protease inhibitors, 189

protein chemistry, 22

prothrombin complex (PTC), 216

prothrombin-complex concentrate (PCC), 199, 216

prothrombin time (PT), 216
Protocol 36, 156
psychological counseling, 57, 138–40
p24 antibody, 215
p24 antigen, 215, 218
Public Health Service, U.S., 15, 23, 83,
    109, 124, 126; Blood Safety Council,
    183. *See also specific agencies*
Puget Blood Center Hemophilia Program
    (Seattle), 104, 123
purification methods, 204, 207, 214, 217

Quayle, Dan, 150
Quick, Armand, 18

Rabiner, Fred, 37–39
Raising a Child with Hemophilia
    (Kelley), 166
Rasputin, Grigori, 13, 94
Ratnoff, Oscar, 14, 15, 22, 37, 40, 41,
    57, 66–67, 86, 111, 123, 124, 131–32, 134,
    135, 236
Ravdin, Isidore S., 17
Ray family, 142, 154, 157, 166, 184, 185
Reagan, Ronald, 107, 109, 113, 150, 195
recombinant DNA techniques, 164,
    209, 217
recombinant Factor VIII, 156, 165, 217
Recombinant Factor VIII Study
    Group, 165
Regional Congenital Heart Disease Cen-
    ters, 84
rehabilitative care, 51–53
Republican Party, 170
retroviruses, 210, 213, 217
Rh blood group, 217, 219
Rickles, Frederick, 4, 22, 37, 38, 41, 134,
    164, 186, 226, 228, 236, 237
Ricky Ray Hemophilia Relief Fund Act
    (1995), 184–85
risk reduction programs, 143–46, 157, 159,
    184, 244
Rochester General Hospital, 27
Rochester Hemophilia Treatment Center,
    75, 84–85
Rogers, Paul, 81–82
Romanovs, 12–13, 256nn6,7
Roosevelt, Eleanor, 160
Rosenberg, Charles, 1, 45
Rosenberg, Michael, 174, 176–78,
    181, 273n15

Rosenbloom, Gerald, 22
Rosenthal, Martin, 49, 55, 58
Rosner, Fred, 237, 255–56n1
Russalem, Herbert, 58–59

Sacks, Oliver, 238
safe sex practices, 140, 152–53, 185
Salk, Jonas, 24
Salk Institute, 164
San Francisco Coordinating Committee
    of Gay and Lesbian Services, 126
Sayers, Dorothy L., 256n6
Schnabel, Frank, 18, 108, 236
Schulman, Irving, 37–39
Scripps Clinic (La Jolla, Ca.), 111
Senate, U.S., 80–83, 170; Health Commit-
    tee, 143
seroconversion, 218
serology, 218
serum, 207, 211, 218
Shalala, Donna, 182, 184
Shanbrom, Edward, 48
Shilts, Randy, 112, 131, 267n8
shock, plasma for treatment of, 17
Shrager, David, 182
Shulhan Arukh (Caro), 8–9
Smith, Harry P., 14
Smith, Linda, 159–60, 237
Smith, Nathan, 74, 101–2, 143, 159,
    178, 269n14
Social Security Act, 106
Social Security Administration, 170
*Social Transformation of American Medi-
    cine, The* (Starr), 25
solvent-detergent, 148, 206, 209, 212, 218
Soucie, Mike, 187
specialization, growth of, 28
Special Programs of Regional and Na-
    tional Significance (SPRANS), 106–7
Stanford University, 40
Starr, Paul, 24, 25, 45–46, 87, 256n16
Stevens, Rosemary, 25
Strong Memorial Hospital (Rochester,
    N.Y.), 55, 75
Sullivan, Billie, 126
surrogate markers, 126–28, 218
"Swine Flu" epidemic, 121
synovitis, 91

Taft, Ted, 100
Taha-Cissé, Ashaki, 161

Taylor, F. H. L., 14, 256n13
Thelin, Murray, 47
Thompson, Paul, 221
Thoreau, Henry David, 192
thrombin, 13, 203, 218
thrombocytes. *See* platelets
thrombocytopenia, 38
thromboplastin generation test, 23
Titmuss, Richard, 31–32
T lymphocytes, 202, 219
total hip replacement, 49
toxic shock syndrome, 117
transfusion, 27, 35, 41, 202, 219; AIDS
    and, 119, 127, 142, 147, 174, 182; blood
    banks and, 31; childhood experiences
    of, 18, 19, 29, 44; earliest attempts at, 9,
    12; hemolytic reaction in, 208; home,
    79; nosocomial infections from, 215; of
    plasma, 14, 27; spread of hepatitis
    through, 209; technology of, 17
Transkaryotic Therapies, Inc., 273n33
Tri-Agency Leadership Model, 141–48, 157
Turner's syndrome, 6

Universal Data Collection System, 187
U.S. Surgeon General's Catalogue, 13

Vaccine Injury Compensation Fund,
    U.S., 174
vaccines, 211, 219; HBV, 209; polio, 24
Vehar, Gordon, 112
Verman, Inder M., 164
Veterans Administration (VA) Hospital
    System, 26
"Victor, Marcus," 55, 58, 69, 71, 73–75,
    78–80, 84, 88, 95, 97, 118–20, 129, 236,
    260n2, 263n4, 265n12, 269n14

Victoria, Queen of England, 12, 256n8;
    descendants of (figure), 10–11
viruses, 201, 202, 204, 206, 211, 219; core
    proteins of, 204; envelope proteins of,
    205; inactivation of, 156, 183, 212, 215,
    218. *See also* retroviruses; *specific viruses*
von Willebrand's disease, 67, 111, 189,
    205, 219

Wadleigh, Jonathan, 155–56, 174, 176, 178,
    179, 181, 271n9
Wagner, Robert, 47, 48
Wales, blood donation program in, 31
Wasserman, Louis, 49
Weinstein, Mark, 186
Weisman, Carol, 159
Western Blot Test, 136
Whipple, George H., 14
White, Ryan, 142, 157
white blood cells, 202, 219–20
Williams, Harrison, 80, 81
World Federation of Hemophilia (WFH),
    18, 46, 58, 104–6, 108, 154, 220, 223, 227
World War II, 17, 18, 24–26, 32, 126

X chromosome, 5, 6, 220

Yale University Hospital, 127
Y chromosome, 5, 220

Zimmerman, Theodore, 67–68, 111, 112
ZY Index, 225

Text:	10/14 Galliard
Display:	Officina Sans
Composition:	BookMasters, Inc.
Printing and Binding:	BookCrafters, Inc.